Molecular and Translational Medicine

Series Editors

William B. Coleman
American Society for Investigative Pathology
Rockville, MD, USA

Gregory J. Tsongalis
Department of Pathology and Laboratory Medicine
Dartmouth-Hitchcock Medical Center
Lebanon, NH, USA

As we enter into this new era of molecular medicine with an expanding body of knowledge related to the molecular pathogenesis of human disease and an increasing recognition of the practical implications for improved diagnostics and treatment, there is a need for new resources to inform basic scientists and clinical practitioners of the emerging concepts, useful applications, and continuing challenges related to molecular medicine and personalized treatment of complex human diseases. This series of resource/reference books entitled Molecular and Translational Medicine is primarily concerned with the molecular pathogenesis of major human diseases and disease processes, presented in the context of molecular pathology, with implications for translational molecular medicine and personalized patient care.

More information about this series at http://www.springer.com/series/8176

Christoph W. Michalski • Jonas Rosendahl
Patrick Michl • Jörg Kleeff
Editors

Translational Pancreatic Cancer Research

From Understanding of Mechanisms to Novel Clinical Trials

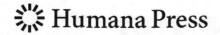 Humana Press

Editors
Christoph W. Michalski
Department of Visceral, Vascular and
Endocrine Surgery
University Hospital Halle (Saale)
Halle (Saale)
Sachsen-Anhalt
Germany

Patrick Michl
Department of Internal Medicine I
University Hospital Halle (Saale)
Halle (Saale)
Sachsen-Anhalt
Germany

Jonas Rosendahl
Department of Internal Medicine I
University Hospital Halle (Saale)
Halle (Saale)
Sachsen-Anhalt
Germany

Jörg Kleeff
Department of Visceral, Vascular and
Endocrine Surgery
University Hospital Halle (Saale)
Halle (Saale)
Sachsen-Anhalt
Germany

ISSN 2197-7852   ISSN 2197-7860   (electronic)
Molecular and Translational Medicine
ISBN 978-3-030-49478-0   ISBN 978-3-030-49476-6   (eBook)
https://doi.org/10.1007/978-3-030-49476-6

This Humana imprint is published by the registered company Springer Nature Switzerland AG
The registered company address is: Gewerbestrasse 11, 6330 Cham, Switzerland

Preface

Recent years have yielded significant progress in better understanding the pathobiology of pancreatic cancer. As a result, novel biomarkers have emerged, as have potentially effective new therapies. Translation of these results into daily clinical practice has been particularly challenging in pancreatic cancer, and large-scale, multinational efforts are only emerging.

This text has been designed in a multi-disciplinary approach to present how research results can be translated into clinical trials. It starts out with parts on variants of pancreatic cancer, precursor lesions and groups of people at risk to developing the disease. There is a particular focus on intraductal papillary mucinous neoplasia as a large-scale clinical challenge in pancreatology. This is followed by a part on (early) diagnosis, biomarkers and stratification. Here, there is a focus on various approaches to biomarker development which will be important both as prognostic and predictive tools. There is hope that the results of such research may in the near future translate into meaningful tools to aid clinical decision-making. This holds particularly true for the rapidly emerging field of multimodality and perioperative treatment of resectable, borderline-resectable and locally advanced pancreatic cancers.

Finally, there is a large section on personalized treatment approaches. As a starting chapter, preclinical models of pancreatic cancer are described, followed by chapters on stromal, epigenetic and metabolism targeting as promising approaches to be translated into early phase clinical trials. Finally, there are three chapters dealing with approaches that are close to be implemented in clinical practice or are already being tested in (early) clinical trials. These include approaches targeting the immune systems and strategies to overcome immunotherapy resistance, phase 1 clinical trials and translational approaches in surgical treatment.

Written by experts in each of the fields, these texts will not only give an overview of ongoing research efforts but will also provide an outlook towards future directions. Integrating information both from basic and clinical research, we hope that this book – through demonstrating pathways to better understanding pancreatic cancer and current approaches to translating these into clinical practice – will be used to conceive smart, more personalized treatment schemes.

Halle (Saale), Sachsen-Anhalt, Germany   Christoph W. Michalski
Halle (Saale), Sachsen-Anhalt, Germany   Jonas Rosendahl
Halle (Saale), Sachsen-Anhalt, Germany   Patrick Michl
Halle (Saale), Sachsen-Anhalt, Germany   Jörg Kleeff

Contents

Contributors

Hana Algül, MD Department of Internal Medicine II, Klinikum rechts der Isar, Technische Universitat München, Munich, Germany

Peter Bailey, BSc, PhD, MIP CRUK Beatson Institute of Cancer Research, Glasgow, UK

Department of General Surgery, Institute of Cancer Sciences, University of Glasgow, Glasgow, UK

A. Balduzzi, MD Department of Surgery, Pancreas Institute Verona, Verona, Italy

Lawrence Barrera, MD Department of Molecular and Clinical Cancer Medicine, University of Liverpool, Liverpool, UK

Andreas W. Berger, MD Department of Gastroenterology, Gastrointestinal Oncology and Interventional Endoscopy, Vivantes Klinikum Im Friedrichshain, Berlin, Germany

Department of Internal Medicine I, Ulm University, Ulm, Germany

M. G. Besselink, MD Department of Surgery, Cancer Center Amsterdam, Amsterdam UMC, University of Amsterdam, Amsterdam, The Netherlands

Alica Beutel, MD Department of Internal Medicine I, Gastroenterology-Endocrinology-Nephrology-Nutrition and Metabolic Diseases, Ulm University Hospital, Ulm, Germany

Manish S. Bhandare, MS, Mch (Surgical Oncology) Gastrointestinal and Hepato-Pancreato-Biliary Surgical Service, Department of Surgical Oncology, Tata Memorial Hospital, Mumbai, India

Holly Brunton, BSc, MSc, PhD CRUK Beatson Institute of Cancer Research, Glasgow, UK

Giuseppina Caliguri, BSc, MSc Institute of Cancer Sciences, University of Glasgow, Glasgow, UK

Vikram A. Chaudhari, MS, DNB Gastrointestinal and Hepato-Pancreato-Biliary Surgical Service, Department of Surgical Oncology, Tata Memorial Hospital, Mumbai, India

Eithne Costello, PhD, BSc Department of Molecular and Clinical Cancer Medicine, University of Liverpool, Liverpool, UK

Koushik K. Das, MD Division of Gastroenterology, Washington University School of Medicine, Saint Louis, MO, USA

M. Engelbrecht, MD Department of Radiology and Nuclear Medicine, Amsterdam Gastroenterology and Metabolism, Amsterdam UMC, University of Amsterdam, Amsterdam, The Netherlands

Irene Esposito, MD Institute of Pathology, Heinrich-Heine University & University Hospital of Düsseldorf, Düsseldorf, Germany

Thomas Ettrich, MD Department of Internal Medicine I, Gastroenterology-Endocrinology-Nephrology-Nutrition and Metabolic Diseases, Ulm University Hospital, Ulm, Germany

Anthony E. Evans, PhD, BSc Department of Molecular and Clinical Cancer Medicine, University of Liverpool, Liverpool, UK

P. Fockens, MD Department of Gastroenterology and Hepatology, Amsterdam Gastroenterology and Metabolism, Amsterdam UMC, University of Amsterdam, Amsterdam, The Netherlands

Helmut Friess, MD Department of Surgery, Klinikum rechts der Isar, School of Medicine, Technical University of Munich (TUM), Munich, Germany

Lena Häberle, MD Institute of Pathology, Heinrich-Heine University & University Hospital of Düsseldorf, Düsseldorf, Germany

Stephen Hasak, MD, MPH Division of Gastroenterology, Washington University School of Medicine, Saint Louis, MO, USA

Alina Hasanain, MD Division of Surgical Oncology, Johns Hopkins Medical Institution, Baltimore, MD, USA

Hanna Heikenwälder, PhD Department of General, Visceral and Transplantation Surgery, Heidelberg University Hospital, Heidelberg, Germany

Luisa Ingenhoff, MD Institute of Pathology, Heinrich-Heine University & University Hospital of Düsseldorf, Düsseldorf, Germany

Gareth J. Inman, BSc, MSc, PhD CRUK Beatson Institute of Cancer Research, Glasgow, UK

Institute of Cancer Sciences, University of Glasgow, Glasgow, UK

D. Kabacaoglu, MD Department of Internal Medicine II, Klinikum rechts der Isar, Technische Universitat München, Munich, Germany

Beate Kamlage, MD Metanomics Health GmbH, Berlin, Germany

Angelika Kestler, MD Departments of Internal Medicine and Gastroenterology, Ulm University, Ulm, Germany

Alexander Kleger, MD Department of Internal Medicine I, Ulm University, Ulm, Germany

Bo Kong, MD, PhD Department of Surgery, Klinikum rechts der Isar, School of Medicine, Technical University of Munich (TUM), Munich, Germany

Department of Gastroenterology, Affiliated Drum Tower Hospital of Nanjing University, Medical School, Nanjing, China

Markus M. Lerch, MD Department of Medicine A, University Medicine, Ernst-Moritz-Arndt-University Greifswald, Greifswald, Germany

Qi Li, MD Medical Department II, University Hospital, LMU, Munich, Germany

Ujjwal Mukund Mahajan, PhD Medical Department II, University Hospital, LMU, Munich, Germany

G. Marchegiani, MD, PhD Department of Surgery, Pancreas Institute Verona, Verona, Italy

Julia Mayerle, MD Medical Department II, University Hospital, LMU, Munich, Germany

Albrecht Neesse, MD, PhD Department of Gastroenterology and Gastrointestinal Oncology, University Medical Center Göttingen, Center Göttingen, Georg-August-University, Göttingen, Germany

John Neoptolemos, MD, MB, BChir, MD, FRCS, FMedSci Department of General, Visceral and Transplantation Surgery, University of Heidelberg, Heidelberg, Germany

Lucy Oldfield, MChem, MSc, PhD Department of Molecular and Clinical Cancer Medicine, University of Liverpool, Liverpool, UK

Lukas Perkhofer, MD Department of Internal Medicine I, Gastroenterology-Endocrinology-Nephrology-Nutrition and Metabolic Diseases, Ulm University Hospita, Ulm, Germany

Svenja Pichlmeier, MD Department of Medicine II, University Hospital, LMU, Munich, Germany

Ivonne Regel, MD Department of Medicine II, University Hospital, LMU, Munich, Germany

Susanne Roth, MD, PhD Department of General, Visceral and Transplantation Surgery, Heidelberg University Hospital, Heidelberg, Germany

D. A. Ruess, MD Department of Surgery, Faculty of Medicine, Medical Center, University of Freiburg, Freiburg, Germany

Thomas Seufferlein, MD Department of Internal Medicine I, Gastroenterology-Endokrinolopgy-Nephrology-Nutrition and Metabolic Diseases, Ulm University Hospital, Ulm, Germany

Shailesh V. Shrikhande, MS, MD, FRCS (HON) Gastrointestinal and Hepato-Pancreato-Biliary Surgical Service, Department of Surgical Oncology, Tata Memorial Hospital, Mumbai, India

J. Stoker, MD Department of Radiology and Nuclear Medicine, Amsterdam Gastroenterology and Metabolism, Amsterdam UMC, University of Amsterdam, Amsterdam, The Netherlands

Yoshiaki Sunami, PhD Department of Visceral, Vascular and Endocrine Surgery, Martin-Luther-University Halle-Wittenberg, University Medical Center Halle, Halle (Saale), Germany

J. E. van Hooft, MD Department of Gastroenterology and Hepatology, Amsterdam Gastroenterology and Metabolism, Amsterdam UMC, University of Amsterdam, Amsterdam, The Netherlands

N. C. M. van Huijgevoort, MD Department of Gastroenterology and Hepatology, Amsterdam Gastroenterology and Metabolism, Amsterdam UMC, University of Amsterdam, Amsterdam, The Netherlands

J. Verheij, MD, PhD Department of Pathology, Cancer Center Amsterdam, Amsterdam UMC, University of Amsterdam, Amsterdam, The Netherlands

Dylan Williams, BSc (Hons), MRes Department of Molecular and Clinical Cancer Medicine, University of Liverpool, Liverpool, UK

Christopher L. Wolfgang, MD, MS, PhD Division of Surgical Oncology, Department of Surgery, Pathology and Oncology, Johns Hopkins Medical Institution, Baltimore, MD, USA

Part I
PDAC Variants and Risk of Disease

Chapter 1
Subtypes of Pancreatic Adenocarcinoma

Luisa Ingenhoff, Lena Häberle, and Irene Esposito

Pancreatic cancers of exocrine origin are mostly represented by pancreatic ductal adenocarcinoma (PDAC) [1]. PDAC is an epithelial neoplasm with a ductal phenotype, which is reflected by strong and diffuse expression of ductal cytokeratins (CKs), such as CK7 and CK19. A few histopathological variants of PDAC are recognized and distinguished on the basis of morphology and marker profiles according to the WHO criteria [2]. PDAC subtypes partially reflect different carcinogenesis pathways, i.e., the development from different precursor lesions following different molecular pathways. Although some of these subtypes display a different biological behavior and harbor a different prognosis, the clinical relevance of such subclassifications remains limited. In particular, a correlation between morphologic and recently identified molecular subtypes is still lacking.

Tumor heterogeneity was first described in association with macroscopic and microscopic observation. Intertumor heterogeneity refers to the histological appearance of different tumors (i.e., of different patients). Intratumor heterogeneity focuses on different growth patterns, cytological characteristics, grade of differentiation, and stromal characteristics in different areas of the same tumor [3]. There are several factors determining phenotypical intratumor heterogeneity: epigenetics, hierarchical organization of cancer cell population, and heterogeneity in the microenvironment (pH, hypoxia, modulation of cell signalling, interaction between stromal and tumor cells) [4, 5]. Tumor heterogeneity is not limited to morphological features of the tumor, and genomic tumor heterogeneity exists. In PDAC, tumor heterogeneity is particularly distinct compared to other human cancers and possibly represents a prominent contributor to drug resistance and therapy failure [4, 5].

L. Ingenhoff · L. Häberle · I. Esposito (✉)
Institute of Pathology, Heinrich-Heine University
& University Hospital of Düsseldorf, Düsseldorf, Germany
e-mail: irene.esposito@med.uni-duesseldorf.de

© Springer Nature Switzerland AG 2020
C. W. Michalski et al. (eds.), *Translational Pancreatic Cancer Research,*
Molecular and Translational Medicine,
https://doi.org/10.1007/978-3-030-49476-6_1

3

PDAC and Morphological Subtypes

Classical PDAC (Pancreatobiliary Type)

PDAC usually presents as a white-yellow firm mass infiltrating the normal, soft, lobular structure of the pancreas (Fig. 1.1). Cystic areas may occur, usually in the form of retention cysts, sometimes being part of the tumor or displaying precursor lesions, rarely because of necrosis and/or hemorrhage. Most PDACs (70%) are located in the head of the pancreas as solitary lesions with a mean size of about 3 cm [6]. This gross aspect is usually common to most subtypes of PDAC; large areas of necrosis and hemorrhage are more common in poorly differentiated tumors. Conventional PDAC forms glandular, duct-like structures infiltrating the pancreatic parenchyma. Tumor cells are cuboidal to tall columnar and usually produce mucins of sialo-type and sulfated acid-type that accumulate in the cytoplasm or in the lumina and can be highlighted by the Alcian-blue periodic-acid-Schiff (AB-PAS) stain. A prominent clear cell differentiation is often seen. Ductal cytokeratins (CK7,

Fig. 1.1 Gross morphology. (**a**) Classical ductal adenocarcinoma of the head of the pancreas presenting as a solid, white-yellowish mass. (**b**) Colloid carcinoma of the head of the pancreas with small, cystic, mucinous areas. (**c**) Adenosquamous carcinoma of the tail of the pancreas, macroscopically not distinguishable from classical PDAC

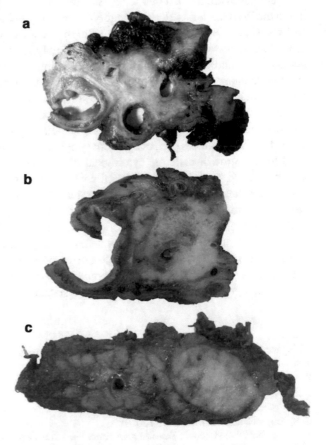

CK8, CK18, and CK19) and the mucin proteins MUC 1, MUC 4, and MUC5AC are positive in most cases. CK20 expression is observed in about 30–75% and does not necessarily reflect an intestinal differentiation [7]. Moreover, CEA, CA19–9, and CA12.5 (MUC 16) are expressed in about 92%, 94%, and 48%, respectively [8–10]. Furthermore, about 75% of PDAC show strong expression of p53 [11, 12], which correlates with mutation of the *TP53* gene, and 55% display loss of SMAD4/DPC4 protein, also correlating with alteration of the corresponding gene [13].

Classical PDAC usually shows a quite high level of intratumoral heterogeneity concerning histological grading and pattern of growth (Fig. 1.2). The grading is assessed according to the criteria of the WHO. Briefly, *well-differentiated* PDACs display a tubular architecture with minimal nuclear enlargement, intact or slight reduced mucin production, and rare mitoses (up to 5/high-power field, HPF) [2] (Fig. 1.2a). *Moderately differentiated* PDAC shows more medium-sized duct-like structures as well as polymorph small tubular glands (Fig. 1.2b). Nuclear size, structure, and shape are more variable. Mitoses are observed more frequently

Fig. 1.2 Histology and grading. (**a**) Well-differentiated PDAC with a tubular architecture and minimal nuclear enlargement, HE 20×. (**b**) Moderately differentiated PDAC with medium-sized tubular structures and polymorph small tubular glands, as well as an abundant desmoplastic stromal response, HE 20×. (**c**) Poorly differentiated PDAC with a solid sheet structure, individual cell budding, and almost no desmoplastic stromal response, HE 20×

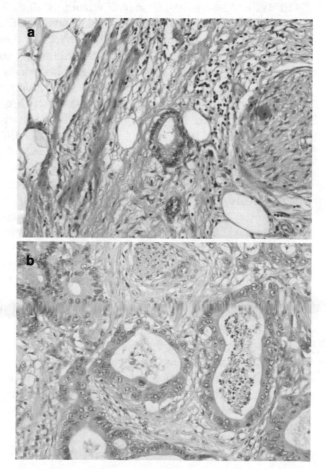

Fig. 1.2 (continued)

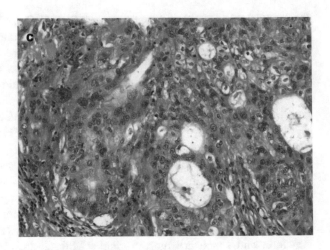

(5–10/HPF). Well- and moderately differentiated PDACs are typically accompanied by an abundant desmoplastic stromal response, which consists of dense fibrosis with activated fibroblasts and myofibroblasts, as well as leucocytes. *Poorly differentiated* PDAC is characterized by a solid sheet structure, sometimes with dense small polymorph glands with higher mitotic activity (>10/HPF) and individual cell budding (Fig 1.2c). Necrosis and hemorrhage are more common, whereas the desmoplastic stromal reaction is usually less developed to absent [2]. Tumor grading represents one of the most important prognostic indicators in PDAC [14], underlying the importance of an accurate evaluation of this parameter. This task can be particularly difficult to accomplish due to the high degree of intratumoral heterogeneity. For instance, in the periphery of the tumor, often in areas of infiltration of surrounding tissues, less differentiated areas may be present. Conventionally, the highest (=poorest) grading is assigned in the tumor classification; however, it may be useful to describe and semi-quantify any relevant component for better clinical correlation, especially concerning therapy response. Among the growth patterns, in addition to the classical tubular form, cribriform, gyriform, complex, micropapillary, large duct and papillary patterns have been described, which share the same genetic profile of the classical PDAC and appear to have no prognostic significance [15].

In addition to the above described growth pattern, homogenous variants of PDAC, defined as those containing at least 30% of a distinct histologic pattern, also exist. They include adenosquamous, colloid, undifferentiated (with or without osteoclastic giant cells), medullary, hepatoid, and signet ring cell carcinomas [2]. Many of these variants display the same genetic profile as the classical PDAC; however, some peculiarities concerning genetics and development from specific subgroups of precursor lesions, as well as regarding prognosis, exist and are briefly outlined in the following.

Adenosquamous carcinomas represent up to 10% of PDAC and have a worse prognosis compared to classical PDAC with a median survival of 7–11 months and a 3-year survival rate of 14% after surgery [2, 16–19] (Table 1.1). This variant

Table 1.1 Variants of pancreatic ductal adenocarcinoma

PDAC variant (frequency)	Histomorphology	Immunohistochemical/ molecular characteristics	Prognosis
Conventional PDAC[a] (85%)	Glandular, duct-like patterns Mucin production intracellularly and/or luminally (AB-PAS) Desmoplastic stroma	CEA+,CA19-9+,CA125+,p53+,SMAD4-	Poor (overall survival rate 6%) [40]
Adenosquamous carcinoma[a] (<10%)	Ductal as well as squamous (at least 30%) differentiation Ductal component: Similar to conventional PDAC Squamous component: Sheet-like tissue with polygonal cells, keratinization	Squamous cells: p53+, p63+p40+,CK5/6+p16-,SMAD4-	Poor (median survival time 7–11 months)
Colloid carcinoma[a] (2%)	Large, well-demarcated tumor masses with large extracellular mucin pools partially lined by atypical epithelial cells Associated with an IPMN of intestinal-type differentiation	CDX2+, MUC2+ High frequency of GNAS1 mutation	Good (5-year survival rate up to 85%)
Undifferentiated carcinoma[a] (<1%)	Extensive loss of differentiation Minimally cohesive, scant stroma Nuclear pleomorphisms High mitotic rate Variants: Sarcomatoid, pleomorphic, rhabdoid	High level of mutant KRAS allele-specific imbalance Rhabdoid variant: Often KRAS wild type	Poor (5-year survival rate 15%) [41]
Undifferentiated carcinomas with osteoclast-like giant cells[a] (<1%)	Highly pleomorphic, round to spindle-shaped mononuclear neoplastic Non-neoplastic reactive, multinucleated, large histiocytic giant cells often in areas of hemorrhage/necrosis	Often accompanied by MCN or in situ PDAC	Good (5-year survival rate 60%)

(continued)

Table 1.1 (continued)

PDAC variant (frequency)	Histomorphology	Immunohistochemical/molecular characteristics	Prognosis
Hepatoid carcinoma[a] (<1%)	Hepatocellular differentiation Large polygonal cells with abundant eosinophilic cytoplasm May be accompanied by conventional PDAC, acinar carcinoma, or neuroendocrine neoplasm	AFP+, HepPar1+, CEA+, CD10+ Transposon-induced Fign mutation found recently	Unknown
Medullary carcinoma[a] (<1%)	Poorly differentiated, scarce gland formation Pushing borders Syncytial growth pattern Tumor tissue infiltrated by CD3+ lymphocytes	Loss of expression of DNA mismatch repair genes and microsatellite instability Sporadically or in lynch syndrome	Unknown
Signet ring cell carcinoma[a] (<1%)	Mucinous differentiation Poorly cohesive, individual neoplastic cells with intracytoplasmic mucin accumulation		Poor
Tubular carcinoma (unknown)	Well-differentiated open tubules	Scarce mutational events	Very good

[a]Listed in the WHO classification

displays a ductal as well as a squamous differentiation (Fig. 1.3a, b). The WHO definition of adenosquamous carcinoma requires at least 30% of the tumor mass to be squamous, whereas even a minimal ductal component warrants the classification of a given PDAC as adenosquamous variant [2]. Squamous cells are usually easily recognized by their eosinophilic cytoplasm with prominent intercellular junctions and, in some cases, by keratinization. In doubtful cases, p63 and/or p40 immunostaining can be applied to highlight a squamous component [20, 21]. Molecular studies, including a recent whole-genome and whole-exome sequencing study of a series of 17 adenosquamous carcinomas, have revealed numerous similarities to classical PDAC, the only exception being the higher frequency of *TP53* mutations [22].

Undifferentiated carcinomas represent less than 1% of PDAC and are characterized by an extensive loss of differentiation accompanied by severe cellular and nuclear pleomorphism [16]. Several subtypes of undifferentiated carcinomas (e.g., sarcomatoid, pleomorphic, rhabdoid) are recognized with distinct morphologic features but have common clinical characteristics (Fig. 1.3c, d). Undifferentiated carcinomas have been shown to bear a high level of mutant *KRAS* allele-specific imbalance compared to classical PDAC, which correlate with aggressive clinical behavior [23, 24]. The rhabdoid variant often has a *KRAS* wild-type status and bears on the other hand alterations of the *SMARCB1* gene

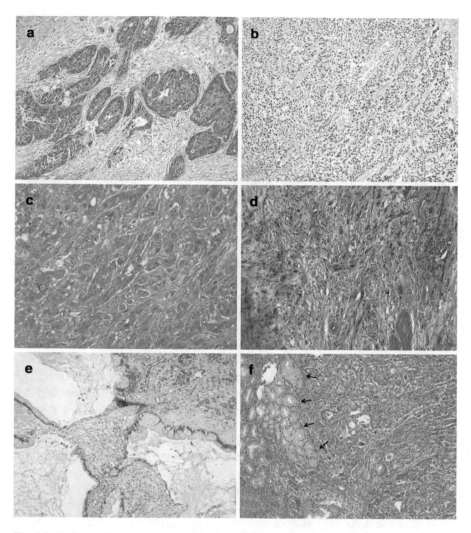

Fig. 1.3 Variants of PDAC. (**a**) Adenosquamous PDAC showing squamous as well as ductal tumor components accompanied by an abundant desmoplastic stromal response, HE, 10×. (**b**) Squamous component in adenosquamous PDAC is positive for p40, 10×. (**c**) Anaplastic pleomorphic PDAC with giant tumor cells growing in a solid sheet pattern, HE 10×. (**d**) Anaplastic PDAC, sarcomatoid variant, showing spindle-shaped sarcoma-like cells, HE 10× (**e**) Colloid carcinoma showing mucin pools partially lined with atypical cuboidal epithelium, HE 10×. (**f**) Medullary carcinoma showing poorly differentiated tumor cells growing in a syncytial pattern and "pushing borders" phenomenon (arrows), HE, 10×

with loss of expression of the corresponding protein at the immunohistochemical level [25].

Signet ring cell carcinoma is very rare variant of cancer with mucinous differentiation and aggressive clinical behavior. It displays poorly cohesive, individual neoplastic epithelial cells with intracytoplasmic mucin accumulation [2].

A few homogeneous variants of PDAC show a better prognosis compared to the conventional pancreatobiliary subtype. However, survival data are for some entities too limited to allow confident statements.

Undifferentiated carcinoma with osteoclast-like giant cells is characterized by the presence of multinuclear histiocytic giant cells often residing in areas of hemorrhage and necrosis. Although previous data have ascribed a particularly aggressive behavior of this variant, a recent large series has identified relevant clinical peculiarities of this PDAC subtype, such as the frequent occurrence in a younger population compared to classical PDAC (mean age 57 vs. 70 yrs.) and a better prognosis with a 5-year overall survival of 60% [26]. An interesting aspect is the peculiar association with mucinous cystic neoplasms or PanIN (pancreatic intraepithelial neoplasm) but not with other PDAC precursors [27].

Colloid (mucinous non-cystic) carcinoma represents up to 2% pancreatic cancers and is usually associated with main duct intraductal papillary mucinous neoplasms of the intestinal subtype. Colloid carcinomas usually form large, well-demarcated tumor masses characterized by large extracellular mucin pools partially lined by atypical epithelial cells [16] (Fig. 1.3e). In addition, groups of tumor cells can be found floating in the mucin pools. Intestinal-type IPMNs (intraductal papillary mucinous neoplasms) are characterized by the expression of markers of intestinal differentiation, like MUC2 and CDX2, which can be also detected in the cells of colloid carcinoma but are uncommon in other PDAC variants [28]. Both intestinal IPMN and colloid carcinomas are characterized by a high frequency of *GNAS1* mutations, underscoring the existence of an intestinal-type progression model in addition to the conventional, *KRAS*-driven pancreatobiliary carcinogenesis [29]. Mucinous carcinomas have a good prognosis with a 5-year-survival rate up to 83% [30].

Medullary carcinomas are poorly differentiated epithelial neoplasms displaying scarce gland formation. Typically, the tumor mass has "pushing" anatomical borders and shows a syncytial growth pattern with numerous infiltrating T lymphocytes (Fig. 1.3f). Medullary carcinomas can occur sporadically or in the context of Lynch syndrome and often display microsatellite instability with loss of expression of mismatch repair proteins at immunohistochemistry [31]. Their prognosis appears more favorable than that of conventional PDAC [32, 33], but the mean survival time is unknown because of its rarity [34].

Recently, a rare variant of well-differentiated tubular adenocarcinoma, morphologically resembling tubular carcinoma of the breast, has been described. This variant shows paucity of mutational events and has a very good prognosis [15].

Hepatoid carcinoma is a very rare epithelial neoplasm with a component of hepatocellular differentiation with large polygonal cells with abundant eosinophilic cytoplasms and HepPar1 immunolabeling. AFP, CD10, and CEA with canalicular pattern may be expressed [35, 36]. Hepatoid PDACs develop along different molecular pathways compared to the conventional subtype [37, 38]. These pathways, which have been partially disclosed using transposon-induced mutagenesis, include alterations of *Fign* gene in the form of *Fign* insertions demonstrated in a recent mouse model study. *Fign* insertion leads to *Fign* overexpression which was found in hepatoid pancreatic cancer [39] . Survival data of hepatoid carcinoma are lacking so far (Table 1.1) [40, 41].

Stromal Heterogeneity in PDAC

An abundant stroma, consisting of various extracellular matrix proteins and cancer-associated (myo-)fibroblasts, termed pancreatic stellate cells (PSCs), is a hallmark of PDAC. While some studies imply that the stroma can have a protective effect in PDAC [42, 43], many data suggest that the stromal reaction promotes the aggressive tumor biology of PDAC as well as its chemoresistance [44–46].

It has been shown that both the desmoplastic stroma and PSC are characterized by marked heterogeneity. The stroma itself can be characterized into histomorphological subgroups according to its composition, e.g., in dense (mature), intermediate, and loose (immature) stroma. Some studies imply that a dense collagen-rich stroma is linked to a better outcome of PDAC patients, compared to a loose mucin-rich stroma characterized by dynamic stromal remodeling, which is correlated with poorer prognosis [47–49]. In addition, the heterogeneous expression of PSC markers in PDAC tissue specimens suggests the presence of PSC at different levels of activation or differentiation or even the presence of different PSC subpopulations [50]. Here, the presence of α-SMA-positive PSC seems to be correlated with worse survival [47, 50, 51].

While these histomorphological subtypes of PDAC stroma have been recapitulated by molecular analyses in part [52], an association of these stromal subtypes to the various histomorphological epithelial subtypes has not been established yet.

PDAC and Molecular Subtypes

With high-throughput techniques becoming more and more readily available, a new concept of molecular subtyping of PDAC has emerged in recent years.

In 2011, Collisson and colleagues proposed three molecular subtypes of PDAC: the *classical*, the *quasi-mesenchymal*, and the *exocrine-like subtype* [53].These subtypes seem to be relevant for survival, with the classical subtype displaying the best prognosis and the quasi-mesenchymal subtype the worst [53]. Moreover, Collisson's subtypes are suggested to be correlated with therapy resistance and sensitivity [53].

Five years later, Bailey et al. suggested the existence of four molecular PDAC subtypes, which overlap in part with the subtypes proposed by Collisson's group: the *squamous subtype*, corresponding to Collisson's quasi-mesenchymal subtype, the *aberrantly differentiated endocrine exocrine (ADEX) subtype*, recapitulating Collisson's exocrine-like subtype, the *pancreatic progenitor subtype*, which seems to be linked to Collisson's classical subtype, and, lastly, the *immunogenic subtype* [54].

In addition to identifying a more favorable "classical" and a prognostically adverse "basal-like" epithelial *subtype* of PDAC, Moffitt and colleagues also proposed two molecular subtypes of PDAC stroma: the "normal" and the "activated" PDAC stromal subtype, with the "activated" subtype being linked to worse prognosis [52].

Taking into consideration the mutational burden, the histomorphological stroma subtype, and the immune infiltrate, the group around Knudsen defined four new molecular PDAC subtypes. *Cluster 1* includes PDACs with low mutational burden, low stromal volume, immature stromal type, and a high number of macrophages ("mutationally cold"), while *Cluster 2* describes PDACs with high mutational activity and high levels of all immune cell types ("hot"), *Cluster 3* is defined as "mutationally active," displaying a high mutational burden, an intermediate stromal type, higher numbers of tumor-infiltrating lymphocytes (TILs), and peritumoral lymphocytes but relatively low levels of macrophages, and *Cluster 4* includes PDACs with low mutational burden, high stromal volume, mature stromal type, and low immune cell levels ("cold") [49]. In this study, Cluster 4 PDACs seem to display improved overall survival compared to all other "immunosubtypes" of PDAC [49].

Although these subtypes described by different authors seem to display some similarities between each other, there is no complete overlap. This may be partially due to methodological imperfections of the studies performed so far. PDAC characteristically consists of dispersed tumor glands embedded in a prominent desmoplastic stroma. This may have led to the contamination of tumor tissue samples with stromal cells during microdissection. Very recently, evidence has also been found that that Collisson's exocrine-like subtype (Bailey's ADEX subtype) may have been a result of contamination of tumor tissues with normal acinar cells of the pancreas [55].

Some molecular subtypes can be recapitulated by immunohistochemistry. For example, immunohistochemical positivity for CK81 identifies PDACs of Collisson's quasi-mesenchymal, Bailey's squamous, and Moffitt's basal-like subtype, while HNF1alpha positivity identifies "non-quasi-mesenchymal," "non-squamous," and "non-basal-like" PDACs [56]. The relevance of these immunohistochemical subtypes for survival has been validated in different patient cohorts, with HNF1alpha-positive PDACs showing the best survival and CK81-positive PDACs the worst [56]. This seems like a big step in integrating molecular subtyping into routine diagnostics. However, the correlation between molecular and immunophenotypical subtypes and histomorphological subtypes is still lacking in PDAC. Most surprisingly, even though the adenosquamous histomorphological variant of PDAC is also associated with especially poor prognosis, no correlation could be established between the histomorphological (adeno-) squamous phenotype and the molecular quasi-mesenchymal/squamous/basal-like subtype yet. Nevertheless, certain links between histomorphological and molecular features of PDAC have been found in the past. For example, *KRAS* mutations are significantly more common in classical PDACs than in its histomorphological variants [15].

While establishing clear associations between histomorphology and molecular profiles, as it has been done in other tumor entities such as lung cancer, proves utterly challenging in PDAC, this still seems to be the next step to take in order to translate molecular findings into viable clinical applications.

Conclusion

Intra- and intertumoral heterogeneity is an emerging concept in PDAC. In addition to histomorphological subtypes, molecular subtypes, even of PDAC stroma, have been proposed. The prognostic and therapeutic relevance of PDAC subtyping is currently under investigation and has delivered promising results. However, the WHO classification has not yet adapted the whole morphological and molecular spectrum and is based mainly on tumor morphology and marker profiles. A correlation between histomorphologic and molecular subtypes is still lacking.

A major task in future studies is to find consensus about the newly described molecular subtypes and to integrate them with morphological features to generate a universal classification that can be easily applied in everyday practice.

References

1. Klimstra DS. Nonductal neoplasms of the pancreas. Mod Pathol. 2007;20(Suppl 1):S94–112.
2. Bosman FT, editor. WHO classification of tumours of the digestive system: Reflects the views of a working group that convened for an editorial and consensus conference at the International Agency for Research on Cancer (IARC), Lyon, December 10–12, 2009; third volume of the 4th edition of the WHO series on histological and genetic typing of human tumours. 4th ed., 1. print run. Lyon: IARC; 2010. (World Health Organization classification of tumours3 (der 4. ed.)).
3. Stanta G, Jahn SW, Bonin S, Hoefler G. Tumour heterogeneity: principles and practical consequences. Virchows Arch. 2016;469(4):371–84.
4. Burrell RA, Swanton C. Tumour heterogeneity and the evolution of polyclonal drug resistance. Mol Oncol. 2014;8(6):1095–111.
5. Verbeke C. Morphological heterogeneity in ductal adenocarcinoma of the pancreas - does it matter? Pancreatology. 2016;16(3):295–301.
6. Ryan DP, Hong TS, Bardeesy N. Pancreatic adenocarcinoma. N Engl J Med. 2014;371(11):1039–49.
7. Matros E, Bailey G, Clancy T, Zinner M, Ashley S, Whang E, et al. Cytokeratin 20 expression identifies a subtype of pancreatic adenocarcinoma with decreased overall survival. Cancer. 2006;106(3):693–702.
8. Loy TS, Quesenberry JT, Sharp SC. Distribution of CA 125 in adenocarcinomas. An immunohistochemical study of 481 cases. Am J Clin Pathol. 1992;98(2):175–9.
9. Hornick JL, Lauwers GY, Odze RD. Immunohistochemistry can help distinguish metastatic pancreatic adenocarcinomas from bile duct adenomas and hamartomas of the liver. Am J Surg Pathol. 2005;29(3):381–9.
10. Loy TS, Sharp SC, Andershock CJ, Craig SB. Distribution of CA 19-9 in adenocarcinomas and transitional cell carcinomas. An immunohistochemical study of 527 cases. Am J Clin Pathol. 1993;99(6):726–8.
11. Li D, Xie K, Wolff R, Abbruzzese JL. Pancreatic cancer. Lancet. 2004;363(9414):1049–57.

12. Weissmueller S, Manchado E, Saborowski M, Morris JP, Wagenblast E, Davis CA, et al. Mutant p53 drives pancreatic cancer metastasis through cell-autonomous PDGF receptor β signaling. Cell. 2014;157(2):382–94.

13. Blackford A, Serrano OK, Wolfgang CL, Parmigiani G, Jones S, Zhang X, et al. SMAD4 gene mutations are associated with poor prognosis in pancreatic cancer. Clin Cancer Res. 2009;15(14):4674–9.

14. Rochefort MM, Ankeny JS, Kadera BE, Donald GW, Isacoff W, Wainberg ZA, et al. Impact of tumor grade on pancreatic cancer prognosis: validation of a novel TNMG staging system. Ann Surg Oncol. 2013;20(13):4322–9.

15 Schlitter AM, Segler A, Steiger K, Michalski CW, Jäger C, Konukiewitz B, et al. Molecular, morphological and survival analysis of 177 resected pancreatic ductal adenocarcinomas (PDACs): identification of prognostic subtypes. Sci Rep. 2017;7:41064.

16. Borazanci E, Millis SZ, Korn R, Han H, Whatcott CJ, Gatalica Z, et al. Adenosquamous carcinoma of the pancreas: molecular characterization of 23 patients along with a literature review. World J Gastrointest Oncol. 2015;7(9):132–40.

17. Hsu J-T, Yeh C-N, Chen Y-R, Chen H-M, Hwang T-L, Jan Y-Y, et al. Adenosquamous carcinoma of the pancreas. Digestion. 2005;72(2–3):104–8.

18. Madura JA, Jarman BT, Doherty MG, Yum MN, Howard TJ. Adenosquamous carcinoma of the pancreas. Arch Surg. 1999;134(6):599–603.

19. Boyd CA, Benarroch-Gampel J, Sheffield KM, Cooksley CD, Riall TS. 415 patients with adenosquamous carcinoma of the pancreas: a population-based analysis of prognosis and survival. J Surg Res. 2012;174(1):12–9.

20. Brody JR, Costantino CL, Potoczek M, Cozzitorto J, McCue P, Yeo CJ, et al. Adenosquamous carcinoma of the pancreas harbors KRAS2, DPC4 and TP53 molecular alterations similar to pancreatic ductal adenocarcinoma. Mod Pathol. 2009;22(5):651–9.

21. Basturk O, Khanani F, Sarkar F, Levi E, Cheng JD, Adsay NV. DeltaNp63 expression in pancreas and pancreatic neoplasia. Mod Pathol. 2005;18(9):1193–8.

22. Fang Y, Su Z, Xie J, Xue R, Ma Q, Li Y, et al. Genomic signatures of pancreatic adenosquamous carcinoma (PASC). J Pathol. 2017;243(2):155–9.

23. Mueller S, Engleitner T, Maresch R, Zukowska M, Lange S, Kaltenbacher T, et al. Evolutionary routes and KRAS dosage define pancreatic cancer phenotypes. Nature. 2018;554(7690):62–8.

24. Krasinskas AM, Moser AJ, Saka B, Adsay NV, Chiosea SI. KRAS mutant allele-specific imbalance is associated with worse prognosis in pancreatic cancer and progression to undifferentiated carcinoma of the pancreas. Mod Pathol. 2013;26(10):1346–54.

25. Agaimy A, Haller F, Frohnauer J, Schaefer I-M, Ströbel P, Hartmann A, et al. Pancreatic undifferentiated rhabdoid carcinoma: KRAS alterations and SMARCB1 expression status define two subtypes. Mod Pathol. 2015;28(2):248–60.

26. Muraki T, Reid MD, Basturk O, Jang K-T, Bedolla G, Bagci P, et al. Undifferentiated carcinoma with osteoclastic giant cells of the pancreas: clinicopathologic analysis of 38 cases highlights a more protracted clinical course than currently appreciated. Am J Surg Pathol. 2016;40(9):1203–16.

27. Bergmann F, Esposito I, Michalski CW, Herpel E, Friess H, Schirmacher P. Early undifferentiated pancreatic carcinoma with osteoclastlike giant cells: direct evidence for ductal evolution. Am J Surg Pathol. 2007;31(12):1919–25.

28. Mostafa ME, Erbarut-Seven I, Pehlivanoglu B, Adsay V. Pathologic classification of "pancreatic cancers": current concepts and challenges. Chin Clin Oncol. 2017;6(6):59.

29. Tan MC, Basturk O, Brannon AR, Bhanot U, Scott SN, Bouvier N, et al. GNAS and KRAS mutations define separate progression pathways in intraductal papillary mucinous neoplasm-associated carcinoma. J Am Coll Surg. 2015;220(5):845–854.e1.

30. Liszka L, Zielinska-Pajak E, Pajak J, Gołka D. Colloid carcinoma of the pancreas: review of selected pathological and clinical aspects. Pathology. 2008;40(7):655–63.

31. Wilentz RE, Goggins M, Redston M, Marcus VA, Adsay NV, Sohn TA, et al. Genetic, immuno-histochemical, and clinical features of medullary carcinoma of the pancreas: a newly described and characterized entity. Am J Pathol. 2000;156(5):1641–51.
32. Yamamoto H, Itoh F, Nakamura H, Fukushima H, Sasaki S, Perucho M, et al. Genetic and clinical features of human pancreatic ductal adenocarcinomas with widespread microsatellite instability. Cancer Res. 2001;61(7):3139–44.
33. Goggins M, Offerhaus GJ, Hilgers W, Griffin CA, Shekher M, Tang D, et al. Pancreatic adeno-carcinomas with DNA replication errors (RER+) are associated with wild-type K-ras and char-acteristic histopathology. Poor differentiation, a syncytial growth pattern, and pushing borders suggest RER+. Am J Pathol. 1998;152(6):1501–7.
34. Stauffer JA, Asbun HJ. Rare tumors and lesions of the pancreas. Surg Clin North Am. 2018;98(1):169–88.
35. Su J-S, Chen Y-T, Wang R-C, Wu C-Y, Lee S-W, Lee T-Y. Clinicopathological character-istics in the differential diagnosis of hepatoid adenocarcinoma: a literature review. World J Gastroenterol. 2013;19(3):321–7.
36. Stamatova D, Theilmann L, Spiegelberg C. A hepatoid carcinoma of the pancreatic head. Surg Case Rep. 2016;2(1):78.
37. Chang JM, Katariya NN, Lam-Himlin DM, Haakinson DJ, Ramanathan RK, Halfdanarson TR, et al. Hepatoid carcinoma of the pancreas: case report, next-generation tumor profiling, and literature review. Case Rep Gastroenterol. 2016;10(3):605–12.
38. Kuo P-C, Chen S-C, Shyr Y-M, Kuo Y-J, Lee R-C, Wang S-E. Hepatoid carcinoma of the pan-creas. World J Surg Oncol. 2015;13:185.
39. Rad R, Rad L, Wang W, Strong A, Ponstingl H, Bronner IF, et al. A conditional piggyBac transposition system for genetic screening in mice identifies oncogenic networks in pancreatic cancer. Nat Genet. 2015;47(1):47–56.
40. Späth C, Nitsche U, Müller T, Michalski C, Erkan M, Kong B, et al. Strategies to improve the outcome in locally advanced pancreatic cancer. Minerva Chir. 2015;70(2):97–106.
41. Paniccia A, Hosokawa PW, Schulick RD, Henderson W, Kaplan J, Gajdos C. A matched-cohort analysis of 192 pancreatic anaplastic carcinomas and 960 pancreatic adenocarcinomas: a 13-year North American experience using the National Cancer Data Base (NCDB). Surgery. 2016;160(2):281–92.
42. Özdemir BC, Pentcheva-Hoang T, Carstens JL, Zheng X, Wu C-C, Simpson TR, et al. Depletion of carcinoma-associated fibroblasts and fibrosis induces immunosuppression and accelerates pancreas cancer with reduced survival. Cancer Cell. 2014;25(6):719–34.
43. Rhim AD, Oberstein PE, Thomas DH, Mirek ET, Palermo CF, Sastra SA, et al. Stromal ele-ments act to restrain, rather than support, pancreatic ductal adenocarcinoma. Cancer Cell. 2014;25(6):735–47.
44. Apte MV, Park S, Phillips PA, Santucci N, Goldstein D, Kumar RK, et al. Desmoplastic reac-tion in pancreatic cancer: role of pancreatic stellate cells. Pancreas. 2004;29(3):179–87.
45. Esposito I, Penzel R, Chaib-Harrireche M, Barcena U, Bergmann F, Riedl S, et al. Tenascin C and annexin II expression in the process of pancreatic carcinogenesis. J Pathol. 2006;208(5):673–85.
46. Olive KP, Jacobetz MA, Davidson CJ, Gopinathan A, McIntyre D, Honess D, et al. Inhibition of Hedgehog signaling enhances delivery of chemotherapy in a mouse model of pancreatic cancer. Science. 2009;324(5933):1457–61.
47. Erkan M, Michalski CW, Rieder S, Reiser-Erkan C, Abiatari I, Kolb A, et al. The activated stroma index is a novel and independent prognostic marker in pancreatic ductal adenocarci-noma. Clin Gastroenterol Hepatol. 2008;6(10):1155–61.
48. Wang JP, Wu C-Y, Yeh Y-C, Shyr Y-M, Wu Y-Y, Kuo C-Y, et al. Erlotinib is effective in pan-creatic cancer with epidermal growth factor receptor mutations: a randomized, open-label, prospective trial. Oncotarget. 2015;6(20):18162–73.

49. Knudsen ES, Vail P, Balaji U, Ngo H, Botros IW, Makarov V, et al. Stratification of pancreatic ductal adenocarcinoma: combinatorial genetic, stromal, and immunologic markers. Clin Cancer Res. 2017;23(15):4429–40.
50. Haeberle L, Steiger K, Schlitter AM, Safi SA, Knoefel WT, Erkan M, Esposito I. Stromal heterogeneity in pancreatic cancer and chronic pancreatitis [published online ahead of print, 2018 May 12]. Pancreatology. 2018;S1424-3903(18)30109–1. https://doi:10.1016/j.pan.2018.05.004.
51. Fujita T, Nakagohri T, Gotohda N, Takahashi S, Konishi M, Kojima M, et al. Evaluation of the prognostic factors and significance of lymph node status in invasive ductal carcinoma of the body or tail of the pancreas. Pancreas. 2010;39(1):e48–54.
52. Moffitt RA, Marayati R, Flate EL, Volmar KE, Loeza SGH, Hoadley KA, et al. Virtual microdissection identifies distinct tumor- and stroma-specific subtypes of pancreatic ductal adenocarcinoma. Nat Genet. 2015;47(10):1168–78.
53. Collisson EA, Sadanandam A, Olson P, Gibb WJ, Truitt M, Gu S, et al. Subtypes of pancreatic ductal adenocarcinoma and their differing responses to therapy. Nat Med. 2011;17(4):500–3.
54. Bailey P, Chang DK, Nones K, Johns AL, Patch A-M, Gingras M-C, et al. Genomic analyses identify molecular subtypes of pancreatic cancer. Nature. 2016;531(7592):47–52.
55. Puleo F, Nicolle R, Blum Y, Cros J, Marisa L, Demetter P, et al. Stratification of pancreatic ductal adenocarcinomas based on tumor and microenvironment features. Gastroenterology. 2018;155(6):1999–2013.e3.
56. Muckenhuber A, Berger AK, Schlitter AM, Steiger K, Konukiewitz B, Trumpp A, et al. Pancreatic ductal adenocarcinoma subtyping using the biomarkers hepatocyte nuclear factor-1A and cytokeratin-81 correlates with outcome and treatment response. Clin Cancer Res. 2018;24(2):351–9.

Part II
PDAC Precursors and Early Diagnosis

Chapter 2
Surveillance and Intervention in IPMN

A. Balduzzi, N. C. M. van Huijgevoort, G. Marchegiani, M. Engelbrecht,
J. Stoker, J. Verheij, P. Fockens, J. E. van Hooft, and M. G. Besselink

More frequent use of high-quality cross-sectional imaging, increased life expectancy, and the trend for healthy individuals to undergo "health checkups," including full-body magnetic resonance imaging (MRI), have increased the detection of intraductal papillary mucinous neoplasm of the pancreas (IPMN) [1]. IPMN is a heterogeneous group of pancreatic cystic neoplasm arising from the proliferation of mucin-producing cells within the pancreatic ducts [2]. IPMN can be morphologically divided into main duct IPMN (MD-IPMN), branch duct IPMN (BD-IPMN) and mixed-type IPMN (MT-IPMN) on the basis of the anatomical distribution of duct(s) dilatation in the pancreatic gland [3, 4].

IPMN represents 20–50% of all pancreas cystic neoplasms and 1–3% of the exocrine pancreatic neoplasms [5–7]. The male to female ratio reported for IPMN in the population is 3:1 (2:1 for BD-IPMN) [8]. Surprisingly, these ratios seem to vary between countries/regions. A male predominance was observed in Korea and

A. Balduzzi · G. Marchegiani
Department of Surgery, Pancreas Institute Verona, Verona, Italy

N. C. M. van Huijgevoort · P. Fockens · J. E. van Hooft
Department of Gastroenterology and Hepatology, Amsterdam Gastroenterology and
Metabolism, Amsterdam UMC, University of Amsterdam, Amsterdam, The Netherlands

M. Engelbrecht · J. Stoker
Department of Radiology and Nuclear Medicine, Amsterdam Gastroenterology and
Metabolism, Amsterdam UMC, University of Amsterdam, Amsterdam, The Netherlands

J. Verheij
Department of Pathology, Cancer Center Amsterdam, Amsterdam UMC, University of
Amsterdam, Amsterdam, The Netherlands

M. G. Besselink (✉)
Department of Surgery, Cancer Center Amsterdam, Amsterdam UMC, University of
Amsterdam, Amsterdam, The Netherlands
e-mail: m.g.besselink@amc.nl

© Springer Nature Switzerland AG 2020
C. W. Michalski et al. (eds.), *Translational Pancreatic Cancer Research*,
Molecular and Translational Medicine,
https://doi.org/10.1007/978-3-030-49476-6_2

Japan, while a more even distribution between male and female was observed in the United States and in Europe. The mean age of presentation is in the fifth to seventh decade [9], and the prevalence increases with increasing age of the population [10].

Due to the potential for progression to invasive cancer, patients with IPMN are routinely monitored. The primary goal is to prevent malignancy and/or alleviate symptoms while avoiding unnecessary surgery. Currently, four guidelines, the 2015 American Gastroenterological Association (AGA) [11], the 2017 International Association of Pancreatology (IAP) [10], the 2018 American College of Gastroenterology (ACG) [12], and the 2018 European Study Group on Cystic Tumours of the Pancreas (European) [13], provide recommendations on surveillance and surgical resection based on symptoms and perceived risk of malignancy (Table 2.1).

Classification of IPMN

Radiological Classification

The morphological classification of IPMN in MD-, BD-, and MT-IPMN is based on radiological characteristics. These subtypes harbor a different risk of malignancy, and therefore each requires a specific therapeutic approach (Fig. 2.1).

MD-IPMN can be recognized by the abrupt dilatation of the pancreatic main duct and the presence of mucus together with villous neoplastic component. The dilatation of the pancreatic main duct can be segmental or along the entire duct. For resected MD-IPMN, the mean frequency of advanced neoplasia (invasive cancer or HGD) is 61.6% (range 36–100%), and the mean frequency of invasive cancer is 43.1% (range 11–82%) [14–26].

BD-IPMN is characterized by a "grape-like" dilatation of pancreatic side branch ducts. For resected BD-IPMN, the mean frequency for invasive carcinoma and high-grade dysplasia (HGD) is 31.1% (range 14.4–47.9%), and the frequency of invasive cancer is 18.5% (range 6.1–37.7%) [27–33].

MT-IPMN presents radiological characteristics of both MD- and BD-IPMN. For resected MT-IPMN, the mean frequency of HGD and invasive carcinoma is the same as for MD-IPMN.

Histological Classification

Histologically, IPMN can be divided on the basis of the epithelium in different histologic phenotypes: intestinal, gastric, oncocytic, and pancreatobiliary type. Typically, these distinctions can only be made reliably based on surgical specimens, thus limiting their value in the diagnostic process [34].

Table 2.1 Absolute and relative indications for surgical resection by 2015 AGA, 2017 IAP, 2018 European, and 2018 ACG guidelines

Guidelines	Cyst type	Absolute indications for surgery	Relative indications for surgery
2015 AGA guideline	IPMN	PD ≥ 5 mm (on MRI *and* EUS) *and* solid component *or* cytology positive for malignancy	
2017 IAP guideline	IPMN	Cytology suspicious or positive for malignancy Jaundice (IPMN related) Enhancing mural nodule (≥5 mm) PD dilatation ≥ 10 mm	Grow rate ≥ 5 mm/2 years Increased levels of serum CA 19.9 PD dilatation between 5 and 9 mm Cyst diameter ≥ 30 mm Acute pancreatitis (caused by IPMN) Enhancing mural nodule (<5 mm) Abrupt change in caliber of PD with distal pancreatic atrophy Lymphadenopathy Thickened/enhancing cyst walls
2018 European guideline	IPMN	Positive cytology for malignancy/HGD Solid mass Jaundice (IPMN related) Enhancing mural nodule (≥5 mm) PD dilatation ≥ 10 mm	Grow rate ≥ 5 mm/year Increased levels of serum CA 19.9 (>37 U/m) * PD dilatation between 5 and 9.9 mm Cyst diameter ≥ 40 mm New onset of diabetes mellitus Acute pancreatitis (caused by IPMN) Enhancing mural nodule (<5 mm)
2018 ACG guideline	IPMN	Decided by multidisciplinary team Referral in case of: Jaundice (IPMN related) Acute pancreatitis (caused by IPMN) Increased levels of serum CA 19.9 Mural nodule/solid component PD dilatation > 5 mm Cyst diameter ≥ 30 mm Positive cytology for malignancy/HGD	

ACG American College of Gastroenterology, *AGA* American Gastroenterological Association, *CA 19.9* cancer antigen 19.9, *EUS* endoscopic ultrasound, *HGD* high-grade dysplasia, *IAP* International Association of Pancreatology, *IPMN* intraductal papillary mucinous neoplasm, *MRI* magnetic resonance imaging, *PD* pancreatic duct

*The 2015 AGA guideline suggests to discontinue the follow-up after 5 years, if there is no change in size or characteristics of the cyst

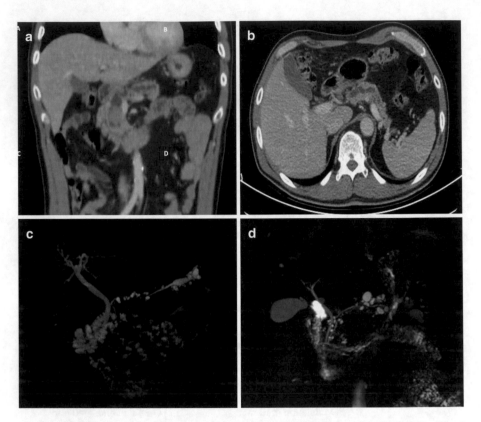

Fig. 2.1 Different types of IPMN. (**a**) BD-IPMN with slender MPD in the tail. (**b**) Both dilated MPD and BD in the pancreatic tail, image matching a MT-IPMN. (**c**) Dilated MPD in the head of the pancreas. (**d**) Image matching a MD-IPMN with solid component as a sign of a possible malignant degeneracy

Further distinction is based on cytological and architectural atypia in noninvasive IPMN. Currently, the World Health Organization (WHO) classification recommends a three-tiered system for grading of dysplasia in IPMN, from low- to high-grade dysplasia [35].

Low-grade dysplasia (LGD) is characterized by cells with oriented nuclei with small variability in nuclear size, shape, and retained polarity. *Moderate-grade* dysplasia is defined by nuclear pleomorphism, increased nucleus-to-cytoplasm ratio, and nuclear pseudostratification. *High-grade* dysplasia (HGD) features architectural complexity and marked variability in nuclear size and shape [36]. In order to improve the concordance of reporting and alignment with practical consequences, a two-tiered grading system has been proposed (low- versus high-grade dysplasia) [37].

Regarding the histological classification of IPMN, *gastric*-type IPMN is characterized by low-grade dysplasia and abundant cytoplasmic mucin that expresses *MUC-5AC*. When the gastric type has invasive characteristics and is localized in the pancreatic main duct, it is more likely a more aggressive tubular carcinoma [38].

The *intestinal epithelial* type [39] is the most common in IPMN and resembles normal intestinal epithelial cells with expression of *MUC-2* and *CDX-2*. The *pancreatobiliary*-type IPMNs express MUC-1, and in this type, cells are organized as complex papillae. This subtype is associated with invasive carcinoma in 90% of patients. The pancreatobiliary subtype is also associated with invasive tubular adenocarcinoma, and both morphology and prognosis are similar to PDAC (pancreatic ductal adenocarcinoma) [40–42]. The *oncocytic*-type IPMN is characterized by cells with abundant eosinophil cytoplasm rich in mitochondria organized in complex papillae or solid sheets and severe high-grade dysplasia [43].

IPMN can contain more than one subtype, and it is recommended to report the dominant subtype and/or the subtype exhibiting the highest degree of dysplasia. The oncocytic type occurs only in a "pure" form, without mixing with other different histological subtypes [40, 41]. A 2011 study classified 283 surgically resected IPMNs: 137 BD-IPMNs, 102 MD-IPMNs, and 44 MT-IPMNs. Among these, 139 patients had gastric type (90 patients with BD-IPMN, 34 with MD-IPMN, and 15 with MT-IPMN), 101 patients had intestinal type (28 patients with BD-IPMN, 54 with MD-IPMN, and 19 with MT-IPMN), 24 patients had oncocytic type (12 patients with BD-IPMN, 8 with MD-IPMN, and 4 with MT-IPMN), and 19 had pancreatobiliary type (7 with BD-IPMN, 6 with MD-IPMN, and 6 with MT-IPMN) [41]. These findings are supported by other studies [40, 44] and demonstrate that the gastric and intestinal subtypes are the most common and that all histopathological subtypes can be found in the three morphological imaging-based subtypes (BD-, MD-, MT-IPMN).

Intraductal tubulopapillary neoplasm (ITPN) is a rare intraductal epithelial neoplasm of the pancreas recently recognized as a distinct entity by the WHO classification in 2010. It accounts less than 1% of all pancreatic exocrine neoplasms and the 3% of intraductal pancreatic neoplasms. Compared to IPMN, they are less often cystic, typically mass forming, without overt production of mucin. ITPNs typically have uniform high-grade dysplasia, and approximately 40–50% of the cases are associated with invasive cancer [45, 46]. ITPN is often difficult to differentiate histologically from IPMN, especially the pancreatobiliary and oncocytic subtype. ITPNs showed positive for cytokeratin, CK19, MUC1, and MUC6 at the immunohistochemistry analysis [47].

Diagnosis

Symptoms

Most IPMNs do not cause symptoms. In case of symptoms, the most common are weight loss, pancreatitis, jaundice, palpable mass, and postprandial fullness according to a study from a high-volume center. Only pancreatitis and jaundice could be related to the presence of IPMN [48]. Main duct IPMN is more often symptomatic than branch duct IPMN. This can be related to the massive production of mucin in MD-IPMN;

mucin plugs may occlude the pancreatic duct and lead to acute pancreatitis with epigastric discomfort. These symptoms have been reported in approximately 25% of patients with MD-IPMN [49, 50]. The chronic obstruction of the outflow of pancreatic juice can lead to pancreatic endocrine and exocrine insufficiency and resulting diabetes, diarrhea, and steatorrhea. Jaundice can be secondary to mucin plugs in the distal bile duct or direct tumor invasion in case of malignant progression.

Symptoms, such as acute pancreatitis, jaundice, or new-onset of diabetes mellitus, are mostly associated with high-grade dysplasia or invasive carcinoma [51, 52]. These symptoms in the presence of an IPMN have been part of the IAP and European criteria in the predictive factors for malignant IPMN [9, 46, 53].

Imaging Techniques

Currently, cross-sectional imaging plays a central role in lesion detection and differentiation of IPMN. The presence and extent of IPMN can be assessed with computed tomography (CT), magnetic resonance imaging (MRI), and endoscopic ultrasound (EUS). Gadolinium-enhanced magnetic resonance imaging (MRI) with magnetic resonance cholangiopancreatography (MRCP) is the modality of choice, because of its superiority in identifying a connection between the MDP and the lesion and mural nodules and septations, as well as cyst differentiation [10, 54]. In addition, studies have shown that repeated exposure to ionizing radiation following CT increases the risk of malignancy. Therefore MRI/MRCP, avoiding the ionizing radiations, is the preferred method for surveillance of PCN (pancreatic cystic neoplasm) [1]. By definition, branch duct IPMNs have a communication to the main pancreatic duct that can be best assessed with either MRI (90–100%) or EUS (80–90%) [55]. For MD-IPMN and MT-IPMN, a focal or diffuse involvement of the main pancreatic duct can easily be assessed by MRI/MRCP and EUS. A systematic review reported that CT is able to correctly differentiate benign from malignant cysts with 71–80% accuracy and a presence of a communication between the cyst and the pancreatic duct with 80% accuracy; for MRI and MRCP, these were 55–76% and 96% [56]. Another systematic review including 37 studies observed a pooled 81% sensitivity and 76% specificity for risk features predictive of malignancy on CT/MRI [57]. Higher accuracy can be observed with EUS, with a 65–96% accuracy to detect benign from malignant cyst, but due to its invasive nature, it should be reserved for selected cases [58].

Cyst Fluid Analysis and Biomarkers

EUS allows fine needle aspiration (FNA) of the cyst fluid. EUS-FNA is a safe procedure. In a retrospective study in two experienced academic institutions, the complication rate of EUS in 603 patients was 2.2% with pancreatitis, abdominal pain, retroperitoneal bleeding, infection, and bradycardia as main complications [59].

A cyst fluid CEA (carcinoembryonic antigen) with a cutoff of 192–200 ng/ml [4, 60], as well as amylase, can be helpful in the differential diagnosis of pancreatic cysts and grade of dysplasia. CEA level showed to have 52–78% of sensitivity and 63–91% of specificity for identifying IPMN and MCN [13, 61, 62].

Cytology may report on low- and intermediate-grade dysplasia, high-grade dysplasia, or invasive carcinoma [63]. It is, however, common to find different grades of atypia within the same lesion; therefore the cytological examination of IPMN is not enough to assess the entire cytological pattern of the cystic lesion. Matthaei et al. [64] reported that the analysis of cells in the cystic fluid allowed to detect invasive carcinoma and HGD with 72% of sensitivity and positive predictive value (80% accuracy).

DNA-based testing of pancreatic cyst fluid seems to be a promising adjunct for the differentiation between mucinous and non-mucinous PCN, between mucinous PCNs (IPMN versus MCN), and between premalignant PCNs and those with advanced neoplasia. Many genetic mutations have been reported regarding IPMN: KRAS (~80% of IPMN), GNAS (~70% of IPMN), RNF43, PIK3CA, p16/CDKN2A, SMAD4, and Tp53 [65, 66]. The mutation of GNAS and KRAS is seen in >90% of IPMN [66, 67], and GNAS mutation is more common in intestinal-type IPMN [66, 68].

From recent genetic studies, it is clear that both invasive and noninvasive components tend to harbor identical mutations [65, 66]. In the near future, micro-RNA might be the key to distinguish IPMN from other cysts of the pancreas and even discern low-grade IPMN from high-grade dysplasia IPMN [68–70]. Moreover glycoprotein altered expression in the cystic fluid might be useful as well in differentiating IPMN with low-grade dysplasia from high-grade IPMN [71–73].

New Developments in Imaging Techniques

Recent evidence suggests that MRCP (thick and thin T2 slices, centered on the main pancreatic duct at the head and body/tail level) or CT scan with slices <2 mm width (three phases: no iodine IV contrast, arterial, and portal phases) should be used when evaluating a pancreatic cyst [1, 10]. EUS should remain a third option for those cases in whom the radiographic characterization of the pancreatic lesion is unclear [74]. Nevertheless, EUS is very useful to detect mural nodules, especially when the examination is integrated with a contrast-enhanced endoscopic ultrasound (CH-EUS) [75]. Contrast-enhanced EUS (CE-EUS) can be used to better differentiate a mucin plug and mural nodule using echo-Doppler during the examination, and even better definition can be assessed with tissue harmonic echo (THE) [76]. Nevertheless, EUS is an operator-dependent procedure that relies on the specialist's experience and ability.

More recently, a new endoscopic modality has been described, the needle-based confocal laser endomicroscopy (nCLE) that can provide a real-time in vivo optical biopsy with the use of a fluorescent dye [77]. The nCLE has been proven feasible and reliable in differentiating SCN from mucinous lesions [78–82].

The micro-forceps biopsy (MFB) is showing good results in the assessment of the nature of pancreatic cysts. The device can be inserted in a 19 gauge needle during the endoscopy procedure and allow a "micro-biopsy" from the cyst wall or septations for histological evaluation of the cyst architecture and subepithelial stroma. The MFB can be used in addition to the pancreatic cyst fluid (PCF) examination and in a recent paper by Zhang et al. [83] has proven good result in diagnosing specific type of pancreatic cyst, with consequent important implications regarding the management of the patients. The presence of epithelial stroma in the biopsy performed with the micro-forceps can help the pathologist in the differential diagnosis between MCN and IPMNs [83].

Another technique to identify and characterize pancreatic IPMNs is the peroral pancreatoscopy (POPS) [84]. The added value of this technique appears to lie in the ability to identify pancreatic duct skip lesions (reported in about 6–19% of the patients [85]) in order to reduce recurrences after pancreatic surgery [86]. In addition, POPS allows collection of pancreatic juice for cytopathological examination and for biopsy using the mini-forceps.

Clinical and Radiological Characteristics Associated with Advanced Neoplasia

Many guidelines have been published on management of pancreatic cystic neoplasms (PCNs): the IAP (2017) guideline for the management of IPMN of the pancreas [10], the European evidence-based guideline (2018) on pancreatic cystic neoplasms [54], the AGA guideline (2015) [87], and the ACG clinical guideline (2018) [88].

According to both the IAP and European guidelines, jaundice, the presence of an enhancing mural nodule ≥5 mm, the presence of a solid component, positive cytology, and a dilated PD ≥ 10 mm are highly predictive of advanced neoplasia and therefore an absolute indication for resection in surgically fit patients. According to both the 2017 IAP and the 2018 European guidelines, acute pancreatitis caused by IPMN, an enhancing mural nodule <5 mm, a dilated PD between 5 and 9.9 mm, and an increased level of serum CA19.9 without jaundice are associated with advanced neoplasia in IPMN and therefore a relative indication for surgery in patients fit for surgery.

According to the 2017 IAP guideline, a thickened or enhancing cyst wall, lymphadenopathy, an abrupt change in caliber of PD with distal pancreatic atrophy, grow rate of the cyst of 5 mm or more in 2 years, and a cyst diameter of 30 mm or more are also associated with advanced neoplasia in IPMN. According to the 2018 European guideline, a cyst growth rate of 5 mm or more in 1 year, new onset of diabetes mellitus, and a cyst diameter of 40 mm or more are associated with advanced neoplasia in IPMN. Increased risks of high-grade dysplasia or cancer are also a MPD (main pancreatic duct) between 5 and 9.9 mm, a cystic growth rate

>5 mm/year, serum CA19-9 > 37 U/mL, symptoms, enhancing mural nodules (<5 mm), and/or a cystic diameter >40 mm.

Treatment

When an IPMN at high(er) risk of malignancy is characterized, the treatment of choice is surgery, in surgically fit patients. All guidelines recommend that surgical resection for IPMN should only be performed by experienced surgeons in high-volume centers after consultation by a multidisciplinary team with pancreatic expertise. Standard treatment recommended is pancreatoduodenectomy or left pancreatectomy according to the site and the extent of the disease with lymphadenectomy [10]. Minimally invasive surgery, especially when distal pancreatectomy is indicated, is mostly feasible with good outcome. Most guidelines consider a total pancreatectomy unnecessarily aggressive, especially considering the total endocrine and exocrine insufficiency. For MD-IPMN there is no consensus regarding the best surgical option (total pancreatectomy and partial pancreatectomy followed by close surveillance are possible strategies) [89–93]. In patients with multifocal BD-IPMN, only high-risk BD-IPMN should be resected during surgery, while the other cystic lesions can undergo follow-up. Every cyst should be evaluated individually regarding the presence of sign of degeneration and/or malignancy [13]. The risk of degeneration in multifocal BD-IPMN seems not to be higher compared to the unifocal BD-IPMN (conflicting results can be seen in published literature [14, 94]); therefore a more aggressive approach might be beneficial only in patients with a family history of PDAC [95].

All current guidelines emphasize the importance of intraoperative frozen section. IPMNs originate from pancreatic ducts, both MPD or peripheral ducts; thus the anatomopathological analysis of resection margins and confirmation of disease-free margins are mandatory for radical surgery. This aspect relates very well for those patients with MT-IPMN misdiagnosed as BD-IPMN before surgery, showing involvement of MPD in the pathological examination. When low-grade dysplasia is present in the frozen section, no further resection is required [96]. Obviously, a frozen section will not compensate for potential skip lesions in the MPD [86, 97, 98].

Surveillance After Pancreatectomy

After surgical resection of IPMN, lifelong follow-up and surveillance are recommended because both new IPMN and concomitant PDAC might occur after surgical resection. Resected IPMN-associated cancer should be followed up in the same way as patients with PDAC after pancreatectomy [99].

The main risks of recurrence in patient undergoing surgery for IPMN are HGD (17% of recurrence after surgery [92]) and family history of PDAC (23% of recurrences vs 7% in patients without family history of PDAC [92]). The debate regarding the surgical margins is still open: while Marchegiani et al. [18] found a significantly higher incidence of recurrence in patients with positive margins after surgical resection, He et al. [92] and Kang et al. [100] didn't report any difference in recurrence rate in the positive margins. The risk of recurrence might be correlated not only to other surgical technique but also to the nature of the IPMN and the subtype of the cystic lesion [101–103].

The IAP guideline recommends follow-up at least twice a year for patients with family history of PDAC, surgical resection margin with HGD, and non-intestinal subtype of IPMN. In all other patients with resected IPMN, follow-up every 6–12 months is mandatory. In contrast, the European guideline advises follow-up every 6 months for the first 2 years, followed by yearly surveillance for IPMN with HGD or main duct involvement. All the others should be followed up in the same way as non-resected IPMN.

Recent series underline the increasing risk of recurrence during the surveillance: 4% after 1 year, 25% after 5 years, and 62% after 10 years [92]; the risks of developing a new invasive IPMN are 0%, 8%, and 38% after 1-, 5-, and 10-year follow-up [100]; concomitant PDACs have a cumulative 5- and 10-year incidence of developing of 4.5% and 5.9%, respectively [103]. Therefore, most of the guidelines agree that the surveillance of the patients should not be discontinued if the patient remains fit for surgery.

In some cases, synchronous and metachronous malignancies can be observed during the follow-up of patients with IPMN (20–30% [104]), but the incidence of extra-pancreatic malignancies might be the same with the incidence of cancer in the general population since the percentage of incidence differs from region to region [105].

Surveillance

Follow-up is recommended for all the patients feasible for surgery, without hard indications for resection. Timing of follow-up and the best radiological examination are still a matter of debate. Therefore, the guidelines vary somewhat in their advice.

According to the revised IAP guidelines, an additional EUS is indicated for further inspection of the PCN in patients with clinical or radiological characteristics associated with advanced neoplasia (relative indications for resection) [10]. If on endoscopic ultrasound, hard indications for resection can be ruled out (i.e., enhancing nodule ≥5 mm, PD ≥ 10 mm, cytology suspicious for HGD/invasive cancer), follow-up is advised. The surveillance interval is established on the basis of the main cyst size (Table 2.2): for cyst <1 cm, CT/MRI in 6 months and then every 2 years if there is no change in cyst characteristics and for cyst 1–2 cm, CT/MRI every 6 months for 1 year, then yearly for 2 years, and every 2 years if no change is seen; patients with cyst of 2–3 cm should undergo EUS in 3–6 months and then 1

Table 2.2 Surveillance interval of non-resected PCN stratified by AGA, IAP, and the European guidelines

Guidelines	Cyst type	Cyst size	Surveillance interval	Surveillance modalities
2015 AGA	IPMN	<3 cm	Yearly for 1 year Every 2 years[a]	MRI/MRCP
2017 IAP	IPMN	<1 cm	In 6 months Every 2 years	CT or MRI/MRCP CT or MRI/MRCP
		1–2 cm	Every 6 months for 1 year Yearly for 2 years Every 2 years	CT or MRI/MRCP CT or MRI/MRCP CT or MRI/MRCP
		2–3 cm	3–6 months Yearly	EUS Alternating MRI with EUS
2018 European	IPMN	<4 cm	Every 6 months for 1 year Yearly	CA 19.9, EUS and/or MRI
2018 ACG	IPMN	<1 cm	Every 2 years	MRI
		1–2 cm	Yearly	MRI
		2–3 cm	6–12 months	MRI or EUS

ACG American College of Gastroenterology, *AGA* American Gastroenterological Association, *CA 19.9* cancer antigen 19.9, *CT* computed tomography, *EUS* endoscopic ultrasound, *IAP* International Association of Pancreatology, *IPMN* intraductal papillary mucinous neoplasm, *MRI* magnetic resonance imaging
[a]The 2015 AGA guideline suggests to discontinue the follow-up after 5 years, if there is no change in size or characteristics of the cyst

per year (EUS and MRI can be eventually alternated), and surgery should be considered for young and fit patients who require a prolonged follow-up.

The European guideline [13] recommends follow-up for BD-IPMN < 4 cm without other risk factors with CA19.9 and MRI/MRCP or EUS every 6 months the first year after diagnosis and yearly thereafter.

The best surveillance modality and timing should be evaluated in a large prospective study, possibly within the scope of the PACYFIC study. The PACYFIC study is an international, prospective cohort study aiming to optimize pancreatic cystic neoplasm surveillance (clinical trial number: NTR4505).

During follow-up the 5-year cumulative incidence of developing a concomitant PDAC in patients with IPMN ranges from 2.2% to 8.8% [10]. The follow-up of the patients should be performed with the same radiological technique if possible in order to lower the bias of interobserver measurement of the pancreatic cyst [106].

Conclusions and Recommendations

The detection of pancreatic IPMNs due to the higher rate of radiological examinations and increased life expectancy in the population has led to a global awareness of this entity. Current diagnostic techniques allow to detect and characterize pancreatic cysts, but the natural history of this pathology is still mainly unknown.

Many guidelines have been published and revised in recent years, but the management and surveillance for patients with IPMN remain contradictory.

IPMNs represent a true challenge nowadays, and due to the heterogeneity of these cysts, we truly believe that a multidisciplinary team, and a referred institute, should be mandatory in the decision-making process for these patients. The risk is to underestimate the potential of malignancy of some cystic lesions, leading to a progression of the cyst degeneration with consequent metastasis or invasion of adjacent organs; on the other hand, a too aggressive policy might expose the patients to unnecessary risks of undergoing surgery (morbidity and mortality rates up to 50% and 6.7%, respectively, in high-volume centers) [107] instead of a surveillance program.

Nowadays many questions are still unsolved. For instance, what are the optimal surveillance program and the timing for radiological examination in patients with IPMNs? Which size of BD-IPMN should be considered as indication for surgery and for which size surveillance should not be mandatory? When is better to perform a total pancreatectomy rather than partial pancreatectomy for MD-IPMN?

Further studies and randomized controlled trial are needed to enlighten these aspects since most literature on IPMN is based only on surgical series.

References

1. Del Chiaro M, et al. European evidence-based guidelines on pancreatic cystic neoplasms. Gut. 2018; https://doi.org/10.1136/gutjnl-2018-316027.
2. Adsay NV, et al. Pathologically and biologically distinct types of epithelium in intraductal papillary mucinous neoplasms: delineation of an 'intestinal' pathway of carcinogenesis in the pancreas. Am J Surg Pathol. 2004; https://doi.org/10.1097/00000478-200407000-00001.
3. Bosman FT, Carneiro F, Hruban RH, Theise ND. WHO classification of tumours of the digestive system. Lyon: International Agency for Research on Cancer (IARC); 2010.
4. Tanaka M, et al. International consensus guidelines 2012 for the management of IPMN and MCN of the pancreas. Pancreatology. 2012; https://doi.org/10.1016/j.pan.2012.04.004.
5. Allen PJ, et al. A selective approach to the resection of cystic lesions of the pancreas: results from 539 consecutive patients. Ann Surg. 2006; https://doi.org/10.1097/01.sla.0000237652.84466.54.
6. Kosmahl M, et al. Cystic neoplasms of the pancreas and tumor-like lesions with cystic features: a review of 418 cases and a classification proposal. Virchows Arch. 2004; https://doi.org/10.1007/s00428-004-1043-z.
7. Lee CJ, et al. Risk of malignancy in resected cystic tumors of the pancreas ≤3 cm in size: is it safe to observe asymptomatic patients? A multi-institutional report. J Gastrointest Surg. 2008; https://doi.org/10.1007/s11605-007-0381-y.
8. Ingkakul T, Warshaw AL, Fernández-Del Castillo C. Epidemiology of intraductal papillary mucinous neoplasms of the pancreas: sex differences between 3 geographic regions. Pancreas. 2011; https://doi.org/10.1097/MPA.0b013e31821f27fb.
9. Khalid A, Brugge W. ACG practice guidelines for the diagnosis and management of neoplastic pancreatic cysts. Am J Gastroenterol. 2007; https://doi.org/10.1111/j.1572-0241.2007.01516.x.
10. Tanaka M, et al. Revisions of international consensus Fukuoka guidelines for the management of IPMN of the pancreas. Pancreatology. 2017;17:738–53.

11. Vege SS, Ziring B, Jain R, Moayyedi P. American gastroenterological association institute guideline on the diagnosis and management of asymptomatic neoplastic pancreatic cysts. Gastroenterology. 2015; https://doi.org/10.1053/j.gastro.2015.01.015.
12. Elta GH, Enestvedt BK, Sauer BG, Lennon AM. ACG clinical guideline: diagnosis and management of pancreatic cysts. Am J Gastroenterol. 2018; https://doi.org/10.1038/ajg.2018.14.
13. Unit PS, Institutet K. European evidence-based guidelines on pancreatic cystic neoplasms. Gut. 2018; https://doi.org/10.1136/gutjnl-2018-316027.
14. Schmidt CM, et al. Intraductal papillary mucinous neoplasms: predictors of malignant and invasive pathology. Ann Surg. 2007; https://doi.org/10.1097/SLA.0b013e318155a9e5.
15. Nagai K, et al. Intraductal papillary mucinous neoplasms of the pancreas: Clinicopathologic characteristics and long-term follow-up after resection. World J Surg. 2008; https://doi.org/10.1007/s00268-007-9281-2.
16. Ohno E, et al. Intraductal papillary mucinous neoplasms of the pancreas: differentiation of malignant and benign tumors by endoscopic ultrasonography findings of mural nodules. Ann Surg. 2011; https://doi.org/10.1097/SLA.0b013e31819edle5.
17. Nara S, et al. Preoperative evaluation of invasive and noninvasive intraductal papillary-mucinous neoplasms of the pancreas: clinical, radiological, and pathological analysis of 123 cases. Pancreas. 2009; https://doi.org/10.1097/MPA.0b013e318181b90d.
18. Marchegiani G, et al. IPMN involving the main pancreatic duct: biology, epidemiology, and long-term outcomes following resection. Ann Surg. 2015; https://doi.org/10.1097/SLA.0000000000000813.
19. Hwang DW, et al. Clinicopathologic analysis of surgically proven intraductal papillary mucinous neoplasms of the pancreas in SNUH: a 15-year experience at a single academic institution. Langenbeck's Arch Surg. 2012; https://doi.org/10.1007/s00423-010-0674-6.
20. Waters JA, et al. CT vs MRCP: optimal classification of IPMN type and extent. J Gastrointest Surg. 2008; https://doi.org/10.1007/s11605-007-0367-9.
21. Crippa S, et al. Mucin-producing neoplasms of the pancreas: an analysis of distinguishing clinical and epidemiologic characteristics. Clin Gastroenterol Hepatol. 2010; https://doi.org/10.1016/j.cgh.2009.10.001.
22. Salvia R, et al. Main-duct intraductal papillary mucinous neoplasms of the pancreas: clinical predictors of malignancy and long-term survival following resection. Ann Surg. 2004; https://doi.org/10.1097/01.sla.0000124386.54496.15.
23. Suzuki Y, et al. Cystic neoplasm of the pancreas: a Japanese multiinstitutional study of intraductal papillary mucinous tumor and mucinous cystic tumor. Pancreas. 2004; https://doi.org/10.1097/00006676-200404000-00005.
24. Lee S-Y, et al. Long-term follow up results of intraductal papillary mucinous tumors of pancreas. J Gastroenterol Hepatol. 2005;20:1379–84.
25. Schnelldorfer T, et al. Experience with 208 resections for intraductal papillary mucinous neoplasm of the pancreas. Arch Surg. 2008; https://doi.org/10.1001/archsurg.143.7.639.
26. Kim SC, et al. Intraductal papillary mucinous neoplasm of the pancreas: clinical characteristics and treatment outcomes of 118 consecutive patients from a single center. J Hepato-Biliary-Pancreat Surg. 2008; https://doi.org/10.1007/s00534-007-1231-8.
27. Sahora K, et al. Branch duct intraductal papillary mucinous neoplasms: does cyst size change the tip of the scale? A critical analysis of the revised international consensus guidelines in a large single-institutional series. Ann Surg. 2013; https://doi.org/10.1097/SLA.0b013e3182a18f48.
28. Goh BKP, et al. Evaluation of the Sendai and 2012 international consensus guidelines based on cross-sectional imaging findings performed for the initial triage of mucinous cystic lesions of the pancreas: a single institution experience with 114 surgically treated patient. Am J Surg. 2014;208:202–9.
29. Aso T, et al. 'High-risk stigmata' of the 2012 international consensus guidelines correlate with the malignant grade of branch duct intraductal papillary mucinous neoplasms of the pancreas. Pancreas. 2014; https://doi.org/10.1097/MPA.0000000000000199.

30. Roch AM, et al. International consensus guidelines parameters for the prediction of malignancy in intraductal papillary mucinous neoplasm are not properly weighted and are not cumulative. HPB. 2014; https://doi.org/10.1111/hpb.12305.
31. Jang JY, et al. Validation of international consensus guidelines for the resection of branch duct-type intraductal papillary mucinous neoplasms. Br J Surg. 2014;101:686–92.
32. Fritz S, et al. Pancreatic main-duct involvement in branch-duct IPMNs: an underestimated risk. Ann Surg. 2014; https://doi.org/10.1097/SLA.0000000000000980.
33. Nguyen AH, et al. Current recommendations for surveillance and surgery of intraductal papillary mucinous neoplasms may overlook some patients with cancer. J Gastrointest Surg. 2015; https://doi.org/10.1007/s11605-014-2693-z.
34. Schaberg KB, Dimaio MA, Longacre TA. Intraductal papillary mucinous neoplasms often contain epithelium from multiple subtypes and/or are unclassifiable. Am J Surg Pathol. 2016; https://doi.org/10.1097/PAS.0000000000000528.
35. Carr NJ, Robin LH. WHO classification of tumors of the digestive system. 4th ed. Lyon: IARC; 2010. https://doi.org/10.6061/clinics/2018/e499.
36. Beger HG, Nakao A, Neoptolemos JP, Shu You Peng MGS. Pancreatic cancer cystic neoplasms and endocrine tumors: Wiley-Blackwell; 2015.
37. Basturk O, et al. A revised classification system and recommendations from the Baltimore consensus meeting for neoplastic precursor lesions in the pancreas. Am J Surg Pathol. 2015; https://doi.org/10.1097/PAS.0000000000000533.
38. Terris B, et al. Mucin gene expression in intraductal papillary-mucinous pancreatic tumours and related lesions. J Pathol. 2002; https://doi.org/10.1002/path.1146.
39. Adsay NV, et al. Colloid (mucinous noncystic) carcinoma of the pancreas. Am J Surg Pathol. 2001; https://doi.org/10.1097/00000478-200101000-00003.
40. Distler M, et al. Pathohistological subtype predicts survival in patients with intraductal papillary mucinous neoplasm (IPMN) of the pancreas. Ann Surg. 2013; https://doi.org/10.1097/SLA.0b013e318287ab73.
41. Furukawa T, et al. Prognostic relevance of morphological types of intraductal papillary mucinous neoplasms of the pancreas. Gut. 2011;60:509–16.
42. Yopp AC, et al. Invasive carcinoma arising in intraductal papillary mucinous neoplasms of the pancreas: a matched control study with conventional pancreatic ductal adenocarcinoma. Ann Surg. 2011; https://doi.org/10.1097/SLA.0b013e318214bcb4.
43. Volkan Adsay N, Adair CF, Heffess CS, Klimstra DS. Intraductal oncocytic papillary neoplasms of the pancreas. Am J Surg Pathol. 1996; https://doi.org/10.1097/00000478-199608000-00007.
44. Del Chiaro M, Verbeke C. Intraductal papillary mucinous neoplasms of the pancreas: reporting clinically relevant features. Histopathology. 2017; https://doi.org/10.1111/his.13131.
45. Kölby D, Thilén J, Andersson R, Sasor A, Ansari D. Multifocal intraductal tubulopapillary neoplasm of the pancreas with total pancreatectomy: report of a case and review of literature. Int J Clin Exp Pathol. 2015;8:9672.
46. Suda K, et al. Variant of intraductal carcinoma (with scant mucin production) is of main pancreatic duct origin: a clinicopathological study of four patients. Am J Gastroenterol. 1996; https://doi.org/10.1016/j.meatsci.2005.09.014.
47. Rooney SL, Shi J. Intraductal tubulopapillary neoplasm of the pancreas an update from a pathologist's perspective. Arch Pathol Lab Med. 2016; https://doi.org/10.5858/arpa.2016-0207-RA.
48. Fernández-del Castillo C, et al. Incidental pancreatic cysts: clinicopathologic characteristics and comparison with symptomatic patients. Arch Surg. 2003; https://doi.org/10.1001/archsurg.138.4.427.
49. Sakorafas GH, Sarr MG. Cystic neoplasms of the pancreas; What a clinician should know. Cancer Treat Rev. 2005; https://doi.org/10.1016/j.ctrv.2005.09.001.
50. Stark A, Donahue TR, Reber HA, Joe Hines O. Pancreatic cyst disease a review. J Am Med Assoc. 2016; https://doi.org/10.1001/jama.2016.4690.

51. Tsutsumi K, et al. A history of acute pancreatitis in intraductal papillary mucinous neoplasms of the pancreas is a potential predictive factor for malignant papillary subtype. Pancreatology. 2010; https://doi.org/10.1159/000320696.
52. Ingkakul T, et al. Predictors of the presence of concomitant invasive ductal carcinoma in intraductal papillary mucinous neoplasm of the pancreas. Ann Surg. 2010; https://doi.org/10.1097/SLA.0b013e3181c5ddc3.
53. Tanaka M, et al. International consensus guidelines for management of intraductal papillary mucinous neoplasms and mucinous cystic neoplasms of the pancreas. Pancreatology. 2006; https://doi.org/10.1159/000090023.
54. Del Chiaro M, et al. European experts consensus statement on cystic tumours of the pancreas. Dig Liver Dis. 2013;45:703–11.
55. Kim YC, et al. Comparison of MRI and endoscopic ultrasound in the characterization of pancreatic cystic lesions. AJR Am J Roentgenol. 2010; https://doi.org/10.2214/AJR.09.3985.
56. Jones MJ, et al. Imaging of indeterminate pancreatic cystic lesions: a systematic review. Pancreatology. 2013; https://doi.org/10.1016/j.pan.2013.05.007.
57. Sultana A, et al. What is the best way to identify malignant transformation within pancreatic IPMN: a systematic review and meta-analyses. Clin Transl Gastroenterol. 2015; https://doi.org/10.1038/ctg.2015.60.
58. Tirkes T, et al. Cystic neoplasms of the pancreas; findings on magnetic resonance imaging with pathological, surgical, and clinical correlation. Abdom Imaging. 2014; https://doi.org/10.1007/s00261-014-0138-5.
59. Lee LS, et al. EUS-guided fine needle aspiration of pancreatic cysts: a retrospective analysis of complications and their predictors. Clin Gastroenterol Hepatol. 2005; https://doi.org/10.1016/S1542-3565(04)00618-4.
60. Brugge WR, et al. Diagnosis of pancreatic cystic neoplasms: a report of the cooperative pancreatic cyst study. Gastroenterology. 2004; https://doi.org/10.1053/j.gastro.2004.02.013.
61. Thornton GD, et al. Endoscopic ultrasound guided fine needle aspiration for the diagnosis of pancreatic cystic neoplasms: a meta-analysis. Pancreatology. 2013; https://doi.org/10.1016/j.pan.2012.11.313.
62. Ngamruengphong S, Bartel MJ, Raimondo M. Cyst carcinoembryonic antigen in differentiating pancreatic cysts: a meta-analysis. Dig Liver Dis. 2013; https://doi.org/10.1016/j.dld.2013.05.002.
63. Pitman MB, Centeno BA, Ali SZ, Genevay M, Stelow E, Mino-Kenudson M, Castillo C F-d, Schmidt CM, Brugge W, Layfield L. Standardized terminology and nomenclature for pancreatobiliary cytology: the Papanicolaou Society of Cytopathology Guidelines. Diagn Cytopathol. 2014;42:338–50.
64. Matthaei H, et al. miRNA biomarkers in cyst fluid augment the diagnosis and management of pancreatic cysts. Clin Cancer Res. 2012; https://doi.org/10.1158/1078-0432.CCR-12-0035.
65. Wu J, et al. Whole-exome sequencing of neoplastic cysts of the pancreas reveals recurrent mutations in components of ubiquitin-dependent pathways. Proc Natl Acad Sci. 2011; https://doi.org/10.1073/pnas.1118046108.
66. Amato E, et al. Targeted next-generation sequencing of cancer genes dissects the molecular profiles of intraductal papillary neoplasms of the pancreas. J Pathol. 2014; https://doi.org/10.1002/path.4344.
67. Wu J, et al. Recurrent GNAS mutations define an unexpected pathway for pancreatic cyst development. Sci Transl Med. 2011; https://doi.org/10.1126/scitranslmed.3002543.
68. Dal Molin M, et al. Clinicopathological correlates of activating gnas mutations in intraductal papillary mucinous neoplasm (IPMN) of the pancreas. Ann Surg Oncol. 2013; https://doi.org/10.1245/s10434-013-3096-1.

69. Ryu JK, et al. Elevated microRNA miR-21 levels in pancreatic cyst fluid are predictive of mucinous precursor lesions of ductal adenocarcinoma. Pancreatology. 2011; https://doi.org/10.1159/000329183.

70. Caponi S, et al. The good, the bad and the ugly: a tale of miR-101, miR-21 and miR-155 in pancreatic intraductal papillary mucinous neoplasms. Ann Oncol. 2013; https://doi.org/10.1093/annonc/mds513.

71. Grüner BM, et al. MALDI imaging mass spectrometry for in situ proteomic analysis of pre-neoplastic lesions in pancreatic cancer. PLoS One. 2012; https://doi.org/10.1371/journal.pone.0039424.

72. Mann BF, Goetz JA, House MG, Schmidt CM, Novotny MV. Glycomic and proteomic profiling of pancreatic cyst fluids identifies Hyperfucosylated Lactosamines on the N -linked Glycans of overexpressed glycoproteins. Mol Cell Proteomics. 2012; https://doi.org/10.1074/mcp.M111.015792.

73. Corcos O, et al. Proteomic assessment of markers for malignancy in the mucus of intraductal papillary mucinous neoplasms of the pancreas. Pancreas. 2012; https://doi.org/10.1097/MPA.0b013e3182289356.

74. Lévy P, Rebours V. The role of endoscopic ultrasound in the diagnosis of cystic lesions of the pancreas. Visc Med. 2018;34:192–6.

75. Yamashita Y, et al. Usefulness of contrast-enhanced endoscopic sonography for discriminating mural nodules from mucous clots in intraductal papillary mucinous neoplasms a single-center prospective study. J Ultrasound Med. 2013; https://doi.org/10.7863/jum.2013.32.1.61.

76. Matsumoto K, et al. Performance of novel tissue harmonic echo imaging using endoscopic ultrasound for pancreatic diseases. Endosc Int Open. 2016; https://doi.org/10.1055/s-0034-1393367.

77. Tsujino T, et al. In vivo identification of pancreatic cystic neoplasms with needle-based confocal laser endomicroscopy. Best Pract Res Clin Gastroenterol. 2015; https://doi.org/10.1016/j.bpg.2015.06.006.

78. Napoléon B, et al. A novel approach to the diagnosis of pancreatic serous cystadenoma: needle-based confocal laser endomicroscopy. Endoscopy. 1998; https://doi.org/10.1055/s-0034-1390693.

79. Napoleon B, et al. In vivo characterization of pancreatic cystic lesions by needle-based confocal laser endomicroscopy (nCLE): proposition of a comprehensive nCLE classification confirmed by an external retrospective evaluation. Surg Endosc Other Interv Tech. 2016; https://doi.org/10.1007/s00464-015-4510-5.

80. Kadayifci A, Atar M, Basar O, Forcione DG, Brugge WR. Needle-based confocal laser endomicroscopy for evaluation of cystic neoplasms of the pancreas. Dig Dis Sci. 2017; https://doi.org/10.1007/s10620-017-4521-2.

81. Krishna SG, et al. *In vivo* and *ex vivo* confocal endomicroscopy of pancreatic cystic lesions: a prospective study. World J Gastroenterol. 2017; https://doi.org/10.3748/wjg.v23.i18.3338.

82. Jais B, Rebours V, Malleo G, Salvia R, Fontana M, Maggino L, Bassi C, Manfredi R, Moran R, Lennon AM, Zaheer A, Wolfgang C, Hruban R, Marchegiani G, Fernández Del Castillo C, Brugge W, Ha Y, Kim MH, Oh D, Hirai I, Kimura W, Jang JY, Kim SW, Jung W, Kang HLP. Serous cystic neoplasm of the pancreas: a multinational study of 2622 patients under the auspices of the International Association of Pancreatology and European Pancreatic Club (European Study Group on Cystic Tumors of the Pancreas). Gut. 2015;65:1–8.

83. Zhang ML, et al. Moray micro forceps biopsy improves the diagnosis of specific pancreatic cysts. Cancer Cytopathol. 2018; https://doi.org/10.1002/cncy.21988.

84. Yamaguchi T, Kita E, Mikata RHT. Peroral Pancreatoscopy (POPS): Springer; 2019. https://doi.org/10.1007/978-4-431-56009-8_31.

85. Sauvanet A, Couvelard A, Belghiti J. Role of frozen section assessment for intraductal papillary and mucinous tumor of the pancreas. World J Gastrointest Surg. 2010; https://doi.org/10.4240/wjgs.v2.i10.352.

86. Eguchi H, et al. Role of intraoperative cytology combined with histology in detecting continuous and skip type intraductal cancer existence for intraductal papillary mucinous carcinoma of the pancreas. Cancer. 2006; https://doi.org/10.1002/cncr.22301.
87. Vege SS, Ziring B, Jain R, Moayyedi P. American gastroenterological association institute guideline on the diagnosis and management of asymptomatic neoplastic pancreatic cysts. Gastroenterology. 2015;148:819–22.
88. Rubio-Tapia A, et al. ACG clinical guidelines: diagnosis and management of celiac disease. Am J Gastroenterol. 2013; https://doi.org/10.1038/ajg.2013.79.
89. Scholten L, et al. Surgical management of intraductal papillary mucinous neoplasm with main duct involvement: an international expert survey and case-vignette study. Surgery (United States). 2018; https://doi.org/10.1016/j.surg.2018.01.025.
90. Ito T, et al. The distribution of atypical epithelium in main-duct type intraductal papillary mucinous neoplasms of the pancreas. J Hepatobiliary Pancreat Sci. 2011; https://doi.org/10.1007/s00534-010-0337-6.
91. Watanabe Y, et al. Validity of the management strategy for intraductal papillary mucinous neoplasm advocated by the international consensus guidelines 2012: a retrospective review. Surg Today. 2016; https://doi.org/10.1007/s00595-015-1292-2.
92. He J, et al. Is it necessary to follow patients after resection of a benign pancreatic intraductal papillary mucinous neoplasm? J Am Coll Surg. 2013; https://doi.org/10.1016/j.jamcollsurg.2012.12.026.
93. Tamura K, et al. Treatment strategy for main duct intraductal papillary mucinous neoplasms of the pancreas based on the assessment of recurrence in the remnant pancreas after resection: a retrospective review. Ann Surg. 2014; https://doi.org/10.1097/SLA.0b013e3182a690ff.
94. Fritz S, et al. Clinicopathologic characteristics of patients with resected multifocal intraductal papillary mucinous neoplasm of the pancreas. Surgery. 2012; https://doi.org/10.1016/j.surg.2012.05.025.
95. Shi C, et al. Increased prevalence of precursor lesions in familial pancreatic cancer patients. Clin Cancer Res. 2009; https://doi.org/10.1158/1078-0432.CCR-09-0004.
96. First GO. European evidence-based guidelines on pancreatic cystic neoplasms. Gut. gutjnl-2018-316027. 2018; https://doi.org/10.1136/gutjnl-2018-316027.
97. Raut CP, et al. Intraductal papillary mucinous neoplasms of the pancreas: effect of invasion and pancreatic margin status on recurrence and survival. Ann Surg Oncol. 2006; https://doi.org/10.1245/ASO.2006.05.002.
98. Farrell JJ, Fernández-Del Castillo C. Pancreatic cystic neoplasms: management and unanswered questions. Gastroenterology. 2013; https://doi.org/10.1053/j.gastro.2013.01.073.
99. Kang MJ, et al. Long-term prospective cohort study of patients undergoing pancreatectomy for intraductal papillary mucinous neoplasm of the pancreas. Ann Surg. 2014; https://doi.org/10.1097/SLA.0000000000000470.
100. Kang MJ, et al. Long-term prospective cohort study of patients undergoing pancreatectomy for intraductal papillary mucinous neoplasm of the pancreas implications for postoperative surveillance. Ann Surg. 2014; https://doi.org/10.1097/SLA.0000000000000470.
101. Ideno N, et al. Intraductal papillary mucinous neoplasms of the pancreas with distinct pancreatic ductal adenocarcinomas are frequently of gastric subtype. Ann Surg. 2013; https://doi.org/10.1097/SLA.0b013e3182828cd008.
102. Hirono S, et al. Long-term surveillance is necessary after operative resection for intraductal papillary mucinous neoplasm of the pancreas. Surgery (United States). 2016; https://doi.org/10.1016/j.surg.2016.04.007.
103. Miyasaka Y, et al. Predictive factors for the metachronous development of high-risk lesions in the remnant pancreas after partial pancreatectomy for intraductal papillary mucinous neoplasm. Ann Surg. 2016; https://doi.org/10.1097/SLA.0000000000001368.
104. Yamaguchi K, et al. Intraductal papillary neoplasm of the pancreas: a clinical review of 13 benign and four malignant tumours. Eur J Surg. 1999; https://doi.org/10.1080/110241599750007081.

105. Reid-Lombardo KM, Mathis KL, Wood CM, Harmsen WS, Sarr MG. Frequency of extrapan-
     creatic neoplasms in intraductal papillary mucinous neoplasm of the pancreas: implications
     for management. Ann Surg. 2010; https://doi.org/10.1097/SLA.0b013e3181b5ad1e.
106. Elta GH, Enestvedt BK, Sauer BG, Marie Lennon A. ACG clinical guideline: diagnosis and
     management of pancreatic cysts. Am J Gastroenterol. 2018:1–16. https://doi.org/10.1038/
     ajg.2018.14.
107. Macedo FIB, et al. The impact of surgeon volume on outcomes after pancreaticoduodenec-
     tomy: a meta-analysis. J Gastrointest Surg. 2017;21:1723–31.

Chapter 3
Novel Biomarkers of Invasive IPMN

Stephen Hasak and Koushik K. Das

With the ubiquitous use and high resolution of cross-sectional imaging, pancreatic cystic lesions (PCL) are common incidental findings, detected in up to 20% of abdominal MRI scans in adults [1, 2]. The overall prevalence of PCL in asymptomatic patients undergoing abdominal CT scans is estimated to be 2.6%, with progressive increasing incidence with age, up to 8.7% of patients above 80 [3, 4]. While PCL, especially mucinous PCL, have the capacity to develop into invasive carcinoma, it is increasingly being recognized that their malignant potential is neither uniform nor certain. Indeed, while data from long-term cohorts of PCL have identified a small but ongoing risk to the development of carcinoma [5, 6], this must be balanced against the increasing data demonstrating low yield and high potential morbidity of surgical intervention in elderly patients with non-worrisome PCL [7, 8]. As pancreatic resection remains an effective modality but continues to carry a 1–2% mortality and 30–60% morbidity [9], there remains an unmet need for molecular tools to stratify high-risk/malignant from low-risk lesions.

PCL can be broadly divided into nonmucinous and mucinous lesions, with mucinous lesions (intraductal papillary mucinous neoplasms (IPMN) and mucinous cystic neoplasm (MCN)), accounting for 10–50% and harboring malignant potential [10–12]. Even within these mucinous lesions, in surgical resection cohorts, main-duct and mixed-type IPMNs have a 48% or 42% chance of harboring invasive carcinoma in comparison to branch-duct lesions (BD-IPMN) with only an 11% chance [13, 14]. While imaging characteristics, including cyst size (typically greater than 3 or 4 cm), main pancreatic duct dilation (typically greater than 5 mm or 10 mm), and the presence of solid components or mural nodules, may predict the presence of high-grade dysplasia (HGD) or invasive disease on surgical resection, all of these

S. Hasak · K. K. Das (✉)
Division of Gastroenterology, Washington University School of Medicine,
Saint Louis, MO, USA
e-mail: k.das@wustl.edu

© Springer Nature Switzerland AG 2020
C. W. Michalski et al. (eds.), *Translational Pancreatic Cancer Research*,
Molecular and Translational Medicine,
https://doi.org/10.1007/978-3-030-49476-6_3

clinical features alone have poor overall accuracy in predicting this important outcome [15–18]. Overall, morphology on endoscopic ultrasound (EUS) is not accurate in distinguishing nonmucinous from mucinous cysts without fluid analysis, let alone assessing dysplastic grade [19]. As discussed in detail in the previous chapter, evidence-based criteria and clinical guidelines have been developed to aid in the appropriate surveillance and management of PCL [16–18, 20]. Despite widespread clinical adoption, these guidelines are imperfect, as the clinical/imaging features they rely upon are themselves imperfect [21, 22]. As a whole, earlier iterations of the guidelines like the Sendai criteria while highly sensitive (97–100%) were not specific (20–30%) for BD-IPMN harboring advanced neoplasia, and while subsequent guidelines like the Fukuoka and AGA guidelines improve the specificity (34.5–45.6%), it was at the cost of reduced sensitivity (7.3–35.2%) [23–25]. Furthermore, these guidelines rely on static assessments of clinical features and do not take into account cyst biology, which may be highly variable.

Ultimately, the objective of any surveillance program is to identify lesions at a preinvasive state or, at most, with HGD/carcinoma in situ (CIS), when curative therapy can be rendered. In the case of pancreatic ductal adenocarcinoma (PDAC), precursor lesions are generally considered to be IPMN or pancreatic intraepithelial neoplasia (PanIN). PanIN are classified into three grades: PanIN-1 and PanIN-2, which are low-grade lesions, and PanIN-3 demonstrating pronounced cytologic and architectural atypia, equivalent to in situ carcinoma [26]. However, given their microscopic nature and heterogeneous distribution, PanIN-3 are not reliably imaged on cross-sectional or ultrasonographic imaging. For example, in a cohort ($n = 125$) of patients who are at high risk for pancreatic cancer due to strong family histories, among those patients who underwent surgical resection for multifocal IPMN ($n = 5$), the location of the most dysplastic histologic lesions (PanIN-3) did not correlate with the preoperatively visualized lesion [27]. This illustrates both the limitations of imaging for resolving microcellular changes and the "field defect" that is apparent in patients with high-risk pancreatic lesions. That said, IPMNs are the only clinically readily appreciated precursor lesions to PDAC [28], and thus the segregation of IPMNs that are at high risk for transformation represents an opportunity for resection before the development of invasive cancer with improved overall survival [29, 30]. However, the last 20 years of clinical experience has continued to demonstrate that the resection of cysts with low risk of malignant transformation carries significant up-front surgical morbidity and mortality, even in high-volume centers, without significant long-term benefit [31, 32].

PCL are readily imaged with ultrasound, CT, and MRI and are relatively safely sampled utilizing EUS-guided FNA with cyst aspiration. The current standard approach is for cyst fluid to be submitted for cytologic analysis and biochemical analysis for carcinoembryonic antigen (CEA) and amylase. Overall, FNA is safe, but the diagnostic yield with currently available clinical testing is limited with poor sensitivity, but high specificity (sensitivity 27–48%, specificity 83–100%) [33–35]. As such, there has been varying enthusiasm for EUS FNA, driven by the dearth of biomarkers and inadequacy of cytology to reliably assess risk in these PCL [33]. The hope of many researchers, including ourselves, is that a new generation of biomarkers together in concert with clinical parameters may influence future guidelines and establish cyst fluid analysis as critical for clinical risk stratification of PCL.

In this chapter, we will review the published data on biomarkers at varying stages of investigation used to risk stratify IPMN and detect invasive carcinoma arising from IPMN. We will first outline the data for routinely used, clinically available fluid studies (Table 3.1) and review the data on novel DNA-, RNA-, and protein-based cyst fluid biomarkers and biomarkers from other sources (circulating cells, pancreatic juice, etc.).

Biomarkers in Current Clinical Practice for the Evaluation of PCL

Amylase

Cyst fluid amylase indicates a connection between the cyst and the ductal system with high specificity [11]. However, the level cannot differentiate between pseudocyst, IPMN, or MCN [36]. In one study, cyst fluid amylase levels decreased with increasing levels of dysplasia in MCN, but these levels were not significantly different [37]. As such, amylase cannot be used to adequately rule out malignancy or assess risk of malignant transformation. Interestingly, in one study, serum levels of amylase were significantly lower in patients with surgically resected invasive IPMN in comparison to matched controls (OR 9.6, 2.99–35.1) [38].

CEA

CEA is a glycoprotein on the cell surface of mucin-producing epithelium. CEA is primarily useful for differentiating mucinous from nonmucinous PCL [11]. Various cutoff values have been explored for CEA in pancreatic cyst fluid with varying sensitivity and specificity. Using the original, traditional cutoff of 192 ng/ml, the area under the curve for differentiating mucinous vs nonmucinous cysts was 0.79 with a likelihood ratio of 4.37 [19, 35]. However, subsequent studies have utilized a cutoff of 30.7 ng/mL (sensitivity 88.3, specificity 77.8%) or 105 ng/mL (sensitivity 70%, specificity 63%) [39, 40]. CEA may be best used for predicting a nonmucinous PCL, as a level below 5 ng/ml effectively rules out a mucinous tumor with a positive predictive value of 94% [41]. Importantly, CEA cannot differentiate IPMN from other mucin-producing cyst types (i.e., MCN).

Beyond differentiating cyst type, studies have evaluated using CEA to detect malignant transformation and dysplasia. While early studies using a cyst CEA cutoff of 200 ng/ml resulted in a sensitivity of 90% and specificity of 72% in identifying HGD or invasive carcinoma on surgical pathology in IPMN [42], subsequent

Table 3.1 Biomarkers in current clinical practice for PCL risk stratification

Biomarker	Study	Year	Sample size	Definition of advanced neoplasia	Sensitivity	Specificity	Other
Cyst amylase	Scourtas et al. [37]	2017	136 MCN	Surgical pathology from resection			Mean amylase lower for invasive MCN than MCN with intermediate-grade dysplasia, which was lower than MCN with low-grade dysplasia
Serum amylase	Yagi et al. [38]	2016	142 surgically resected IPMN	Surgical pathology – invasive IPMN			Low serum amylase (<16 IU/L) associated with higher risk of invasive IPMN. OR 9.6 (2.99–35.1)
Cyst CEA	Brugge et al. [19]	2005	112	Mucinous vs nonmucinous	75%	83.6%	CEA > 192 ng/ml Accuracy: 79%
Cyst CEA	Maire et al. [42]	2008	41	IPMN with HGD or invasive carcinoma	90%	71%	CEA ≥ 200 ng/ml PPV 50%, NPV 96%
Cyst CEA	Correa-Gallego et al. [43]	2009	197	IPMN with carcinoma in situ or invasive carcinoma	47%	40%	CEA ≥ 200 ng/ml PPV 20%, NPV 70%
Cyst CEA	Kucera et al. [44]	2012	47	IPMN with HGD or invasive carcinoma	52.4%	42.3%	CEA ≥ 200 ng/ml PPV 42.3%, NPV 52.4%
Cyst CEA	Thornton et al. [35]	2013	1438	Mucinous vs nonmucinous	63%	88%	Meta-analysis
Cyst CEA	Ngamruengphong et al. [45]	2013	504	All malignant pancreatic cystic lesions (HGD or invasive cancer)	63% 65% for mucinous only	63% 66% for mucinous only	Meta-analysis of studies of pancreatic cysts
Cyst CEA	Gaddam et al. [39]	2015	226	Mucinous vs nonmucinous	105 ng/ml: 70% 192 ng/ml: 61%	105 ng/ml: 63% 192 ng/ml: 77%	Tested various cutoffs

Cyst CEA	Jin et al. [40]	2015	86	Mucinous vs nonmucinous	88.3%	77.8%	CEA > 30.7 ng/ml
Serum CEA	Fritz et al. [49]	2011	142	Surgically resected IPMN – invasive vs noninvasive	40%	92.4%	CEA of 5 ug/l, PPV 74.1%, NPV 73.9%
Cyst Ca19-9	Pais et al. [51]	2007	74	Malignant IPMN on surgical pathology	60%	75%	Ca19-9 of 10,000 U/ml PPV 75% NPV 60% Mean Ca19-9 not different between malignant and benign cysts
Serum Ca19-9	Fritz et al. [49]	2011	142	Surgically resected IPMN – invasive vs noninvasive	74%	85.9%	CA19-9 of 37 u/ml PPV 74% NPV 85.9%
Serum Ca19-9	Kim et al. [52]	2015	367	HGD and invasive IPMN on surgical pathology	34.2%	92.4%	"Elevated Ca19-9"
Serum Ca19-9	Wang et al. [53]	2015	1629	Malignant or invasive IPMN	Malignant: 40% Invasive: 52%	Malignant: 89% Invasive: 88%	Ca19-9 35 ng/ml Meta-analysis
Cyst cytology	Sedlack et al. [64]	2002	111	Malignant/potentially malignant vs benign cysts	27%	100%	Accuracy: 55%
Cyst cytology	Brugge et al. [19]	2005	112	Mucinous vs nonmucinous	34.5%	83.3%	Accuracy: 58.7%
Cyst cytology – atypical epithelial cells	Pitman et al. [59]	2008	20	Invasive or malignant IPMN	Malignant: 83% Invasive: 88%%	Malignant: 67%, Invasive: 59%	Addition of CEA > 2500 ng/ml improves sensitivity, but decreases specificity
Cyst cytology	Morris-Stiff et al. [58]	2010	121	Mucinous vs nonmucinous	38%	90%	PPV: 90% NPV: 31%

(continued)

Table 3.1 (continued)

Biomarker	Study	Year	Sample size	Definition of advanced neoplasia	Sensitivity	Specificity	Other
Cyst cytology	Cizinger et al. [56]	2011	198	Mucinous vs nonmucinous Subgroup with malignant pathology	Mucinous: 43% Malignant: 37.5%	Mucinous: 96.2%, Malignant: 96%	Mucinous accuracy: 58%, Malignant accuracy: 74.7%
Cyst cytology	de Jong et al. [55]	2012	32	Mucinous vs nonmucinous	48%	100%	
Cytopathology KRAS GNAS	Bournet [79]	2016	37	HGD and invasive carcinoma	Cytology: 55% KRAS: 66% GNAS: 19% Cytology+ KRAS: 92% Cytology+ GNAS: 62% Cytology+ KRAS+ GNAS 92%	Cytology: 100%, KRAS: 50% GNAS: 70%, Cytology+ KRAS: 50% Cytology+ GNAS: 70%, Cytology+ KRAS+ GNAS: 50%	
Cyst cytology	Tanaka et al. [65]	2019	743	IPMN with HGD, CIS, invasive carcinoma	57%	84%	Systematic review
Pancreatic juice cytology	Tanaka et al. [65]	2019	537	IPMN with HGD, CIS, invasive carcinoma	54%	91%	Systematic review
Pancreatic juice cytology	Kawada et al. [165]	2016	50	Malignant IPMN without mural nodule	94% without mural nodule vs 53% with mural nodule		

studies in mucinous cystic neoplasm and IPMN have shown that CEA levels in benign and malignant cysts overlap significantly, with poor test characteristics [37, 43–45]. This result has been demonstrated in multiple studies, suggesting that CEA alone should not be used to detect invasive PCL or IPMN [19, 41, 46, 47]. Serum CEA is elevated in 60% of patients with pancreatic ductal adenocarcinoma. While serum CEA has a high specificity for invasive IPMN, the sensitivity of serum CEA for malignant and invasive IPMN is only 18% [48, 49].

CA19-9

Carbohydrate antigen 19-9 (CA19-9) is a tumor-associated glycoprotein that is elevated in the serum of 85% of patients with PDAC [48]. However about 5–10% of the population is unable to produce Ca19-9 due to lack of an enzyme needed for epitope production, which does limit its use as biomarker [50]. In cyst fluid, Ca19-9 performs worse than CEA for differentiating mucinous from nonmucinous cysts [19]. Cyst fluid Ca19-9 is also not useful in differentiating malignant from benign IPMN with one study showing no difference in levels between these groups [51]. Serum Ca19-9 may be useful in ruling in invasive IPMN with reasonable specificities and poor sensitivities [49, 52]. In a meta-analysis, the sensitivity and specificity of Ca19-9 level of 35 ng/ml measured in serum were 52% and 88%, respectively, for detecting invasive IPMN [53].

Cytology

While routinely performed, standard cytological evaluation of cyst fluid is hampered by low cellular content, the focal nature of dysplasia, and high interobserver variability [54]. The overall performance of cytology in PCL diagnosis ranges with low sensitivities of 27–48% and high specificities of 83–100% [19, 33, 55–58]. The pooled sensitivity and specificity in a systematic review and meta-analysis were 54% and 93%, respectively, in differentiating mucinous from nonmucinous cysts [35]. To improve the clinical utility of cyst fluid cytology, the inclusion of atypical epithelial cells has been suggested and this improved the sensitivity and specificity to 72% and 85%, respectively, for identifying malignant cysts [59, 60]. However, the clinical utility of this system is limited as interobserver agreement is poor without significant experience [61, 62]. Yield may also be increased by cyst wall biopsy or other technical maneuvers, but there remains a significant need for improvement [36, 63, 64]. Cytologic analysis of pancreatic juice collected during ERCP in patients with IPMN has similar test characteristic to EUS FNA acquired cyst fluid cytology with recent systematic review showing a sensitivity of 54% and specificity of 91% [65].

Overall, with a low diagnostic accuracy of 8–59%, cytology from FNA while highly predictive if positive has too poor a negative predictive value to exclude advanced neoplastic change in a PCL [19, 33, 56, 64].

DNA Testing

DNA testing has emerged as a potential adjunct to risk stratifying IPMN in part as DNA from lysed or exfoliated epithelium from cyst lining is abundant and can be analyzed for genetic mutations [66–68]. In addition to differentiating mucinous from nonmucinous cysts, it has also been proposed for use in detecting advanced neoplasia in IPMN as we review below (Table 3.2).

KRAS

Mutations in KRAS, an oncogene that encodes a membrane-bound guanosine triphosphate (GTP) binding protein upstream of MAPK signaling pathways [69], are present in more than 90% of pancreatic adenocarcinomas. Furthermore, successive accumulation of alterations in cancer-associated genes including *KRAS*, *p16/ CDKN2A*, *TP53*, and *SMAD4/DPC4* has been noted in the progression from PanIN-1/2 lesions to high-grade PanIN-3 lesions [70]. Given the ubiquity and critical nature of KRAS in pancreatic cancer, its early detection has been seen as a promising target for risk stratification of lesions that have undergone malignant transformation in PCL [71, 72].

Khalid et al. first examined the potential role of evaluating Kras mutations in cyst fluid in a small cohort that included 11 malignant lesions [66]. This was followed by a series of additional studies that studied the presence of KRAS mutations as well as other DNA parameters (quantity, quality, etc.) which showed that the presence of KRAS mutation was specific (80–100%) for mucinous cysts but not sensitive (33–86%) [73–79]. In addition, the majority of these studies did not find KRAS to have significant accuracy in differentiating malignant from premalignant mucinous cysts alone, though they suggested combinations with other parameters like allelic loss to improve sensitivity/specificity (sensitivity of 54% and specificity of 46%) [65]. Of particular note is the multicenter PANDA study, in which the presence of KRAS mutations in pancreatic cyst fluid was useful in differentiating mucinous cysts from nonmucinous cysts with a specificity of 96% but a low sensitivity of 45% [68]. The presence of a Kras mutation along with an allelic loss was only 37% sensitive and 96% specific for a malignant lesion [68]. In a real-world follow-up study of prospectively sampled patients utilizing this commercially available technique, KRAS mutation presence had a 42% sensitivity and 90% specificity for mucinous lesion, but did not have adequate accuracy for high-risk lesions [80]. Overall, the test characteristics of KRAS vary on the setting, definition, and design (Table 3.1).

Table 3.2 Novel DNA-based biomarkers

Biomarker	Study	Year	Sample size	Definition of advanced neoplasia	Sensitivity	Specificity	Other
KRAS	Khalid et al. [66]	2005	36	Malignant pathology	91% 91% when followed by allelic loss	86% 93% when followed by allelic loss	MCN
KRAS and LOH	Schoedel et al. [73]	2006	16	HGD/cancer vs LGD/MGD			KRAS plus LOH in 50% HGD/cancer vs 8% in LGD/MGD
KRAS and LOH	Schoedel et al. [73]	2006	16	Carcinoma vs adenoma or borderline IPMN			50% of carcinomas and 8% of others
KRAS, allelic loss, mutational amplitude, mean number of mutations	Khalid et al. [68]	2009	113	Mucinous vs nonmucinous IPMN and MCN	KRAS: 45% KRAS and allelic loss: 19% MALA: 67% Mean number of mutations: 62%	KRAS: 96% KRAS and allelic loss: 100% MALA: 66% Mean number of mutations: 62%	
KRAS, allelic loss, mutational amplitude, DNA quality and quantity	Khalid et al. [68]	2009	113	Malignant vs premalignant IPMN and MCN	KRAS and allelic loss: 37% MALA: 90% DNA quantity: 75% Mean DNA quality: 75%	KRAS and allelic loss: 96% MALA: 67% DNA quantity: 79% Mean DNA quality: 67%	
CEA, molecular analysis, KRAS, allelic imbalance, DNA concentration	Sawney et al. [74]	2009	100	Mucinous vs nonmucinous	CEA: 82% Molecular analysis: 77 KRAS: 11% Allelic imbalance: 70% DNA concentration: 29%	CEA: 100% Molecular analysis: 100% KRAS: 100% Allelic imbalance: 100% DNA concentration: 100%	

(continued)

Table 3.2 (continued)

Biomarker	Study	Year	Sample size	Definition of advanced neoplasia	Sensitivity	Specificity	Other
PathFinder TG KRAS, LOH, DNA quantity/quality	Shen et al. [75]	2009	35	CIS and invasive cancer All cysts	83%	100%	PPV 100%
KRAS	Nikiforova et al. [78]	2013	618	Mucinous vs nonmucinous	54%	100%	
KRAS and GNAS	Siddiqui et al. [95]	2013	25	IPMN vs other cysts	KRAS: 67% GNAS: 44% Either: 100%	KRAS: 69% GNAS: 100% Either: 69%	
KRAS	Al-Haddad et al. [80]	2014	48 surgically resected cysts 38 mucinous cysts 35 IPMN	Mucinous vs nonmucinous	42.1%	90%	
KRAS and GNAS	Singhi et al. [96]	2014	91	IPMN vs other cysts	KRAS: 70% GNAS: 36% Either: 84%	KRAS: 98% GNAS: 100% Either: 98%	
KRAS, elevated DNA, ≥2 LOH, and KRAS and ≥2 LOH	Winner et al. [87]	2015	40	Invasive adenocarcinoma vs benign	KRAS: 44.4% Elevated DNA: 66.7% ≥2 LOH: 62.5% KRAS and ≥LOH: 50%	KRAS: 55.6% Elevated DNA: 77.8% ≥2 LOH: 76.9% KRAS and ≥LOH: 96.2%	Retrospective
KRAS and LOH	Guo et al. [89]	2016	428	Mucinous vs nonmucinous Benign vs malignant cysts	Mucinous vs nonmucinous KRAS: 47%, LOH: 63%; Benign vs malignant KRAS: 59% LOH: 89%	Mucinous vs nonmucinous KRAS: 98% LOH: 76% Benign vs malignant KRAS: 78% LOH: 69%	Systematic review and meta-analysis

				HGD or invasive	89%	100%	
NGS: KRAS/GNAS, *TP53/PIK3CA/PTEN*	Singhi et al. [97]	2018	595 – NGS 159 – KRAS/GNAS				
KRAS	Tanaka et al. [65]	2019	333	HGD, CIS, invasive carcinoma	54%	46%	Systematic review
GNAS	Tanaka et al. [65]	2019	144	HGD, CIS, invasive carcinoma	29%	46%	Systematic review
Telomerase	Hata et al. [101]	2016	119 cysts; 74 IPMN	HGD or invasive cancer	74.2% in all 74.2% in IPMN	93.2% all 86.1% in IPMN	Cystic lesions
TP53	Tanaka et al. [65]	2019	780	HGD, CIS, invasive carcinoma	31%	93%	TP53 from surgical pathology
SMAD4	Tanaka et al. [65]	2019	291	HGD, CIS, invasive carcinoma	14%	99%	
P16	Tanaka et al. [65]	2019	325	HGD, CIS, invasive carcinoma	52%	46%	
Cell-free DNA	Berger et al. [163]	2016	21 IPMN, 38 controls, 24 metastatic PDAC, 26 SCA, 16 borderline IPMN	PDAC vs IPMN vs control	IPMN vs control: 81% PDAC vs control: 83% PDAC vs IPMN: 75%	IPMN vs control: 84% PDAC vs control: 94 PDAC vs IPMN: 71%	

There may be a variety of reasons why KRAS mutations have not proven to be an accurate biomarker for high-risk lesions. KRAS mutations are seen in a significant number of patients with chronic pancreatitis who do not go on to develop pancreatic cancer but have a high prevalence of PanIN lesions [81, 82]. KRAS mutations do not differ by degree of dysplasia as this may be an earlier event in carcinogenesis [83, 84]. In addition, in an autopsy series of 138 patients who died of non-pancreatic-related causes, 38 patients were found with PanIN lesions and 12 were found with oncogenic Kras mutations, suggesting that these mutations may occur outside of the context of clinically significant carcinogenesis [85]. Alternatively, there may be differential presence of the mutations varying by epithelial subtype of IPMN. In one study, KRAS mutations were more common in gastric- and pancreatobiliary-type IPMN than in intestinal or oncocytic subtypes and were more common in tubular and minimally invasive carcinoma than in those with mucinous or oncocytic carcinoma when surgical specimens were stained [86].

DNA Quantity, Loss of Heterozygosity, and Mean Allelic Loss Amplitude (MALA)

DNA quantity can be assessed as a part of molecular analysis of cyst fluid and was routinely included in the abovementioned studies examining KRAS gene mutations in cyst fluid. In one study, the sensitivity and specificity of a DNA level >40 ng/μl for differentiating mucinous from nonmucinous cysts were 29% and 100%, respectively [74]. In two other studies, an elevated DNA level as confirmed by an optical density >10 had sensitivities of 75% and 67% and specificities of 79% and 77.8% for differentiating malignant from premalignant cysts [68, 87]. Overall however, DNA quantity alone, essentially as a surrogate for cellularity in the cyst fluid, has not been felt to be a highly accurate biomarker for high-risk lesions.

Loss of heterozygosity (LOH), the loss of one copy of a tumor suppressor gene, is evaluated with a panel of microsatellite markers [88]. In a meta-analysis, the sensitivity and specificity of LOH in cyst fluid for distinguishing mucinous cysts from nonmucinous cysts were 63% and 76%, respectively [89]. For differentiating malignant from benign cysts, LOH yielded a sensitivity of 89% and specificity of 69% [89]. When KRAS and LOH were combined, the sensitivity for differentiating malignant from benign cysts was 50%, with a specificity of 96% [87]. In another study, the combination of KRAS mutations and LOH was present in 50% of IPMN with high-grade dysplasia and cancer versus 8% of IPMN with low-grade or indeterminate dysplasia [73].

The mean allelic loss amplitude (MALA) is another metric of DNA analysis that has been shown to have a sensitivity and specificity of 90% and 67%, respectively, for detecting malignant cysts in one study [68]. When KRAS was combined with MALA, the specificity for detecting malignant cysts was improved to 96%, but the sensitivity was only 37% [68].

As each of these assessments proved promising but insufficient, investigators have suggested the combination of KRAS gene mutations, DNA concentration, and allelic loss in cyst fluid analysis together. A commercialized version of these assays that combines KRAS analysis, LOH, and DNA quantity for cyst fluid analysis (PathFinder TG, Interpace Diagnostics) demonstrated a sensitivity and specificity of 83% and 100%, respectively, in a single study [75]. A retrospective review of 492 patients utilizing this molecular diagnostic testing, integrated with first-line test results (cytology, fluid chemistry, and imaging), suggested a method called integrated molecular pathology (IMP) and compared the results to real-world decisions and guidelines recommendations [90, 91]. Among the cohort of patients ($n = 209$) with surgical pathology available, IMP demonstrated a sensitivity and specificity of 81.0% and 78.0%, respectively, which was significantly better than the Sendai guidelines.

GNAS

GNAS is an oncogene that encodes the alpha subunit of stimulatory G protein (Gs-α) that is ubiquitously expressed for G-protein stimulatory signaling, especially in several hormonal axes. Germline mutations are associated with McCune-Albright syndrome, and somatic mutations are seen in a variety of endocrine tumors (Leydig tumors, ovarian granular cell tumors, pituitary tumors) [92–94]. Mutations at codon 201 have been shown to be useful in distinguishing IPMN from other pancreatic cyst types, with studies showing that GNAS mutations occur in 44–61% of IPMN, while there were no mutations in other mucinous cysts [83, 95]. In the initial work examining the association of GNAS with cystic lesions of the pancreas, Wu et al. examined 19 IPMN sequenced for 169 genes utilizing massively parallel sequencing to identify even very small cell populations. In this cohort, ~81% had a KRAS mutation (G12D, G12V, or G12R) and ~66% had a GNAS mutation (R201H or R201C) with no expression in serous cyst adenoma and no correlation to grade, size, or prognosis [94]. In a large prospective study on cyst fluid preoperatively, the presence of a mutation in either KRAS or GNAS had a sensitivity of 84% with a specificity of 98% for detecting IPMN [96]. Using next-generation sequencing, KRAS and/or GNAS mutations were present in all IPMN when confirmed by surgical pathology [97]. However, utilizing 86 surgically resected patient specimens, GNAS mutations were found to be more frequently associated with intestinal-type (100%) and pancreatobiliary-type (71%) IPMN as opposed to gastric (51%) and oncocytic (0%) IPMN, but there was no association with location, malignancy, or survival [98]. In a study from 291 pancreatic juice aspirates from high-risk patients, there was no association with GNAS mutations and prognosis or histologic grade of cystic lesions. In fact, the presence of the mutation predicted the subsequent radiologic development of cysts in a small group of patients [99]. In a recent systematic review, the sensitivity and specificity for GNAS alone in differentiating HGD, CIS, and invasive carcinoma from benign cysts were 29% and 46%, respectively [65, 79].

When combined with KRAS testing, the sensitivity and specificity in diagnosing IPMN when either marker was positive in one small pilot study were 100% and 69%, respectively [95]. This finding is supported by mouse models suggesting the cooperation of KRAS and GNAS to promote pancreatic tumorigenesis [100].

Telomerase

Telomerase is a ribonucleoprotein that regulates telomere length which is critical in stem cells and most cancer cells. Telomerase and telomere length has been shown to be associated with IPMN progression, as it is in many cancers [46]. In a study of cyst fluid from 219 patients, telomerase activity was higher in cysts with HGD or invasive cancer and was an independent predictor of high-grade dysplasia or invasive cancer on surgical resection [101]. The sensitivity and specificity for detecting advanced neoplasia in IPMN were 74.2% and 86.1%, respectively [101].

Tumor Suppressor Genes

Loss of heterozygosity of TP53 was seen only in invasive IPMN in one study of 23 patients with surgically resected IPMN [102]. Another tumor suppressor, p16 or cyclin-dependent kinase inhibitor 2a (CDKN2A), may be useful for discriminating IPMN with low to intermediate dysplasia from IPMN with carcinoma [48, 103]. p16 is more commonly inactivated in IPMN with carcinoma than borderline IPMN [104]. In combination with p16 inactivation, inactivation of TP53 is found in 20% of low-grade tumors, 33% of noninvasive carcinomas, and in all invasive carcinomas in IPMN [48, 102]. In another retrospective study of 172 IPMNs, TP53 mutation overexpression was associated with poorer survival in IPMN and worse histologic grade [86]. Overall, estimates of the prevalence of Tp53 and p16 in IPMN vary, and these mutations may occur early in malignant transformation limiting the use of these genes as biomarkers for invasive IPMN [46]. In a recent systematic review, TP53 in 780 IPMNs yielded a sensitivity of 31% and specificity of 93% in differentiating HGD, CIS, and invasive carcinoma from benign IPMN [65]. However, a recent study looking at the combination of mutations in TP53, PIK3CA, and/or PTEN along with KRAS and/or GNAS mutations demonstrated a sensitivity of 89% and specificity of 100% for detecting advanced neoplasia in IPMN [97].

Other Genes

Inactivating mutations in SMAD4 occur late in the progression of precursor lesions to pancreatic cancer, likely working as a critical mediator between the extracellular matrix and the TGF-ß family as a well as a substrate of Erk/MAPK and GSK3 [28]. Mouse models have demonstrated that haploinsufficiency of SMAD4 in association with oncogenic KRAS is associated with macroscopic, mucinous cystic lesions in the body/tail of the pancreas consistent with human MCN [105]. In a retrospective study of 172 IPMNs, SMAD4 loss was associated with worse histologic grade, invasive phenotypes, and worse survival [86]. In the systematic review by Tanaka et al., surgical pathology stained for SMAD4 in 291 IPMNs yielded a sensitivity of 14% and specificity of 99% in differentiating HGD, CIS, and invasive carcinoma from benign IPMN [65].

Brahma-related gene 1 (BRG1) is a member of the SWI/SNF family of proteins with helicase and ATPase activity that can regulate transcription by altering chromatin superstructure [106]. Mutations are common in lung cancer cell lines, medulloblastoma, AML, and pancreatic cancer. In mouse models, acinar-specific deletion of BRG1, in conjunction with oncogenic KRAS mutations, leads to the development of cystic neoplastic lesions reminiscent of MCN vs IPMN in humans [107–109]. In one study, BRG1 was found to be inactivated in 53.3% of IPMN, and mutation was more common in high-grade IPMN than in intermediate- and low-grade IPMN [110]. The role of BRG1 in human IPMN-associated carcinogenesis continues to be investigated.

Next-Generation Sequencing (NGS)/Molecular Panels

NGS allows for high-throughput sequencing that is more sensitive than Sanger sequencing, facilitating rapid detection of mutations even at very low frequencies [97, 111]. In an early study of NGS of cyst fluid using a number of genes previously implicated in tumorigenesis in pancreatic neoplasia, NGS was most valuable in identifying mucinous cysts that were thought to be nonmucinous by CEA level [81]. A study evaluating cyst fluid from IPMN for 51 cancer-associated genes found adequate DNA for analysis in 70% of cysts [112]. GNAS and/or KRAS were present in 92% of IPMN, and TP53, BRAF, and p16 mutations were observed more frequently in high grade IPMN or IPMN-associated carcinomas [112]. Subsequently, in a recent study utilizing a cohort of 102 patients where diagnostic pathology was available, an NGS panel consisting of mutations in TP53, PIK3CA, and/or PTEN with KRAS and/or GNAS mutations had a sensitivity of 89% and specificity of 100% for detecting advanced neoplasia in IPMN using cyst fluid preoperatively [97]. While panel testing is attractive due to the identification of small populations of cells with mutations and overcoming limitations of individual gene analysis, this has to be balanced by the considerable cost as well as complexity in the completion and analysis of this kind of testing. Given these initial promising results, these panels are undergoing prospective validation to establish their utility and assess their precise role in guiding clinical decision-making.

Epigenetic Alterations

There has also been research into DNA methylation as an epigenetic factor related to tumorigenesis for use as a biomarker in IPMN, but this has not been extensively studied for use in pancreatic cyst fluid. Promoter hypermethylation at cytosine-phosphoate-guanine (CpG) islands leads to tumor suppressor gene silencing [48]. In one study of 51 IPMNs, >80% of IPMN exhibited hypermethylation of at least one of seven CpG islands [113]. ppENK and p16 hypermethylation were more common in high-grade IPMN than in low-grade IPMN, and the average number of methylated loci was higher in high-grade than low-grade IPMN [113]. In another study, high-grade IPMNs had a higher number of hypermethylated genes than low-grade IPMNs [114]. The genes BNIP3, PTCHD2, SOX17, NXPH1, and EBF3 were more likely to be hypermethylated in IPMN with high-grade dysplasia than with low-grade dysplasia or normal tissue [114]. Studies testing serum-based cell-free DNA promoter hypermethylation as a marker of pancreatic cancer have been limited by small power, and no studies have been performed using this in IPMN [115].

RNA-Based Biomarkers

MicroRNAs (miRNAs) are small, noncoding RNA molecules that are involved in epigenetic posttranscriptional gene regulation [116]. Variation in miRNA has been shown to be involved in tumorigenesis and progression in pancreatic ductal adenocarcinoma [117]. miRNA-21 has been found to be clinically useful in IPMN differentiation in a few small studies. In cyst fluid, miRNA-21 was able to differentiate mucinous from nonmucinous cysts with a sensitivity of 80% and specificity of 76% [118]. In another study, there was a gradient of increasing miRNA-21 and miRNA-221 expression from benign to premalignant to malignant cysts [119]. Expression of miRNA-155 and miRNA-21 were significantly higher in invasive IPMN compared to noninvasive IPMN in surgically resected lesions, while miRNA-101 was higher in noninvasive IPMN compared to invasive IPMN [120]. miRNA-216 and miRNA-217 expression increased in a gradient from low-grade IPMN to high-grade IPMN to invasive cancer [121]. Finally, in a study of 65 cyst fluid samples, a panel of 18 miRNAs separated high-grade from low-grade IPMN, and a model using a panel of 9 miRNAs could predict cyst pathology improving surgical management versus conservative management with a sensitivity of 89% and a specificity of 100% [122]. Research into the clinical utility of miRNA is still evolving and has been primarily exploratory in small studies, but results are promising (Table 3.3).

Protein-Based Biomarkers

Several protein-based biomarkers as well as large-scale proteomic analyses have been conducted in attempts to identify possible biomarkers for invasive IPMN and are summarized in Table 3.4.

Table 3.3 Novel RNA-based biomarkers

Biomarker	Study	Year	Sample size	Definition of advanced neoplasia	Sensitivity	Specificity	Other
miRNA	Rye et al. [118]	2011	40	Mucinous vs nonmucinous	76%	80%	miRNA 21
miRNA	Matthaei et al. [122]	2012	120	Surgical resection vs conservative management	89%	100%	9 miRNA predicted need for surgical resection (high-grade IPMN, PanNETS and SPNs) vs conservative management (low-grade IPMN, SCA)
miRNA	Farrell et al. [119]	2013	38	Malignant vs premalignant vs benign			miR-221 higher in malignant vs benign cysts miR-21 higher in malignant than premalignant than benign
miRNA	Caponi et al. [120]	2013	86	Invasive vs noninvasive IPMN vs benign cyst			miR-21 and miR-155 were higher in invasive than noninvasive IPMN, miR-101 was higher in noninvasive and benign IPMN than invasive IPMN. Higher miR-21 predicted worse overall survival and independently predicted mortality and disease progression
miRNA	Wang et al. [121]	2015	17	High grade/invasive vs low grade/benign			miR-216 and miR-217 levels increased from low to high grade to cancer

Table 3.4 Novel Protein-Based Biomarkers

Biomarker	Study	Year	Sample size	Definition of advanced neoplasia	Sensitivity	Specificity	Other
SHH	Tanaka et al. [65]	2019	148	HGD, CIS, invasive carcinoma	81%	66%	SHH from surgical pathology
Proteomics	Corcos et al. [125]	2012	43	Low- and moderate-grade dysplasia vs IPMN with severe dysplasia or adenocarcinoma			31 peaks were expressed differentially in IPMN with low to moderate dysplasia versus IPMN with severe dysplasia or invasive adenocarcinoma. 5 unspecified proteins were accurate in differentiating the groups with an AUC of 0.88 on receiver operator curve (ROC) analysis
MUC1 from pancreatic juice from ERCP	Shimamoto et al. [134]	2010	34	IPMN with carcinoma vs IPMN adenoma	88.9%	71.4%	PPV 83.3%, NPV 81.3%, pancreatic juice from ERCP
MUC	Maker et al. [129]	2011	40	LGD IPMN vs HGN/invasive cancer			MUC2 and MUC4 concentrations were higher in cyst fluid in patients with IPMN with high-grade dysplasia or carcinoma compared to IPMN with low- to moderate-grade dysplasia. Serum MUC5 AC was higher in patients with IPMN with high-grade dysplasia
MUC5AC	Cao et al. [127]	2013	44 prevalidation 22 blinded	Mucinous vs nonmucinous	87–89%	100%	
MUC1, MUC2, MUC5 AC, and MUC6	Sai et al. [133]	2013	44	Malignant vs benign branch-duct IPMN	92%	100%	100% PPV, 97% NPV; pancreatic duct lavage cytology from ERCP
MUC1	Jabbar et al. [131]	2014	29	Malignant vs nonmalignant	87.5%	92.3%	89.7% accurate, 92.3% PPV, 85.7% NPV

				Malignant/ premalignant vs benign			
MUC 5 AC and MUC2	Jabbar et al. [130]	2018	68				97% accurate in identifying malignant from premalignant lesions
Plec-1	Bausch et al [147]	2009	37	HGD and invasive carcinoma vs low and moderate dysplasia	84%	83%	
Amphiregulin	Tun et al. [149]	2012	33	HGD/cancer in IPMN or MCN	83%	73%	
Spink 1	Raty et al. [150]	2013	61	Main/mixed-duct IPMN and MCn vs side-branch IPMN and SCA	85%	84%	@ 118 µg/l
Das 1	Das et al. [139]	2014	38	High-risk IPMN = Intestinal IPN with intermediate-grade dysplasia, IPMN-gastric, intestinal, pancreaticobiliary, or oncocytic with HGD, and invasive IPMN	89%	100%	
PGE_2	Yip-Schneider et al. [145]	2017	100	High-grade dysplasia and invasive carcinoma	PGE_2 1.1 pg/µl: 63% CEA > 192 ng/ml and PGE_2 0.5 pg/µl: 78%	PGE_2 1.1 pg/µl: 79% CEA > 192 ng/ml and PGE_2 0.5 pg/µl: 100%	Mean cyst fluid levels higher in HGD/ invasive carcinoma vs low-/moderate-grade IPMNS
Cytokine panel	Maker et al. [148]	2011	40	HGD/invasive IPMN vs LGD/MGD	Il1β: 79%	Il1β: 95%	Il5, Il8, and Il1β levels were higher in advanced IPMN; Il1β remained accurate in differentiating the groups on multivariate analysis

Proteomics

There have been several small studies using proteomics-based approaches to detect differential protein expression in pancreatic cyst fluid to differentiate cyst types. In one study of 59 patients, a cluster of 14 proteins could differentiate serous cystadenomas from IPMN in 92%. Most tested proteins were downregulated in IPMN compared with serous cystadenoma [123]. In a small study of cyst fluid from 10 patients, 12 protein peaks were differentially expressed in pancreatic cyst fluid in patients with pancreatic adenocarcinoma compared to nonmalignant cysts [124]. In a study of surgical samples from IPMN in 43 patients and 952 protein peaks, 31 peaks were expressed differentially in IPMN with low to moderate dysplasia versus IPMN with severe dysplasia or invasive adenocarcinoma [125]. In the same study, results from five unspecified proteins were accurate in differentiating the groups with an AUC of 0.88 on receiver operator curve (ROC) analysis [125]. These data are promising and will hopefully identify targets appropriate for further study.

MUC Proteins

Mucin (MUC) glycoproteins are involved in lubricating and enforcing the epithelial lining of luminal organs, including the pancreatic duct [126]. Interest in MUCs as biomarkers arises from our understanding that MUC expression varies by IPMN histologic subtype, which affects malignant potential. Gastric-type IPMN, comprising the majority of branch-duct IPMN, expresses MUC5AC but not MUC1/2, and rarely exhibits high-grade dysplasia. The intestinal type of IPMN that makes up the majority of the main-duct IPMN expresses MUC2, often exhibits intermediate- to high-grade dysplasia, and is prone to developing invasive carcinoma. Pancreatobiliary-type IPMNs are rare, but typically express MUC1 and demonstrate high-grade dysplasia and often contain invasive or minimally invasive carcinoma [14, 126]. A panel of three glycan alterations on MUC5AC was shown to be able to differentiate mucinous from nonmucinous cysts with sensitivity of 87–89% and specificity of 100% [127]. Direct staining of cyst fluid for mucin expression yielded a sensitivity of 80% and a specificity of 40% for diagnosing mucinous cysts [128]. MUC2 and MUC4 concentrations were higher in cyst fluid in patients with IPMN with high-grade dysplasia or carcinoma compared to IPMN with low- to moderate-grade dysplasia [129]. Similarly, serum MUC5 AC was higher in patients with IPMN with high-grade dysplasia [129]. Overall, these data were collected from small samples of patients, retrospectively. However, in a more recent study with a training cohort followed by a prospective cohort of 68 patients, MUC5 AC and MUC2 expression from cyst fluid could discriminate premalignant and malignant cysts from benign cysts in 97% of cases [130]. In the same study, MUC5 AC and prostate stem-cell antigen could identify high-grade dysplasia and cancer with a 96% accuracy [130]. In another prospective study, proteomic MUC profiling was more accurate than cytology and cyst fluid CEA in identifying lesions with malignant potential and predicting malignant transformation [131].

In addition to MUC subtype expression in cyst fluid, analyses of the DNA methylation status of MUC1, MUC2, and MUC4 in pancreatic juice were useful in differentiating PDAC from gastric- and intestinal-type IPMN in 45 patients [132]. Cytology from pancreatic duct lavage with staining for MUC1, MUC2, MUC5 AC, and MUC6 was useful in differentiating benign and malignant IPMNs with sensitivity and specificity of 92% and 100%, respectively [133]. Finally, MUC1 mRNA expression in pancreatic juice obtained from ERCP was higher in IPMN with carcinoma than in benign IPMN [134].

mAb Das-1

mAb Das-1 is a monoclonal antibody against a colonic epithelial phenotype that is reactive to premalignant conditions of the upper GI tract including Barrett's esophagus/esophageal adenocarcinoma, incomplete type gastric intestinal metaplasia/gastric adenocarcinoma, and small bowel adenomas/small bowel adenocarcinoma [135–138]. The specific antigen reactive to mAb Das-1 remains unknown, limited by its very high molecular weight (>200kd) and extensive glycosylation. Given the recent observations that intestinal-type IPMNs were at particular malignant potential and the utility of this biomarker in identifying colonic-type metaplasia in multiple organs, we sought to investigate the reactivity of this biomarker in patients with IPMN. In an initial study with 94 surgically resected IPMNs, mAb Das-1 was overexpressed in high-risk and malignant IPMN compared with low-risk IPMN (sensitivity 85%, specificity 95%) [139]. In the same study, mAb Das-1 expression was highly reactive in cyst fluid obtained perioperatively from high-risk/malignant IPMN, but minimally reactive in low- and intermediate-grade IPMN, yielding a sensitivity and specificity for detecting high-risk/malignant IPMN of 89% and 100%, respectively [139]. Further multicenter validation studies are currently underway.

Sonic Hedgehog

Sonic Hedgehog (SHH) is detected in IPMN cyst fluid, but not in pancreatic juice associated with chronic pancreatitis [46, 140]. SHH expression was more commonly expressed in surgical specimens with invasive carcinoma or high-grade IPMN than in moderate- or low-grade IPMN [141, 142]. In a systematic review by Tanaka et al., surgical pathology stained for SHH in 148 IPMNs yielded a sensitivity of 81% and specificity of 66% in differentiating HGD, CIS, and invasive carcinoma from benign IPMN [65].

S100

The S100 family is a group of proteins involved in cell signaling with increased expression in PDAC and IPMN associated with PDAC. One member was associated with nodal spread in PDAC [143]. In one study of mRNA expression in bulk tissue and pancreatic juice, S100P, a specific member of the S100 family, was useful for differentiating neoplastic disease from chronic pancreatitis; however, further studies are needed [144].

Prostaglandin E$_2$

Prostaglandin E$_2$ (PGE$_2$) is a product of the inflammatory pathways, and overexpression has been observed in multiple cancer types, including pancreatic cancer [145]. PGE$_2$ in cyst fluid was higher in IPMN than other mucinous cystic neoplasms and increased linearly by dysplastic grade from low-grade through invasive carcinoma [146]. In a larger prospective study of 100 patients with IPMN, PGE$_2$ levels in cyst fluid were higher in high-grade and invasive IPMN than low-/moderate-grade IPMN. In a subset of patients with cyst fluid CEA > 192 ng/ml, PGE$_2$ at a threshold of 0.5 pg/µl yielded a sensitivity of 78%, specificity of 100%, and accuracy of 86% for detecting high-grade or invasive IPMN [145].

Other Protein-Based Biomarkers

Plectin-1 (Plec-1) is highly specific and sensitive for early invasive PDAC [147]. In one small retrospective study, Plec-1 expression had a sensitivity of 84% and a specificity of 83% in differentiating malignant IPMN from benign IPMN, though further studies are required for validation [147].

In an analysis of cytokine expression profiles in IPMN cyst fluid, IL5, IL8, and IL1β concentrations were higher in cyst fluid from patients with HGD or cancer than in patients with low or moderate dysplasia [148]. At a level >1.26 pg/ml, the sensitivity was 79% and specificity was 95% [148]. On multivariate analysis, IL1β remained a significant predictor of high-risk cysts with an AUC of 0.92 [148].

Amphiregulin (AREG), an epidermal growth factor ligand overexpressed in pancreatic cancer, was significantly higher in cyst fluid in pancreatic cysts with cancer in a retrospective, single-center study [149]. At a threshold of 300 pg/ml, AREG had a diagnostic accuracy of 78% for cancer or high-grade dysplasia in cysts of multiple types with a sensitivity of 83% and a specificity of 73% [149].

Serine protease inhibitor Kazal type 1 (Spink1) is a peptide that has been associated with ovarian, bladder, and renal cancers. In a study of 61 surgical patients with various pancreatic cystic lesions, Spink1 levels were higher in surgically recommended lesions (main/mixed-duct IPMN and mucinous cystadenoma) than in benign lesions (side-branch IPMN and serous cystadenoma) [150]. At a cutoff of 118 µg/l, the sensitivity for differentiating surgically recommended lesions from benign lesions was 85% with a specificity of 84% and AUC of 0.94 [150].

Metabolomics

Metabolites in cyst fluid have been measured as a biomarker to differentiate mucinous from nonmucinous cysts. In an exploratory study of 45 cysts, concentrations of glucose and kynurenine, a tryptophan metabolite associated with cancer development, were lower in mucinous cysts with high accuracy (AUC 0.92 and 0.94, respectively) [62, 151]. However, these tests could not distinguish premalignant from malignant cysts [151]. In another study, glucose was lower in mucinous cysts compared to nonmucinous cysts, though this was not examined as a marker of invasiveness [152].

Biomarkers in Other Tissues (Table 3.5)

Blood Parameters

An increased serum neutrophil to lymphocyte ratio (NLR) may be indicative of increased active inflammation in IPMN-derived malignancy as it is associated with tumorigenesis in other systems [48]. In two retrospective studies, the preoperative NLR was higher in patients with IPMN with carcinoma than with IPMN alone [153, 154]. In a recent study of 205 IPMNs, the sensitivity and specificity for NLR in detecting high-grade dysplasia and invasive carcinoma were 35.3% and 87% [155]. Even when combined with CEA and Ca19-9, the combination assay yielded a modest sensitivity of 58.8% and a specificity of 76.8% [155].

Pancreatic Juice

Analysis of pancreatic juice is attractive as it potentially represents a sampling of the entire network of pancreatic ducts. Given the inherent connection and genesis of IPMN from ductal cells of the pancreas, pancreatic juice analysis may allow us to more accurately assess the entire organ and overcome issues of "field defect" that have been well demonstrated in IPMN and IPMN-associated PDAC. Using sampling of pancreatic juice aspirated during ERCP preoperatively for NGS, TP53 was detected in 50% of malignant IPMN [156]. The concentration of SMAD4/TP53 mutations in secretin-stimulated pancreatic juice collected from the duodenum could distinguish PDAC from IPMN with 32.4% sensitivity and 100% specificity [157]. In this study, 50% of the patients who developed cancer despite close surveillance had SMAD4/TP53 mutations detected in pancreatic juice samples 1 year prior to cancer detection [157].

Stool

In a proof-of-concept study to detect gene mutations in stool for early detection of pancreatic cancer, BMP3 detected 51%, KRAS detected 50%, and the combination of mutations in either gene detected 67% of pancreatic cancers [158]. This has not been evaluated prospectively or in invasive IPMN.

Table 3.5 Non-cyst fluid biomarkers

Biomarker	Study	Year	Sample size	Definition of advanced neoplasia	Sensitivity	Specificity	Other
Neutrophil to lymphocyte ratio	Arima et al. [153]	2015	76 IPMN	IPMN with carcinoma vs IPMN with adenoma	NLR > 2.074: 73.1% Combined criteria: 27%	NLR > 2.074: 58% Combined criteria: 96%	NLR > 2.074: PPV 47.5% and NPV of 80.6% for combined criteria of ICCS 2012 guidelines NLR > 2.074 and Ca19-9 > 37 IU/ml: PPV 78% and NPV of 72%
Neutrophil to lymphocyte ratio	Gemenetzis et al. [154]	2016	272	IPMN with carcinoma	NLR > 4: 33.8% NLR > 2.65: 74.1%	NLR > 4: 95% NLR > 2.65: 83.1%	NLR > 4: PPV 70.6% and NPV 80.3% Model including NLR, imaging findings, and jaundice: sensitivity 43.8% to 96.5% and specificity 98% to 50.3%
NLR, CRP to albumin ratio (CAR), CEA, CA19-9	Hata et al. 2019 [155]	2019	205	HGD /invasive carcinoma	NLR > 2.5: 35.3% CAR > 0.03: 31.8% CEA > 5, Ca19-9 > 37, and NLR: 58.8%	NLR > 2.5: 87% CAR > 0.03: 82.6% CEA > 5, Ca19-9 > 37, and NLR: 58.8%	NLR > 2.5: PPV 84.2% CAR > 0.03: PPV 77.8%, CEA > 5, Ca19-9 > 37, and NLR: PPV 83.3%
Pancreatic juice NGS	Yu et al. [157]	2017	115	PDAC vs IPMN	32.4%	100%	NGS of mutant TP53/SMAD4

Stool DNA	Kisiel et al. [158]	2012	57 cases, 62 controls	Pancreatic cancer	BMP3: 51% KRAS: 75% Combination: 67%	BMP3: 90% KRAS: 90% Combination: 90%	
Circulating epithelial cells	Rhim et al. [160]	2014	48	PDAC vs pancreatic cysts vs controls			>3 CECS in 73% with PDAC, 33% with pancreatic cysts and 0 controls
Circulating epithelial cells	Poruk et al. [161]	2017	19 with IPMN without malignancy	IPMN vs other cysts	58%	100%	IPMN with HGD more likely to have dual staining CECs

Circulating Cells

Preclinical mouse models of pancreatic cancer have demonstrated that epithelial to mesenchymal transition is indeed an early event in the development of PDAC, and circulating pancreatic tumor cells may in fact be present in the bloodstream prior to the demonstration of overt metastasis [159]. In a prospective study, 78% of patients with PDAC, 33% of patients with pancreatic cysts, and 0% of the controls undergoing screening colonoscopy had circulating epithelial cells (CECs) [160]. The outcome of those patients or their ultimate pathology was not reported in this study, nor was a threshold of "acceptable" circulating cells. In another study of patients undergoing surgical resection for IPMN, the sensitivity and specificity of cytokeratin-positive CECs for differentiating IPMN from other cysts were 58% and 100%, respectively [161]. In this study, CECs were more likely to be found in patients with high-grade dysplasia [161]. More recently, a group improved the assay and detected CECs in 88% of patients with IPMN regardless of underlying grade [162].

Another potential blood-based biomarker paradigm is analysis of circulating DNA for mutations seen in pancreatic tissues. In a retrospective study, the total amount of cell-free DNA was higher in patients with pancreatic cancer and IPMN than in controls [163]. GNAS mutations were detected in the cell-free DNA from patients with IPMN, but not serous cystadenomas or controls [163]. In a proof-of-concept study, KRAS and TP53 mutations in serum were detected in PDAC and IPMN, and KRAS mutations were detected in chronic pancreatitis patients [164]. While very exciting, these studies remain investigational and will hopefully be able to be integrated with other genetic/protein biomarkers to develop a minimally invasive surveillance tool for patients with pancreatic cysts or who are otherwise at risk for pancreatic cancer.

References

1. de Oliveira PB, Puchnick A, Szejnfeld J, et al. Prevalence of incidental pancreatic cysts on 3 tesla magnetic resonance. PLoS One. 2015;10:e0121317.
2. Zhang XM, Mitchell DG, Dohke M, et al. Pancreatic cysts: depiction on single-shot fast spin-echo MR images. Radiology. 2002;223:547–53.
3. Laffan TA, Horton KM, Klein AP, et al. Prevalence of unsuspected pancreatic cysts on MDCT. AJR Am J Roentgenol. 2008;191:802–7.
4. de Jong K, Nio CY, Hermans JJ, et al. High prevalence of pancreatic cysts detected by screening magnetic resonance imaging examinations. Clin Gastroenterol Hepatol. 2010;8:806–11.
5. Tanno S, Nakano Y, Sugiyama Y, et al. Incidence of synchronous and metachronous pancreatic carcinoma in 168 patients with branch duct intraductal papillary mucinous neoplasm. Pancreatology. 2010;10:173–8.
6. Lawrence SA, Attiyeh MA, Seier K, et al. Should patients with cystic lesions of the pancreas undergo long-term radiographic surveillance?: results of 3024 patients evaluated at a single institution. Ann Surg. 2017;266:536–44.

7. Kwok K, Chang J, Duan L, et al. Competing risks for mortality in patients with asymptomatic pancreatic cystic neoplasms: implications for clinical management. Am J Gastroenterol. 2017;112:1330–6.
8. Crippa S, Bassi C, Salvia R, et al. Low progression of intraductal papillary mucinous neoplasms with worrisome features and high-risk stigmata undergoing non-operative management: a mid-term follow-up analysis. Gut. 2017;66:495–506.
9. Ho CK, Kleeff J, Friess H, et al. Complications of pancreatic surgery. HPB (Oxford). 2005;7:99–108.
10. Al-Haddad M, El H II, Eloubeidi MA. Endoscopic ultrasound for the evaluation of cystic lesions of the pancreas. JOP. 2010;11:299–309.
11. Brugge WR, Lauwers GY, Sahani D, et al. Cystic neoplasms of the pancreas. N Engl J Med. 2004;351:1218–26.
12. Stark A, Donahue TR, Reber HA, et al. Pancreatic cyst disease: a review. JAMA. 2016;315:1882–93.
13. Crippa S, Fernandez-Del Castillo C, Salvia R, et al. Mucin-producing neoplasms of the pancreas: an analysis of distinguishing clinical and epidemiologic characteristics. Clin Gastroenterol Hepatol. 2010;8:213–9.
14. Mino-Kenudson M, Fernandez-del Castillo C, Baba Y, et al. Prognosis of invasive intraductal papillary mucinous neoplasm depends on histological and precursor epithelial subtypes. Gut. 2011;60:1712–20.
15. Scheiman JM, Hwang JH, Moayyedi P. American gastroenterological association technical review on the diagnosis and management of asymptomatic neoplastic pancreatic cysts. Gastroenterology. 2015;148:824–48 e22.
16. Tanaka M, Fernandez-del Castillo C, Adsay V, et al. International consensus guidelines 2012 for the management of IPMN and MCN of the pancreas. Pancreatology. 2012;12:183–97.
17. Vege SS, Ziring B, Jain R, et al. American gastroenterological association institute guideline on the diagnosis and management of asymptomatic neoplastic pancreatic cysts. Gastroenterology. 2015;148:819–22; quize12-3.
18. Tanaka M, Chari S, Adsay V, et al. International consensus guidelines for management of intraductal papillary mucinous neoplasms and mucinous cystic neoplasms of the pancreas. Pancreatology. 2006;6:17–32.
19. Brugge WR, Lewandrowski K, Lee-Lewandrowski E, et al. Diagnosis of pancreatic cystic neoplasms: a report of the cooperative pancreatic cyst study. Gastroenterology. 2004;126:1330–6.
20. Tanaka M, Fernandez-Del Castillo C, Kamisawa T, et al. Revisions of international consensus Fukuoka guidelines for the management of IPMN of the pancreas. Pancreatology. 2017;17:738–53.
21. Singhi AD, Zeh HJ, Brand RE, et al. American Gastroenterological Association guidelines are inaccurate in detecting pancreatic cysts with advanced neoplasia: a clinicopathologic study of 225 patients with supporting molecular data. Gastrointest Endosc. 2016;83:1107–1117 e2.
22. Goh BK, Lin Z, Tan DM, et al. Evaluation of the Fukuoka Consensus Guidelines for intraductal papillary mucinous neoplasms of the pancreas: results from a systematic review of 1,382 surgically resected patients. Surgery. 2015;158:1192–202.
23. Tang RS, Weinberg B, Dawson DW, et al. Evaluation of the guidelines for management of pancreatic branch-duct intraductal papillary mucinous neoplasm. Clin Gastroenterol Hepatol. 2008;6:815–9; quiz 719.
24. Xu MM, Yin S, Siddiqui AA, et al. Comparison of the diagnostic accuracy of three current guidelines for the evaluation of asymptomatic pancreatic cystic neoplasms. Medicine (Baltimore). 2017;96:e7900.
25. Ma GK, Goldberg DS, Thiruvengadam N, et al. Comparing American Gastroenterological Association Pancreatic Cyst Management Guidelines with Fukuoka consensus guidelines as predictors of advanced neoplasia in patients with suspected pancreatic cystic neoplasms. J Am Coll Surg. 2016;223:729–737 e1.

26. Hruban RH, Goggins M, Parsons J, et al. Progression model for pancreatic cancer. Clin Cancer Res. 2000;6:2969–72.
27. Bartsch DK, Dietzel K, Bargello M, et al. Multiple small "imaging" branch-duct type intraductal papillary mucinous neoplasms (IPMNs) in familial pancreatic cancer: indicator for concomitant high grade pancreatic intraepithelial neoplasia? Familial Cancer. 2013;12:89–96.
28. Maitra A, Fukushima N, Takaori K, et al. Precursors to invasive pancreatic cancer. Adv Anat Pathol. 2005;12:81–91.
29. Salvia R, Crippa S, Falconi M, et al. Branch-duct intraductal papillary mucinous neoplasms of the pancreas: to operate or not to operate? Gut. 2007;56:1086–90.
30. Traverso LW. Surgical treatment of intraductal papillary mucinous neoplasms of the pancreas: the aggressive approach. J Gastrointest Surg. 2002;6:662–3.
31. McPhee JT, Hill JS, Whalen GF, et al. Perioperative mortality for pancreatectomy: a national perspective. Ann Surg. 2007;246:246–53.
32. La Torre M, Nigri G, Ferrari L, et al. Hospital volume, margin status, and long-term survival after pancreaticoduodenectomy for pancreatic adenocarcinoma. Am Surg. 2012;78:225–9.
33. European Study Group on Cystic Tumours of the P. European evidence-based guidelines on pancreatic cystic neoplasms. Gut. 2018;67:789–804.
34. Wang KX, Ben QW, Jin ZD, et al. Assessment of morbidity and mortality associated with EUS-guided FNA: a systematic review. Gastrointest Endosc. 2011;73:283–90.
35. Thornton GD, McPhail MJ, Nayagam S, et al. Endoscopic ultrasound guided fine needle aspiration for the diagnosis of pancreatic cystic neoplasms: a meta-analysis. Pancreatology. 2013;13:48–57.
36. Rogart JN, Loren DE, Singu BS, et al. Cyst wall puncture and aspiration during EUS-guided fine needle aspiration may increase the diagnostic yield of mucinous cysts of the pancreas. J Clin Gastroenterol. 2011;45:164–9.
37. Scourtas A, Dudley JC, Brugge WR, et al. Preoperative characteristics and cytological features of 136 histologically confirmed pancreatic mucinous cystic neoplasms. Cancer Cytopathol. 2017;125:169–77.
38. Yagi Y, Masuda A, Zen Y, et al. Predictive value of low serum pancreatic enzymes in invasive intraductal papillary mucinous neoplasms. Pancreatology. 2016;16:893–9.
39. Gaddam S, Ge PS, Keach JW, et al. Suboptimal accuracy of carcinoembryonic antigen in differentiation of mucinous and nonmucinous pancreatic cysts: results of a large multicenter study. Gastrointest Endosc. 2015;82:1060–9.
40. Jin DX, Small AJ, Vollmer CM, et al. A lower cyst fluid CEA cut-off increases diagnostic accuracy in identifying mucinous pancreatic cystic lesions. JOP J Pancreas. 2015;16:271–7.
41. van der Waaij LA, van Dullemen HM, Porte RJ. Cyst fluid analysis in the differential diagnosis of pancreatic cystic lesions: a pooled analysis. Gastrointest Endosc. 2005;62:383–9.
42. Maire F, Voitot H, Aubert A, et al. Intraductal papillary mucinous neoplasms of the pancreas: performance of pancreatic fluid analysis for positive diagnosis and the prediction of malignancy. Am J Gastroenterol. 2008;103:2871–7.
43. Correa-Gallego C, Warshaw AL, Fernandez-del Castillo C. Fluid CEA in IPMNs: a useful test or the flip of a coin? Am J Gastroenterol. 2009;104:796–7.
44. Kucera S, Centeno BA, Springett G, et al. Cyst fluid carcinoembryonic antigen level is not predictive of invasive cancer in patients with intraductal papillary mucinous neoplasm of the pancreas. JOP. 2012;13:409–13.
45. Ngamruengphong S, Bartel MJ, Raimondo M. Cyst carcinoembryonic antigen in differentiating pancreatic cysts: a meta-analysis. Dig Liver Dis. 2013;45:920–6.
46. Kaplan JH, Gonda TA. The use of biomarkers in the risk stratification of cystic neoplasms. Gastrointest Endosc Clin N Am. 2018;28:549–68.
47. Al-Rashdan A, Schmidt CM, Al-Haddad M, et al. Fluid analysis prior to surgical resection of suspected mucinous pancreatic cysts. A single centre experience. J Gastrointest Oncol. 2011;2:208–14.

48. Moris D, Damaskos C, Spartalis E, et al. Updates and critical evaluation on novel biomarkers for the malignant progression of intraductal papillary mucinous neoplasms of the pancreas. Anticancer Res. 2017;37:2185–94.
49. Fritz S, Hackert T, Hinz U, et al. Role of serum carbohydrate antigen 19-9 and carcinoembryonic antigen in distinguishing between benign and invasive intraductal papillary mucinous neoplasm of the pancreas. Br J Surg. 2011;98:104–10.
50. Ballehaninna UK, Chamberlain RS, Serum CA. 19-9 as a biomarker for pancreatic cancer-a comprehensive review. Indian J Surg Oncol. 2011;2:88–100.
51. Pais SA, Attasaranya S, Leblanc JK, et al. Role of endoscopic ultrasound in the diagnosis of intraductal papillary mucinous neoplasms: correlation with surgical histopathology. Clin Gastroenterol Hepatol. 2007;5:489–95.
52. Kim JR, Jang JY, Kang MJ, et al. Clinical implication of serum carcinoembryonic antigen and carbohydrate antigen 19-9 for the prediction of malignancy in intraductal papillary mucinous neoplasm of pancreas. J Hepatobiliary Pancreat Sci. 2015;22:699–707.
53. Wang W, Zhang L, Chen L, et al. Serum carcinoembryonic antigen and carbohydrate antigen 19-9 for prediction of malignancy and invasiveness in intraductal papillary mucinous neoplasms of the pancreas: a meta-analysis. Biomed Rep. 2015;3:43–50.
54. Thosani N, Thosani S, Qiao W, et al. Role of EUS-FNA-based cytology in the diagnosis of mucinous pancreatic cystic lesions: a systematic review and meta-analysis. Dig Dis Sci. 2010;55:2756–66.
55. de Jong K, van Hooft JE, Nio CY, et al. Accuracy of preoperative workup in a prospective series of surgically resected cystic pancreatic lesions. Scand J Gastroenterol. 2012;47:1056–63.
56. Cizginer S, Turner B, Bilge AR, et al. Cyst fluid carcinoembryonic antigen is an accurate diagnostic marker of pancreatic mucinous cysts. Pancreas. 2011;40:1024–8.
57. Sedlack R, Affi A, Vazquez-Sequeiros E, et al. Utility of EUS in the evaluation of cystic pancreatic lesions. Gastrointest Endosc. 2002;56:543–7.
58. Morris-Stiff G, Lentz G, Chalikonda S, et al. Pancreatic cyst aspiration analysis for cystic neoplasms: mucin or carcinoembryonic antigen—which is better? Surgery. 2010;148:638–45.
59. Pitman MB, Michaels PJ, Deshpande V, et al. Cytological and cyst fluid analysis of small (< or =3 cm) branch duct intraductal papillary mucinous neoplasms adds value to patient management decisions. Pancreatology. 2008;8:277–84.
60. Pitman MB, Genevay M, Yaeger K, et al. High-grade atypical epithelial cells in pancreatic mucinous cysts are a more accurate predictor of malignancy than "positive" cytology. Cancer Cytopathol. 2010;118:434–40.
61. Pitman MB, Centeno BA, Genevay M, et al. Grading epithelial atypia in endoscopic ultrasound-guided fine-needle aspiration of intraductal papillary mucinous neoplasms: an international interobserver concordance study. Cancer Cytopathol. 2013;121:729–36.
62. Thiruvengadam N, Park WG. Systematic review of pancreatic cyst fluid biomarkers: the path forward. Clin Transl Gastroenterol. 2015;6:e88.
63. Sendino O, Fernandez-Esparrach G, Sole M, et al. Endoscopic ultrasonography-guided brushing increases cellular diagnosis of pancreatic cysts: a prospective study. Dig Liver Dis. 2010;42:877–81.
64. Sedlack R, Affi A, Vazquez-Sequeiros E, et al. Utility of EUS in the evaluation of cystic pancreatic lesions. Gastrointest Endosc. 2002;56:543–7.
65. Tanaka M, Heckler M, Liu B, et al. Cytologic analysis of pancreatic juice increases specificity of detection of malignant IPMN - a systematic review. Clin Gastroenterol Hepatol. 2019;17:2199.
66. Khalid A, McGrath KM, Zahid M, et al. The role of pancreatic cyst fluid molecular analysis in predicting cyst pathology. Clin Gastroenterol Hepatol. 2005;3:967–73.
67. Theisen BK, Wald AI, Singhi AD. Molecular diagnostics in the evaluation of pancreatic cysts. Surg Pathol Clin. 2016;9:441–56.
68. Khalid A, Zahid M, Finkelstein SD, et al. Pancreatic cyst fluid DNA analysis in evaluating pancreatic cysts: a report of the PANDA study. Gastrointest Endosc. 2009;69:1095–102.

69. Fritz S, Fernandez-del Castillo C, Mino-Kenudson M, et al. Global genomic analysis of intra-ductal papillary mucinous neoplasms of the pancreas reveals significant molecular differences compared to ductal adenocarcinoma. Ann Surg. 2009;249:440–7.
70. Maitra A, Adsay NV, Argani P, et al. Multicomponent analysis of the pancreatic adenocarcinoma progression model using a pancreatic intraepithelial neoplasia tissue microarray. Mod Pathol. 2003;16:902.
71. Eser S, Schnieke A, Schneider G, et al. Oncogenic KRAS signalling in pancreatic cancer. Br J Cancer. 2014;111:817–22.
72. Kanda M, Matthaei H, Wu J, et al. Presence of somatic mutations in most early-stage pancreatic intraepithelial neoplasia. Gastroenterology. 2012;142:730–733 e9.
73. Schoedel KE, Finkelstein SD, Ohori NP. K-Ras and microsatellite marker analysis of fine-needle aspirates from intraductal papillary mucinous neoplasms of the pancreas. Diagn Cytopathol. 2006;34:605–8.
74. Sawhney MS, Devarajan S, O'Farrel P, et al. Comparison of carcinoembryonic antigen and molecular analysis in pancreatic cyst fluid. Gastrointest Endosc. 2009;69:1106–10.
75. Shen J, Brugge WR, Dimaio CJ, et al. Molecular analysis of pancreatic cyst fluid: a comparative analysis with current practice of diagnosis. Cancer. 2009;117:217–27.
76. Sreenarasimhaiah J, Lara LF, Jazrawi SF, et al. A comparative analysis of pancreas cyst fluid CEA and histology with DNA mutational analysis in the detection of mucin producing or malignant cysts. JOP. 2009;10:163–8.
77. Talar-Wojnarowska R, Pazurek M, Durko L, et al. A comparative analysis of K-ras mutation and carcinoembryonic antigen in pancreatic cyst fluid. Pancreatology. 2012;12:417–20.
78. Nikiforova MN, Khalid A, Fasanella KE, et al. Integration of KRAS testing in the diagnosis of pancreatic cystic lesions: a clinical experience of 618 pancreatic cysts. Mod Pathol. 2013;26:1478–87.
79. Bournet B, Vignolle-Vidoni A, Grand D, et al. Endoscopic ultrasound-guided fine-needle aspiration plus KRAS and GNAS mutation in malignant intraductal papillary mucinous neoplasm of the pancreas. Endosc Int Open. 2016;4:E1228–35.
80. Al-Haddad M, DeWitt J, Sherman S, et al. Performance characteristics of molecular (DNA) analysis for the diagnosis of mucinous pancreatic cysts. Gastrointest Endosc. 2014;79:79–87.
81. Jones M, Zheng Z, Wang J, et al. Impact of next-generation sequencing on the clinical diagnosis of pancreatic cysts. Gastrointest Endosc. 2016;83:140–8.
82. Tatarian T, Winter JM. Genetics of pancreatic cancer and its implications on therapy. Surg Clin North Am. 2016;96:1207–21.
83. Wu J, Matthaei H, Maitra A, et al. Recurrent GNAS mutations define an unexpected pathway for pancreatic cyst development. Sci Transl Med. 2011;3:92ra66.
84. Kitago M, Ueda M, Aiura K, et al. Comparison of K-ras point mutation distributions in intraductal papillary-mucinous tumors and ductal adenocarcinoma of the pancreas. Int J Cancer. 2004;110:177–82.
85. Tada M, Ohashi M, Shiratori Y, et al. Analysis of K-ras gene mutation in hyperplastic duct cells of the pancreas without pancreatic disease. Gastroenterology. 1996;110:227–31.
86. Kuboki Y, Shimizu K, Hatori T, et al. Molecular biomarkers for progression of intraductal papillary mucinous neoplasm of the pancreas. Pancreas. 2015;44:227–35.
87. Winner M, Sethi A, Poneros JM, et al. The role of molecular analysis in the diagnosis and surveillance of pancreatic cystic neoplasms. JOP. 2015;16:143–9.
88. Khalid A, Pal R, Sasatomi E, et al. Use of microsatellite marker loss of heterozygosity in accurate diagnosis of pancreaticobiliary malignancy from brush cytology samples. Gut. 2004;53:1860–5.
89. Guo X, Zhan X, Li Z. Molecular analyses of aspirated cystic fluid for the differential diagnosis of cystic lesions of the pancreas: a systematic review and meta-analysis. Gastroenterol Res Pract. 2016;2016:3546085.

90. Loren D, Kowalski T, Siddiqui A, et al. Influence of integrated molecular pathology test results on real-world management decisions for patients with pancreatic cysts: analysis of data from a national registry cohort. Diagn Pathol. 2016;11:5.
91. Al-Haddad MA, Kowalski T, Siddiqui A, et al. Integrated molecular pathology accurately determines the malignant potential of pancreatic cysts. Endoscopy. 2015;47:136–46.
92. Tinschert S, Gerl H, Gewies A, et al. McCune-Albright syndrome: clinical and molecular evidence of mosaicism in an unusual giant patient. Am J Med Genet. 1999;83:100–8.
93. Turan S, Bastepe M. The GNAS complex locus and human diseases associated with loss-of-function mutations or epimutations within this imprinted gene. Horm Res Paediatr. 2013;80:229–41.
94. Wu J, Matthaei H, Maitra A, et al. Recurrent GNAS mutations define an unexpected pathway for pancreatic cyst development. Sci Transl Med. 2011;3:92ra66–6.
95. Siddiqui AA, Kowalski TE, Kedika R, et al. EUS-guided pancreatic fluid aspiration for DNA analysis of KRAS and GNAS mutations for the evaluation of pancreatic cystic neoplasia: a pilot study. Gastrointest Endosc. 2013;77:669–70.
96. Singhi AD, Nikiforova MN, Fasanella KE, et al. Preoperative GNAS and KRAS testing in the diagnosis of pancreatic mucinous cysts. Clin Cancer Res. 2014;20:4381–9.
97. Singhi AD, McGrath K, Brand RE, et al. Preoperative next-generation sequencing of pancreatic cyst fluid is highly accurate in cyst classification and detection of advanced neoplasia. Gut. 2018;67:2131–41.
98. Dal Molin M, Matthaei H, Wu J, et al. Clinicopathological correlates of activating GNAS mutations in intraductal papillary mucinous neoplasm (IPMN) of the pancreas. Ann Surg Oncol. 2013;20:3802–8.
99. Kanda M, Knight S, Topazian M, et al. Mutant GNAS detected in duodenal collections of secretin-stimulated pancreatic juice indicates the presence or emergence of pancreatic cysts. Gut. 2013;62:1024–33.
100. Taki K, Ohmuraya M, Tanji E, et al. GNAS(R201H) and Kras(G12D) cooperate to promote murine pancreatic tumorigenesis recapitulating human intraductal papillary mucinous neoplasm. Oncogene. 2016;35:2407–12.
101. Hata T, Dal Molin M, Suenaga M, et al. Cyst fluid Telomerase activity predicts the histologic grade of cystic neoplasms of the pancreas. Clin Cancer Res. 2016;22:5141–51.
102. Wada K. p16 and p53 gene alterations and accumulations in the malignant evolution of intraductal papillary-mucinous tumors of the pancreas. J Hepato-Biliary-Pancreat Surg. 2002;9:76–85.
103. Biankin AV, Biankin SA, Kench JG, et al. Aberrant p16(INK4A) and DPC4/Smad4 expression in intraductal papillary mucinous tumours of the pancreas is associated with invasive ductal adenocarcinoma. Gut. 2002;50:861–8.
104. Campa D, Pastore M, Gentiluomo M, et al. Functional single nucleotide polymorphisms within the cyclin-dependent kinase inhibitor 2A/2B region affect pancreatic cancer risk. Oncotarget. 2016;7:57011–20.
105. Izeradjene K, Combs C, Best M, et al. KrasG12D and Smad4/Dpc4 haploinsufficiency cooperate to induce mucinous cystic neoplasms and invasive adenocarcinoma of the pancreas. Cancer Cell. 2007;11:229–43.
106. Narayanan R, Tuoc TC. Roles of chromatin remodeling BAF complex in neural differentiation and reprogramming. Cell Tissue Res. 2014;356:575–84.
107. Von Figura G, Fukuda A, Roy N, et al. The chromatin regulator Brg1 suppresses formation of intraductal papillary mucinous neoplasm and pancreatic ductal adenocarcinoma. Nat Cell Biol. 2014;16:255.
108. Roy N, Malik S, Villanueva KE, et al. Brg1 promotes both tumor-suppressive and oncogenic activities at distinct stages of pancreatic cancer formation. Genes Dev. 2015;29:658–71.
109. Dal Molin M, Hong S-M, Hebbar S, et al. Loss of expression of the SWI/SNF chromatin remodeling subunit BRG1/SMARCA4 is frequently observed in intraductal papillary mucinous neoplasms of the pancreas. Hum Pathol. 2012;43:585–91.

110. Dal Molin M, Hong SM, Hebbar S, et al. Loss of expression of the SWI/SNF chromatin remodeling subunit BRG1/SMARCA4 is frequently observed in intraductal papillary mucinous neoplasms of the pancreas. Hum Pathol. 2012;43:585–91.
111. Tsiatis AC, Norris-Kirby A, Rich RG, et al. Comparison of Sanger sequencing, pyrosequencing, and melting curve analysis for the detection of KRAS mutations: diagnostic and clinical implications. J Mol Diagn. 2010;12:425–32.
112. Amato E, Molin MD, Mafficini A, et al. Targeted next-generation sequencing of cancer genes dissects the molecular profiles of intraductal papillary neoplasms of the pancreas. J Pathol. 2014;233:217–27.
113. Sato N, Ueki T, Fukushima N, et al. Aberrant methylation of CpG islands in intraductal papillary mucinous neoplasms of the pancreas. Gastroenterology. 2002;123:365–72.
114. Hong SM, Omura N, Vincent A, et al. Genome-wide CpG island profiling of intraductal papillary mucinous neoplasms of the pancreas. Clin Cancer Res. 2012;18:700–12.
115. Henriksen SD, Madsen PH, Krarup H, et al. DNA hypermethylation as a blood-based marker for pancreatic cancer: a literature review. Pancreas. 2015;44:1036–45.
116. Wang L, Zheng J, Sun C, et al. MicroRNA expression levels as diagnostic biomarkers for intraductal papillary mucinous neoplasm. Oncotarget. 2017;8:58765–70.
117. Lee EJ, Gusev Y, Jiang J, et al. Expression profiling identifies microRNA signature in pancreatic cancer. Int J Cancer. 2007;120:1046–54.
118. Ryu JK, Matthaei H, Dal Molin M, et al. Elevated microRNA miR-21 levels in pancreatic cyst fluid are predictive of mucinous precursor lesions of ductal adenocarcinoma. Pancreatology. 2011;11:343–50.
119. Farrell JJ, Toste P, Wu N, et al. Endoscopically acquired pancreatic cyst fluid microRNA 21 and 221 are associated with invasive cancer. Am J Gastroenterol. 2013;108:1352–9.
120. Caponi S, Funel N, Frampton AE, et al. The good, the bad and the ugly: a tale of miR-101, miR-21 and miR-155 in pancreatic intraductal papillary mucinous neoplasms. Ann Oncol. 2013;24:734–41.
121. Wang J, Paris PL, Chen J, et al. Next generation sequencing of pancreatic cyst fluid microRNAs from low grade-benign and high grade-invasive lesions. Cancer Lett. 2015;356:404–9.
122. Matthaei H, Wylie D, Lloyd MB, et al. miRNA biomarkers in cyst fluid augment the diagnosis and management of pancreatic cysts. Clin Cancer Res. 2012;18:4713–24.
123. Allen PJ, Qin LX, Tang L, et al. Pancreatic cyst fluid protein expression profiling for discriminating between serous cystadenoma and intraductal papillary mucinous neoplasm. Ann Surg. 2009;250:754–60.
124. Scarlett CJ, Samra JS, Xue A, et al. Classification of pancreatic cystic lesions using SELDI-TOF mass spectrometry. ANZ J Surg. 2007;77:648–53.
125. Corcos O, Couvelard A, Dargere D, et al. Proteomic assessment of markers for malignancy in the mucus of intraductal papillary mucinous neoplasms of the pancreas. Pancreas. 2012;41:169–74.
126. Maker AV, Carrara S, Jamieson NB, et al. Cyst fluid biomarkers for intraductal papillary mucinous neoplasms of the pancreas: a critical review from the international expert meeting on pancreatic branch-duct-intraductal papillary mucinous neoplasms. J Am Coll Surg. 2015;220:243–53.
127. Cao Z, Maupin K, Curnutte B, et al. Specific glycoforms of MUC5AC and endorepellin accurately distinguish mucinous from nonmucinous pancreatic cysts. Mol Cell Proteomics. 2013;12:2724–34.
128. Morris-Stiff G, Lentz G, Chalikonda S, et al. Pancreatic cyst aspiration analysis for cystic neoplasms: mucin or carcinoembryonic antigen--which is better? Surgery. 2010;148:638–44; discussion 644-5.
129. Maker AV, Katabi N, Gonen M, et al. Pancreatic cyst fluid and serum mucin levels predict dysplasia in intraductal papillary mucinous neoplasms of the pancreas. Ann Surg Oncol. 2011;18:199–206.

130. Jabbar KS, Arike L, Verbeke CS, et al. Highly accurate identification of cystic precursor lesions of pancreatic cancer through targeted mass spectrometry: a phase IIc diagnostic study. J Clin Oncol. 2018;36:367–75.
131. Jabbar KS, Verbeke C, Hyltander AG, et al. Proteomic mucin profiling for the identification of cystic precursors of pancreatic cancer. J Natl Cancer Inst. 2014;106:djt439.
132. Yokoyama S, Kitamoto S, Higashi M, et al. Diagnosis of pancreatic neoplasms using a novel method of DNA methylation analysis of mucin expression in pancreatic juice. PLoS One. 2014;9:e93760.
133. Sai JK, Nobukawa B, Matsumura Y, et al. Pancreatic duct lavage cytology with the cell block method for discriminating benign and malignant branch-duct type intraductal papillary mucinous neoplasms. Gastrointest Endosc. 2013;77:726–35.
134. Shimamoto T, Tani M, Kawai M, et al. MUC1 is a useful molecular marker for malignant intraductal papillary mucinous neoplasms in pancreatic juice obtained from endoscopic retrograde pancreatography. Pancreas. 2010;39:879–83.
135. Das KM, Sakamaki S, Vecchi M, et al. The production and characterization of monoclonal antibodies to a human colonic antigen associated with ulcerative colitis: cellular localization of the antigen by using the monoclonal antibody. J Immunol. 1987;139:77–84.
136. Das KM, Prasad I, Garla S, et al. Detection of a shared colon epithelial epitope on Barrett epithelium by a novel monoclonal antibody. Ann Intern Med. 1994;120:753–6.
137. Mirza Z, Das K, Slate J, et al. Gastric intestinal metaplasia as detected by a monoclonal antibody is highly associated with gastric adenocarcinoma. Gut. 2003;52:807–12.
138. Onuma EK, Amenta PS, Jukkola AF, et al. A phenotypic change of small intestinal epithelium to colonocytes in small intestinal adenomas and adenocarcinomas. Am J Gastroenterol. 2001;96:2480.
139. Das KK, Xiao H, Geng X, et al. mAb Das-1 is specific for high-risk and malignant intraductal papillary mucinous neoplasm (IPMN). Gut. 2014;63:1626–34.
140. Ohuchida K, Mizumoto K, Fujita H, et al. Sonic hedgehog is an early developmental marker of intraductal papillary mucinous neoplasms: clinical implications of mRNA levels in pancreatic juice. J Pathol. 2006;210:42–8.
141. Jang KT, Lee KT, Lee JG, et al. Immunohistochemical expression of Sonic hedgehog in intraductal papillary mucinous tumor of the pancreas. Appl Immunohistochem Mol Morphol. 2007;15:294–8.
142. Satoh K, Kanno A, Hamada S, et al. Expression of Sonic hedgehog signaling pathway correlates with the tumorigenesis of intraductal papillary mucinous neoplasm of the pancreas. Oncol Rep. 2008;19:1185–90.
143. Huang S, Zheng J, Huang Y, et al. Impact of S100A4 expression on clinicopathological characteristics and prognosis in pancreatic cancer: a meta-analysis. Dis Markers. 2016;2016:8137378.
144. Ohuchida K, Mizumoto K, Egami T, et al. S100P is an early developmental marker of pancreatic carcinogenesis. Clin Cancer Res. 2006;12:5411–6.
145. Yip-Schneider MT, Carr RA, Wu H, et al. Prostaglandin E2: a pancreatic fluid biomarker of intraductal papillary mucinous neoplasm dysplasia. J Am Coll Surg. 2017;225:481–7.
146. Schmidt CM, Yip-Schneider MT, Ralstin MC, et al. PGE(2) in pancreatic cyst fluid helps differentiate IPMN from MCN and predict IPMN dysplasia. J Gastrointest Surg. 2008;12:243–9.
147. Bausch D, Mino-Kenudson M, Fernandez-Del Castillo C, et al. Plectin-1 is a biomarker of malignant pancreatic intraductal papillary mucinous neoplasms. J Gastrointest Surg. 2009;13:1948–54; discussion 1954.
148. Maker AV, Katabi N, Qin LX, et al. Cyst fluid interleukin-1beta (IL1beta) levels predict the risk of carcinoma in intraductal papillary mucinous neoplasms of the pancreas. Clin Cancer Res. 2011;17:1502–8.
149. Tun MT, Pai RK, Kwok S, et al. Diagnostic accuracy of cyst fluid amphiregulin in pancreatic cysts. BMC Gastroenterol. 2012;12:15.

150. Raty S, Sand J, Laukkarinen J, et al. Cyst fluid SPINK1 may help to differentiate benign and potentially malignant cystic pancreatic lesions. Pancreatology. 2013;13:530–3.
151. Park WG, Wu M, Bowen R, et al. Metabolomic-derived novel cyst fluid biomarkers for pancreatic cysts: glucose and kynurenine. Gastrointest Endosc. 2013;78:295–302 e2.
152. Zikos T, Pham K, Bowen R, et al. Cyst fluid glucose is rapidly feasible and accurate in diagnosing mucinous pancreatic cysts. Am J Gastroenterol. 2015;110:909–14.
153. Arima K, Okabe H, Hashimoto D, et al. The neutrophil-to-lymphocyte ratio predicts malignant potential in intraductal papillary mucinous neoplasms. J Gastrointest Surg. 2015;19:2171–7.
154. Gemenetzis G, Bagante F, Griffin JF, et al. Neutrophil-to-lymphocyte ratio is a predictive marker for invasive malignancy in intraductal papillary mucinous neoplasms of the pancreas. Ann Surg. 2017;266:339–45.
155. Hata T, Mizuma M, Motoi F, et al. Diagnostic and prognostic impact of neutrophil-to-lymphocyte ratio for intraductal papillary mucinous neoplasms of the pancreas with high-grade dysplasia and associated invasive carcinoma. Pancreas. 2019;48:99–106.
156. Takano S, Fukasawa M, Kadokura M, et al. Next-generation sequencing revealed TP53 mutations to be malignant marker for intraductal papillary mucinous neoplasms that could be detected using pancreatic juice. Pancreas. 2017;46:1281–7.
157. Yu J, Sadakari Y, Shindo K, et al. Digital next-generation sequencing identifies low-abundance mutations in pancreatic juice samples collected from the duodenum of patients with pancreatic cancer and intraductal papillary mucinous neoplasms. Gut. 2017;66:1677–87.
158. Kisiel JB, Yab TC, Taylor WR, et al. Stool DNA testing for the detection of pancreatic cancer: assessment of methylation marker candidates. Cancer. 2012;118:2623–31.
159. Rhim AD, Mirek ET, Aiello NM, et al. EMT and dissemination precede pancreatic tumor formation. Cell. 2012;148:349–61.
160. Rhim AD, Thege FI, Santana SM, et al. Detection of circulating pancreas epithelial cells in patients with pancreatic cystic lesions. Gastroenterology. 2014;146:647–51.
161. Poruk KE, Valero V 3rd, He J, et al. Circulating epithelial cells in intraductal papillary mucinous neoplasms and cystic pancreatic lesions. Pancreas. 2017;46:943–7.
162. Franses JW, Basar O, Kadayifci A, et al. Improved detection of circulating epithelial cells in patients with intraductal papillary mucinous neoplasms. Oncologist. 2018;23:121–7.
163. Berger AW, Schwerdel D, Costa IG, et al. Detection of hot-spot mutations in circulating cell-free DNA from patients with intraductal papillary mucinous neoplasms of the pancreas. Gastroenterology. 2016;151:267–70.
164. Yang S, Che SP, Kurywchak P, et al. Detection of mutant KRAS and TP53 DNA in circulating exosomes from healthy individuals and patients with pancreatic cancer. Cancer Biol Ther. 2017;18:158–65.
165. Kawada N, Uehara H, Nagata S, et al. Pancreatic juice cytology as sensitive test for detecting pancreatic malignancy in intraductal papillary mucinous neoplasm of the pancreas without mural nodule. Pancreatology. 2016;16:853–8.

Part III
Diagnosis, Biomarkers and Stratification

Chapter 4
Challenges and Opportunities for Early Pancreatic Cancer Detection: Role for Protein Biomarkers

Lucy Oldfield, Lawrence Barrera, Dylan Williams, Anthony E. Evans, John Neoptolemos, and Eithne Costello

The Case for Earlier Detection

Currently, for three out of four PDAC patients, the diagnosis of PDAC comes at a time when the disease is advanced. Late diagnosis severely limits treatment options and contributes to the poor overall 5-year survival of 7%. Reliable diagnostic biomarkers that facilitate earlier diagnosis are much needed [1]. Generally speaking, it is recognised that early detection of cancer increases the opportunities for effective management and treatment (http://www.who.int/cancer/prevention/diagnosis-screening/en). Biomarker development projects aim to introduce diagnostic biomarkers that will permit PDAC detection at a time when therapeutic intervention that leads to improved prognosis is feasible. It is essential to ensure that earlier detection facilitates interventions that both improve outcome and well-being for patients, without simply increasing the time interval between diagnosis and death, known as lead time. Much research supports the benefit of earlier PDAC detection. Patients in whom PDAC is incidentally diagnosed have longer median survival compared with PDACs discovered when patients are symptomatic [2]. Furthermore, patients diagnosed with stage I disease survive markedly better compared to patients with all other stages [2]. Surgery followed by chemotherapy confers a significant survival advantage [3, 4]. In this setting, the 5-year survival is 70% for stage I disease and 22% for stage III disease. The ESPAC-4 trial which compared

L. Oldfield · L. Barrera · D. Williams · A. E. Evans · E. Costello
Department of Molecular and Clinical Cancer Medicine,
University of Liverpool,
Liverpool, UK

J. Neoptolemos (✉)
Department of General, Visceral and Transplantation Surgery,
University of Heidelberg, Heidelberg, Germany
e-mail: john.neoptolemos@med.uni-heidelberg.de

© Springer Nature Switzerland AG 2020
C. W. Michalski et al. (eds.), *Translational Pancreatic Cancer Research*,
Molecular and Translational Medicine,
https://doi.org/10.1007/978-3-030-49476-6_4

gemcitabine to combination gemcitabine/capecitabine therapy in R0/R1 resected PDAC patients demonstrated superior 5-year survival of 28·8% in the gemcitabine/capecitabine arm [5]. By contrast, for patients with locally advanced and metastatic pancreatic cancer randomised to either gemcitabine or gemcitabine/capecitabine, the 1-year survival in the superior arm of gemcitabine/capecitabine was 24% [6]. Thus, detecting PDAC at a time when patients are eligible for potentially curative surgery or for neoadjuvant therapy to downstage locally unresectable disease could significantly improve prognosis. The success of early detection schemes will require education of both the general public and healthcare professionals so that possible warning signs of pancreatic cancer are recognised. Alongside education, effective screening will be a major element in earlier detection of PDAC.

Challenges Associated with Diagnostic PDAC Marker Development

PDAC early detection faces a number of critical challenges (Table 4.1). PDAC is relatively uncommon, and it is therefore difficult for a single group or institution to amass the number and variety of samples required for successful biomarker development. PDAC tumours exhibit both intra-tumour and inter-individual variation [7,

Table 4.1 Challenges and potential solutions to early detection biomarker development for pancreatic cancer

Description	Challenge	Potential solutions
PDAC is a relatively uncommon disease	Large numbers of samples are required for novel biomarker development	National and international collaboration is required for adequate sample availability
PDAC tumours exhibit both intra-tumour and inter-individual variation	Large numbers of samples are required to enable diversity to be captured	National and international collaboration is required Capture as much clinico-pathological data relevant to samples as possible Sub-categorise samples to allow biomarker performance in individual categories to be manifested
PDAC is accompanied by comorbidities	Comorbidities such as obstructive jaundice, new-onset diabetes mellitus and chronic pancreatitis could influence biomarker behaviour or mislead biomarker analysis (e.g. the biomarker detects the comorbidity rather than the principal disease)	Carefully design studies Include groups that control for comorbidities, allowing the biomarkers' power to discriminate cancer from controls to be accurately assessed Be clear about the intended use population

Table 4.1 (continued)

Description	Challenge	Potential solutions
The majority of PDAC patients are diagnosed with late-stage disease	Use of late-stage samples in biomarker discovery and/or validation may lead to the detection of biomarkers capable of detecting late-stage disease, but not necessarily early-stage disease	Include patients with early-stage disease and studies Use pre-diagnostic samples where possible Collect custom-made bespoke cohorts in order to obtain pre-diagnostic samples with pancreatic cancer detection specifically in mind

8]. This heterogeneity is likely to be reflected in a variation in biomarkers from patient to patient, and robust biomarker panels may be required. PDAC is often accompanied by obstructive jaundice, which can lead to false-positive findings in blood-borne biomarker studies [9–11]. Moreover, PDAC-associated diabetes is present in a substantial proportion of individuals with pancreatic cancer [12]. Therefore, it is conceivable that biomarkers appearing to relate to PDAC could be the consequence of diabetes and as such may be present in cancer-free individuals who have diabetes. Finally, PDAC tissue exhibits areas of chronic pancreatitis. Understanding the impact of comorbidities on PDAC biomarkers is essential and requires carefully designed studies. Depending on the intended use population, samples from multiple disease controls may be required.

To date, most studies aimed at identifying early-stage biomarkers of PDAC have used samples from patients already diagnosed with PDAC and are thus compromised by both late changes during tumorigenesis that are not seen in early-stage disease and the general poor health of patients with advanced disease. It is recognised that new lines of early detection research should include relevant early-stage, pre-diagnostic samples in order to validate existing biomarkers and offer chances of discovering new biomarkers of early PDAC. Some of the protein markers discussed below have been discovered or validated in such samples.

How Would a Biomarker Panel Be Used?

The intended use of a biomarker will dictate the required sensitivity and specificity and the patient and control groups required during biomarker development. Individual and tumoural heterogeneity suggests that no single biomarker on its own will give adequate sensitivity and that a panel of two or more protein biomarkers will be required. Moreover, if the biomarker is being used to stratify risk within a population, then it is likely that follow-up screening will be carried out to achieve diagnosis (Fig. 4.1). Thus, while high sensitivities and specificities are desirable, currently it is envisaged that a positive biomarker test will not be used as a stand-alone diagnostic.

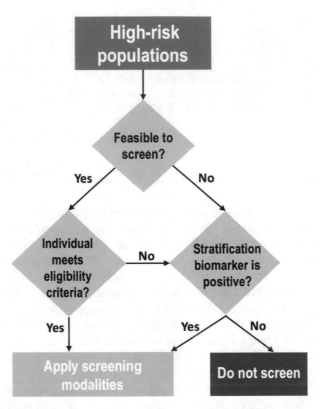

Fig. 4.1 Pathways to screening in high-risk groups; role of biomarkers. Currently there are no biomarkers suitable for screening the general population. Although PDAC is a leading cause of cancer deaths, it is relatively uncommon. A screening test would have to be extremely specific (approaching 100%) in order to avoid large numbers of false positives, and no such screening modality presently exists. For some high-risk populations, it is feasible to screen individuals who meet the eligibility criteria. However, even if individuals in this group do not meet the eligibility criteria, a positive biomarker result may suggest that screening via existing modalities (EUS, CT/MRI scan, biochemistry panels) is warranted. Within some high-risk groups, such as individuals with new-onset diabetes mellitus, subjecting all individuals to screening is not feasible due to the low incidence of PDAC within the population. Biomarkers for early detection of PDAC could select for those at a higher risk of a PDAC diagnosis, creating an enriched group of the highest-risk individuals to be screened. Those with a negative result from the biomarker test and therefore deemed to be at lower risk would be spared the worry and inconvenience of screening, while the healthcare system would avoid the associated burden and costs of unnecessary screening

Barriers to Screening for PDAC

Until relatively recently, cancers, such as breast and cervical cancer, seemed intractable. However, mortality from these cancers has decreased, in part attributed to the introduction of screening programmes which facilitate detection of early lesions or localised tumours that are easier to treat. There are practical barriers to screening the general public for PDAC. Although the mortality rate of PDAC is very high, the disease is relatively uncommon, with an incidence in Europe of 8/100,000 (Age Standardised Rate) [13]. Given the diagnostic accuracy of current detection methods, this is too low to permit screening of the asymptomatic adult population. False positives for this disease are especially serious, as it is not easy to access pancreatic lesions. For some patients, a definitive diagnosis requires surgery, and this carries the risk of significant morbidity and mortality. There are at least two ways in which the accuracy of screening for PDAC could be improved. Firstly, the development of a high-performing screening test could make screening possible. Secondly, restricting screening to those at the highest risk of PDAC would increase the rate of disease detection and reduce the occurrence of false-positive findings. These two options are not mutually exclusive, and implementing a higher-performing screening test in a high-risk population would offer the best chances of increasing accuracy [2]. Effective screening requires many conditions to be met, including that its effectiveness is proven, that it is resourced sufficiently to cover the group being screened, that a pathway exists for confirming diagnoses and for offering treatment and follow-up where tests show abnormal results, and, finally, that the prevalence of the disease should be sufficiently high to justify the costs of screening. The cost-benefit analysis should take into account the cost of the initial screening test as well as the cost of subsequent tests required to confirm the diagnosis. Since, in all cases, abnormal results require confirmatory tests, keeping false positives to a minimum is essential to reduce costs. Thus, great attention needs to be paid to the specificity of the test. Ghatnekar et al. [14] describe a model which enabled them to determine cost and the quality-adjusted life years (QALY) of screening for PDAC using a biomarker panel. According to their model, screening high-risk individuals for PDAC using a serum biomarker panel is highly desirable.

High-Risk Groups

An estimated 10% of patients with PDAC have a family history of the disease. For a proportion of these families, the pattern of risk is consistent with autosomal dominant predisposition [15]. In Europe, the European Registry of Hereditary Pancreatitis and Familial Pancreatic Cancer (EUROPAC) is the largest registry of families with an inherited risk of PDAC. The United States also has successful pancreas screening [16]. Currently, screening is restricted to families with an inherited risk [17]. By contrast, 90% of PDAC cases cannot be predicted by family history and are considered sporadic. No current screening modality exists for sporadic PDAC.

Epidemiological data indicate that PDAC can cause diabetes mellitus [18], with new-onset diabetes an early warning sign of the presence of PDAC [18]. Sharma et al. reported that pancreatic cancer patients are hyperglycaemic for an average duration of 36–30 months before PDAC diagnosis [19]. At the time of PDAC diagnosis, the majority of PDAC patients have diabetes [12, 20]. By contrast, the prevalence of diabetes in individuals with lung, breast, prostate, and colorectal cancers is no higher than non-cancer controls [21]. New-onset diabetes occurs in ~50% of PDAC cases; it is the largest high-risk group for sporadic PDAC. With regard to early detection, distinguishing new-onset diabetes caused by PDAC (known as type 3c) from the more common type 2 form of the disease would allow for earlier diagnosis of PDAC [18]. However, hyperglycaemia and diabetes are common in the general population, and additional factors will need to be considered in order to enrich individuals within this group who are most likely at risk of being diagnosed with PDAC. Based on data from four independent cohorts of patients with new-onset diabetes, Sharma et al. identified three factors which were strongly correlated with PDAC [22], change in weight, change in blood glucose, and age at onset of diabetes. These form the basis of the Enriching New-Onset Diabetes for Pancreatic Cancer (ENDPAC) model. Biomarkers may allow for further enrichment of the new-onset diabetes group for PDAC.

The Need for Better Biomarkers

CA19–9 is the only biomarker in routine use for the management of PDAC [23, 24]. It has a number of limitations including lack of expression in ~5% of the population and elevation in related diseases including chronic pancreatitis and obstructive jaundice [23, 25]. CA19–9 has a sensitivity/specificity of ~85%/~85% for the detection of advanced PDAC [26]. Since PDAC is relatively uncommon, screening the general population with CA19–9 is not feasible because for every true positive identified, several thousand false positives would also be identified. All positives (both true and false) would require additional tests (imaging, biochemical panels) to verify the presence of PDAC. The ratio of true positives to false positives is far too low to justify the costs of additional tests and the potential harm caused to individuals without the disease who test positive for it. Consequently, biomarkers with superior sensitivities and particularly superior specificities are required.

Progress in Protein Biomarker Development

A number of recent studies which reported protein biomarkers are compiled here (Table 4.2). Given the large body of literature to select from, we have prioritised studies which have either used pre-diagnostic samples, included samples from early-stage disease cases, or contained large numbers of subjects. Additionally, we have made subjective decisions about the studies that are most relevant to our own research interests. Liquid biopsy denotes a sample of body fluid collected in a minimally invasive manner [27]. The liquid biopsy most frequently analysed for biomarkers of PDAC is blood (Table 4.2), although other body fluids such as urine and saliva have also been investigated.

Table 4.2 Selected blood-borne protein biomarkers

Protein biomarkers	Analysis included	Performance	Sample source	Reference
CA19–9 and TSP-1	Multiple reaction monitoring (MRM)	AUC of 0.86 to distinguish PDAC (in samples taken between 0 and 24 months prior to diagnosis) from control	Blood; pre-diagnostic PDAC cases (UKCTOCS), chronic pancreatitis, healthy controls, diagnosed PDAC, KPC mice	Jenkinson et al. [28]
ERBB2, ESR1 and TNC	Antibody microarray	AUC of 0.86 for diagnosed PDAC; AUC of 0.68 for the pre-diagnostic samples	Blood; KPC mice, pre-diagnostic plasma samples from women in the Women's health initiative (WHI)	Mirus et al. [29]
CA19–9	ELISA and/or CLIA	At 95% specificity, the sensitivity of CA19–9 (>37 U/mL) was 68% up to 1 year, and 53% up to 2 years prior to diagnosis	Blood; pre-diagnostic PDAC cases (UKCTOCS)	O'Brien et al. [30]
LYVE-1, REG1A, and TFF1	GeLC/MS/MS, ELISA	AUC of 0.92 to distinguish stage I and II PDAC cases from healthy controls	Urine; PDAC samples, including with early stage, healthy control, chronic pancreatitis	Radon et al. [31]
CA19–9 with THBS2	ELISA	AUC >0.84 to distinguish PDAC of all stages from controls	Blood; PDAC samples, including with early stage, healthy control, chronic pancreatitis	Kim et al. [32]
29-protein biomarker panel	Antibody microarray	AUC of 0.96 to distinguish stage I and II PDAC cases from healthy controls	Blood; PDAC samples, including with early stage, healthy control, chronic pancreatitis	Mellby et al. 2018 [33]

AUC area under the curve, *GeLC-MS/MS* SDS-PAGE-Liquid Chromatography-Tandem Mass Spectrometry, *UKCTOCS* United Kingdom Trial of Ovarian Cancer Screening

Future Perspectives

There is no doubt that improvements have been made in the way in which biomarkers are discovered and validated. A key issue for biomarker programs that use samples from individuals already diagnosed with PDAC is gauging whether biomarker alterations, evident at the time of diagnosis, are detectable earlier in the disease pathway. A number of cohort studies containing samples taken from individuals who went on to be diagnosed with PDAC show that certain candidate markers perform poorly in pre-diagnostic samples. Lokshin and co-workers [34] used pre-diagnostic sera from PDAC patients from the Prostate, Lung, Colorectal, and Ovarian Cancer Screening Trial (PLCO) to evaluate the performance of 67 proteins. They concluded that most biomarkers identified in previously conducted case/control studies are ineffective in pre-diagnostic samples, including examples such as MIC-1, TIMP-1, ICAM1, HE4, OPG, MUC1, and MMP9. Jenkinson et al. [35]

similarly reported that ICAM-1 and TIMP-1, promising candidate PDAC diagnostic markers, failed to show significant elevation in samples from the UKCTOCS study taken 0–12 months prior to PDAC diagnosis [35]. Both ICAM-1 and TIMP-1 proteins were significantly elevated in blood from PDAC patients with obstructive jaundice [35], and this finding possibly explains the observed upregulation of these proteins in diagnosed PDAC cases.

The use of existing cohorts for the discovery or validation of PDAC early detection biomarkers is not ideal. Existing cohorts lack important demographic data such as diabetes status, presence of obstructive jaundice, or history of chronic pancreatitis. For this reason bespoke pre-diagnostic cohorts are currently being assembled. In the United States, Chari and colleagues in the Consortium for the Study of Chronic Pancreatitis, Diabetes, and Pancreatic Cancer (CPDPC) have begun to assemble a prospective high-risk cohort of 10,000 individuals with new-onset diabetes mellitus, called NOD [36]. In the United Kingdom, a similar cohort of 2500 individuals, called UK-NOD, is being led at University of Liverpool by the authors of this book chapter, and there are other similar initiatives underway in Europe. Together, these multi-centre collaborative projects have the scale to acquire the high numbers of individuals (with presymptomatic PDAC and new-onset type 2 diabetes mellitus) necessary for rigorous validation of existing biomarkers and the discovery of new early detection biomarkers for PDAC. High-risk registries of familial PDAC will also provide an invaluable resource for the development of early PDAC biomarkers. It is foreseeable that biomarkers for early detection of PDAC will initially be tested and used in high-risk groups. This progress in early detection, along with concurrent advances in treatment, will undoubtedly lead to improvements in outcomes for PDAC patients.

References

1. Oldfield L, Rao R, Barrera LN, Costello E. Development of novel diagnostic pancreatic tumour biomarkers. In: Neoptolemos JP, Urrutia R, Abbruzzese J, Büchler MW, editors. Pancreatic cancer. 2nd ed. New York: Springer; 2018. pp. 1241–72.
2. Poruk KE, Firpo MA, Adler DG, Mulvihill SJ. Screening for pancreatic cancer: why, how, and who? Ann Surg. 2013;257(1):17–26.
3. Conroy T, Hammel P, Hebbar M, Ben Abdelghani M, Wei AC, Raoul JL, et al. FOLFIRINOX or gemcitabine as adjuvant therapy for pancreatic cancer. N Engl J Med. 2018;379(25):2395–406.
4. Neoptolemos JP, Kleeff J, Michl P, Costello E, Greenhalf W, Palmer DH. Therapeutic developments in pancreatic cancer: current and future perspectives. Nat Rev Gastroenterol Hepatol. 2018;15(6):333–48.
5. Neoptolemos JP, Palmer DH, Ghaneh P, Psarelli EE, Valle JW, Halloran CM, et al. Comparison of adjuvant gemcitabine and capecitabine with gemcitabine monotherapy in patients with resected pancreatic cancer (ESPAC-4): a multicentre, open-label, randomised, phase 3 trial. Lancet. 2017;389(10073):1011–24.
6. Cunningham D, Chau I, Stocken DD, Valle JW, Smith D, Steward W, et al. Phase III randomized comparison of gemcitabine versus gemcitabine plus capecitabine in patients with advanced pancreatic cancer. J Clin Oncol. 2009;27(33):5513–8.

7. Campbell PJ, Yachida S, Mudie LJ, Stephens PJ, Pleasance ED, Stebbings LA, et al. The patterns and dynamics of genomic instability in metastatic pancreatic cancer. Nature. 2010;467(7319):1109–13.
8. Yachida S, Jones S, Bozic I, Antal T, Leary R, Fu B, et al. Distant metastasis occurs late during the genetic evolution of pancreatic cancer. Nature. 2010;467(7319):1114–7.
9. Yan L, Tonack S, Smith R, Dodd S, Jenkins RE, Kitteringham N, et al. Confounding effect of obstructive jaundice in the interpretation of proteomic plasma profiling data for pancreatic cancer. J Proteome Res. 2009;8(1):142–8.
10. Tonack S, Jenkinson C, Cox T, Elliott V, Jenkins RE, Kitteringham NR, et al. iTRAQ reveals candidate pancreatic cancer serum biomarkers: influence of obstructive jaundice on their performance. Br J Cancer. 2013;108(9):1846–53.
11. Nie S, Lo A, Wu J, Zhu J, Tan Z, Simeone DM, et al. Glycoprotein biomarker panel for pancreatic cancer discovered by quantitative proteomics analysis. J Proteome Res. 2014;13(4):1873–84.
12. Pannala R, Leirness JB, Bamlet WR, Basu A, Petersen GM, Chari ST. Prevalence and clinical profile of pancreatic cancer-associated diabetes mellitus. Gastroenterology. 2008;134(4):981–7.
13. Bray F, Ferlay J, Soerjomataram I, Siegel RL, Torre LA, Jemal A. Global cancer statistics 2018: GLOBOCAN estimates of incidence and mortality worldwide for 36 cancers in 185 countries. CA Cancer J Clin. 2018;68(6):394–424.
14. Ghatnekar O, Andersson R, Svensson M, Persson U, Ringdahl U, Zeilon P, et al. Modelling the benefits of early diagnosis of pancreatic cancer using a biomarker signature. Int J Cancer. 2013;133(10):2392–7.
15. Petersen GM. Familial pancreatic adenocarcinoma. Hematol Oncol Clin North Am. 2015;29(4):641–53.
16. Canto MI, Almario JA, Schulick RD, Yeo CJ, Klein A, Blackford A, et al. Risk of neoplastic progression in individuals at high risk for pancreatic cancer undergoing long-term surveillance. Gastroenterology. 2018;155(3):740–51.e2.
17. Stoffel EM, McKernin SE, Brand R, Canto M, Goggins M, Moravek C, et al. Evaluating susceptibility to pancreatic cancer: ASCO provisional clinical opinion. J Clin Oncol. 2019;37(2):153–64.
18. Andersen DK, Korc M, Petersen GM, Eibl G, Li D, Rickels MR, et al. Diabetes, pancreatogenic diabetes, and pancreatic cancer. Diabetes. 2017;66(5):1103–10.
19. Sharma A, Smyrk TC, Levy MJ, Topazian MA, Chari ST. Fasting blood glucose levels provide estimate of duration and progression of pancreatic cancer before diagnosis. Gastroenterology. 2018;155(2):490–500.e2.
20. Permert J, Ihse I, Jorfeldt L, von Schenck H, Arnqvist HJ, Larsson J. Pancreatic cancer is associated with impaired glucose metabolism. Eur J Surg. 1993;159(2):101–7.
21. Aggarwal G, Kamada P, Chari ST. Prevalence of diabetes mellitus in pancreatic cancer compared to common cancers. Pancreas. 2013;42(2):198–201.
22. Sharma A, Kandlakunta H, Nagpal SJS, Feng Z, Hoos W, Petersen GM, et al. Model to determine risk of pancreatic cancer in patients with new-onset diabetes. Gastroenterology. 2018;155(3):730–9.e3.
23. Locker GY, Hamilton S, Harris J, Jessup JM, Kemeny N, Macdonald JS, et al. ASCO 2006 update of recommendations for the use of tumor markers in gastrointestinal cancer. J Clin Oncol. 2006;24(33):5313–27.
24. Wong D, Ko AH, Hwang J, Venook AP, Bergsland EK, Tempero MA. Serum CA19-9 decline compared to radiographic response as a surrogate for clinical outcomes in patients with metastatic pancreatic cancer receiving chemotherapy. Pancreas. 2008;37(3):269–74.
25. Marrelli D, Caruso S, Pedrazzani C, Neri A, Fernandes E, Marini M, et al. CA19-9 serum levels in obstructive jaundice: clinical value in benign and malignant conditions. Am J Surg. 2009;198(3):333–9.
26. Huang Z, Liu F. Diagnostic value of serum carbohydrate antigen 19-9 in pancreatic cancer: a meta-analysis. Tumour Biol. 2014;35(8):7459–65.

27. Yadav DK, Bai X, Yadav RK, Singh A, Li G, Ma T, et al. Liquid biopsy in pancreatic cancer: the beginning of a new era. Oncotarget. 2018;9(42):26900–33.
28. Jenkinson C, Elliott VL, Evans A, Oldfield L, Jenkins RE, O'Brien DP, et al. Decreased serum thrombospondin-1 levels in pancreatic cancer patients up to 24 months prior to clinical diagnosis: association with diabetes mellitus. Clin Cancer Res. 2016;22(7):1734–43.
29. Mirus JE, Zhang Y, Li CI, Lokshin AE, Prentice RL, Hingorani SR, et al. Cross-species antibody microarray interrogation identifies a 3-protein panel of plasma biomarkers for early diagnosis of pancreas cancer. Clin Cancer Res. 2015;21(7):1764–71.
30. O'Brien DP, Sandanayake NS, Jenkinson C, Gentry-Maharaj A, Apostolidou S, Fourkala EO, et al. Serum CA19-9 is significantly upregulated up to 2 years before diagnosis with pancreatic cancer: implications for early disease detection. Clin Cancer Res. 2015;21(3):622–31.
31. Radon TP, Massat NJ, Jones R, Alrawashdeh W, Dumartin L, Ennis D, et al. Identification of a three-biomarker panel in urine for early detection of pancreatic adenocarcinoma. Clin Cancer Res. 2015;21(15):3512–21.
32. Kim J, Bamlet WR, Oberg AL, Chaffee KG, Donahue G, Cao XJ, et al. Detection of early pancreatic ductal adenocarcinoma with thrombospondin-2 and CA19–9 blood markers. Sci Transl Med. 2017;9(398):eaah5583.
33. Mellby LD, Nyberg AP, Johansen JS, Wingren C, Nordestgaard BG, Bojesen SE, et al. Serum biomarker signature-based liquid biopsy for diagnosis of early-stage pancreatic cancer. J Clin Oncol. 2018;36(28):2887–94.
34. Nolen BM, Brand RE, Prosser D, Velikokhatnaya L, Allen PJ, Zeh HJ, et al. Prediagnostic serum biomarkers as early detection tools for pancreatic cancer in a large prospective cohort study. PLoS One. 2014;9(4):e94928.
35. Jenkinson C, Elliott V, Menon U, Apostolidou S, Fourkala OE, Gentry-Maharaj A, et al. Evaluation in pre-diagnosis samples discounts ICAM-1 and TIMP-1 as biomarkers for earlier diagnosis of pancreatic cancer. J Proteome. 2014;113C:400–2.
36. Maitra A, Sharma A, Brand RE, Van Den Eeden SK, Fisher WE, Hart PA, et al. A prospective study to establish a new-onset diabetes cohort: from the consortium for the study of chronic pancreatitis, diabetes, and pancreatic cancer. Pancreas. 2018;47(10):1244–8.

Chapter 5
Metabolic Biomarkers of Pancreatic Cancer

Ujjwal Mukund Mahajan, Qi Li, Beate Kamlage, Markus M. Lerch, and Julia Mayerle

The Metabolome: Mirror of Our Organism

Since the completion of sequencing of the human genome, several systemic profiling tools have been developed to provide a more comprehensive picture of tumor development [1]. The acquisition of cancer hallmarks necessitates molecular alterations at multiple levels including genome, epigenome, transcriptome, proteome, and metabolome [2]. The different "-omics" levels vary greatly in their complexity which is largely driven by spatial and temporal dynamics, chemical modifications, and environmental influence. The flow of information from genome to protein and ultimately to metabolites is accompanied by an exponential increase in the complexity [2, 3]. Though functional genomic strategies such as transcriptome and proteome led to the understanding of cancer biology, such as the identification of new tumor subtypes and transcriptional and protein biomarkers for certain types of cancer [4–8], metabolic profiling provides the closest link to the phenotype of an organism. It has been known for almost a century that altered cell metabolism is a characteristic feature of cancers [1, 9, 10]. Aside from well-described changes in nutrient consumption and waste excretion, altered cancer cell metabolism also leads to changes in intracellular metabolite concentrations. Increased levels of metabolites that result directly from genetic mutations and cancer-associated modifications in protein expression can promote cancer initiation and progression [11].

U. M. Mahajan · Q. Li · J. Mayerle (✉)
Medical Department II, University Hospital, LMU, Munich, Germany
e-mail: Julia.Mayerle@med.uni-muenchen.de

B. Kamlage
Metanomics Health GmbH, Berlin, Germany

M. M. Lerch
Department of Medicine A, University Medicine,
Ernst-Moritz-Arndt-University Greifswald, Greifswald, Germany

© Springer Nature Switzerland AG 2020
C. W. Michalski et al. (eds.), *Translational Pancreatic Cancer Research*,
Molecular and Translational Medicine,
https://doi.org/10.1007/978-3-030-49476-6_5

Techniques that monitor and discover metabolic changes in subjects related to disease status or in response to a medical or external intervention have great potential to impact clinical practice [12–14]. Measuring metabolite concentrations is a more sensitive approach than following the rates of chemical reactions directly. Metabolic control analysis has demonstrated that although changes in enzyme concentrations and activities have a small impact on metabolic flux, changes in flux have a significant impact on metabolite concentrations [15, 16]. This is because the control of metabolic flux of a pathway is spread across all enzymes present in the pathway, rather than being controlled by a rate-determining step. Furthermore, there is not necessarily a good quantitative relation between transcription and enzymatic activities. As metabolites are downstream of both transcription and protein synthesis cascade, they are potentially a better indicator of enzyme activity [1, 17]. Thus, metabolic profiling offers a particularly sensitive method to monitor changes in a biological system, through observed changes in the metabolic network.

Metabolic profiling is usually referred to as the quantitative study of a group of metabolites that are associated with a particular pathway [13]. Global metabolic profiling has been referred to as metabolomics. Metabolomics is defined as a quantitative description of all endogenous low-molecular-weight components (<1 kDa) in a biological sample using state-of-the-art analytical instrumentation in conjunction with pattern recognition techniques. Each cell type and biological fluid has a characteristic set of metabolites that reflect the organism under a particular set of environmental conditions and that fluctuate according to physiological demands [12]. Lipidomics is a specialized subset of metabolomics that evaluates lipid profiles [18]. Lipids play many important roles in cancer processes including invasion, migration, and proliferation [19].

Currently, a truly global comprehensive assessment of the metabolome by a single analytical platform is not yet possible, due to the high heterogeneity of the metabolites (chemical structure, physicochemical properties, and concentration) [20]. Although it would be ideal to know the entire metabolic content of a sample, depending on the purpose of analysis, there might be situations where the information provided from only one part would be sufficient; hence, the quantification and identification of "all" metabolites would not be necessary [21, 22].

Application of Metabolomics in Pancreatic Cancer Biomarker Discovery

Pancreatic ductal adenocarcinoma (PDAC) is one of the most aggressive malignancies and burdened with a 5-year survival rate of only 8% [5, 23]. Multiple factors are known to contribute to this dismal prognosis, most prominently delayed diagnosis and resistance to chemo- or radiation therapy [24]. Surgical resection alone, which is feasible in around 20% of patients, results in 5-year survival of around 10% [25]. The use of adjuvant chemotherapy with either 5-fluorouracil-folinic acid (5FU/folinic acid) or gemcitabine increases 5-year survival to around 28%, and the use of

FOLFIRINOX prolongs median survival to 54 months [26]. Even though insights into the molecular pathology of cancer can create opportunities for the development of therapies with substantial clinical benefit [27], for pancreatic cancer such options are currently unavailable [26, 28]. Biomarker-driven treatment strategies are urgently needed for PDAC [27]. Earlier diagnosis is one factor that could alter this trajectory [29].

The ultimate goal of most metabolomics cancer studies is to discover cancer-specific diagnostic, prognostic, or predictive biomarkers for a patient [30]. The National Institutes of Health Biomarkers Definitions Working Group defined a bio-marker as "a characteristic that is measured as an indicator of normal biological processes, pathogenic processes, or responses to exposure or intervention, including therapeutic interventions" [31]. Diagnostic biomarkers are used for the critical determination of whether a patient has a particular medical condition for which treatment may be indicated or whether an individual should be enrolled in a clinical trial studying a particular disease. A prognostic biomarker is one that indicates an increased (or decreased) likelihood of a future clinical event, disease recurrence, or progression in an identified population, while a predictive biomarker is used to iden-tify individuals who are more likely to respond to exposure to a particular medical product or environmental agent. The response could be a symptomatic benefit, improved survival, or an adverse effect [32]. An ideal biomarker should meet vari-ous criteria that include the following: (i) it should be present in readily available and minimally invasive sources (e.g., blood and urine); (ii) it should be highly sensi-tive (allowing early diagnosis) and specific (unaffected by external and comorbid conditions); (iii) it should vary promptly in response to treatment and disease pro-gression; (iv) it should provide a deeper understanding about the disease mecha-nism; and (v) it should be useful in risk stratification and prognosis [33]. Metabolomics has an advantage over other "-omics" and is better suited for this purpose. In fact, as changes in metabolites normally appear in readily available biofluids, such as blood and urine, the translation of metabolomic studies to clinical practice is easier [34]. Biofluids are usually the easiest samples to work with, requir-ing less sample preparation than other biological samples [21].

The metabolome is highly dynamic, reflecting continuous fluxes of both meta-bolic and signaling pathways, and is sensitive to diverse host and environmental factors. These unique features make metabolomics able to capture a plurality of subtle changes. Thus, metabolomics holds the promise for simultaneously evaluat-ing a variety of complex pathways and their consequences [34]. Also, metabolomic experiments are also less expensive than proteomic and transcriptional approaches [21, 30, 35, 36].

Although targeting cancer metabolism is a promising therapeutic strategy, clini-cal success will depend on accurate diagnostic identification of tumor subtypes with specific metabolic requirements. Through broad metabolite profiling, PDAC was successfully categorized into three highly distinct metabolic subtypes, namely, slow proliferating, glycolytic, and lipogenic subtypes [37]. One subtype was defined by reduced proliferative capacity, whereas glycolytic and lipogenic subtypes showed distinct metabolite levels associated with glycolysis, lipogenesis, and redox pathways. The lipogenic subtype associated with the epithelial subtype, whereas the glycolytic subtype strongly associated with the mesenchymal subtype, suggesting functional relevance in disease progression [37, 38]. This identification of distinct metabolic subtypes in PDAC may add to patient selection for investigational metabolic inhibitors and in the selection of new therapeutic targets [37, 39, 40].

Pancreatic Cancer-Specific Metabolic Biomarkers

The only routinely used serum marker for PDAC with demonstrated clinical usefulness for therapeutic monitoring and early detection of recurrent disease after treatment in patients with known PDAC is carbohydrate antigen 19–9 (CA19–9) [41]. Elevation of CA19–9 indicates advanced PDAC and poor prognosis [42, 43]. However, elevation of CA19–9 is observed in only 65% of patients with resectable PDAC [42, 44] and can also be caused by other conditions such as pancreatitis, cirrhosis, and cholestasis [45]. In addition, patients who are negative for Lewis antigen a or b (approximately 10% of patients with PDAC) are unable to synthesize CA19–9 and express undetectable levels, even in advanced stages of the disease. Although measurement of serum CA19–9 levels is useful in patients with known pancreatic cancer, the use of this biomarker as a screening tool has had disappointing results and is not recommended [41, 42, 46].

There are several attempts for metabolomics-based clinical investigations to identify potential biomarkers for diagnosis, stratification of a prognosis, and monitoring of therapy [47]. Table 5.1 summarizes studies that specifically addressed metabolic biomarkers for PDAC.

Table 5.1 Different metabolic biomarkers

Metabolites	Sample matrix	Discrimination group	Sample size	Conclusion	References
Plasma free amino acids					
Arginine ↓, total amino acids ↓	Plasma	PDAC vs control	21/21	Arginine decreased in cancer patients both with and without weight loss, irrespective of tumor type and stage	[48, 49]
PFAA index (serine ↓, asparagine ↑, isoleucine ↓, alanine ↓, histidine ↓, and tryptophan ↓)	Plasma	PDAC vs control	120/600	AUC on ROC analysis of PFAA index to discriminate PDAC from control was 0.89 (95% CI: 0.86–0.93)	[50]

Table 5.1 (continued)

Metabolites	Sample matrix	Discrimination group	Sample size	Conclusion	References
PFAA index (serine ↓, asparagine ↑, isoleucine ↓, alanine ↓, histidine ↓, and tryptophan ↓)	Plasma	PDAC vs CP vs control	240/28/7772	AUC on ROC analysis of PFAA index to discriminate PDAC from control were 0.81 (95% CI: 0.75–0.86) and 0.87 (95%CI: 0.80–0.93) to discriminate PDAC from CP	[50]
Total amino acids ↓	Plasma	PDAC vs CP vs control	12/12/12.	A significant deficit in circulating amino acid levels in pancreatic cancer patients	[51]
Xylitol ↓, 1,5-anhydro-D-glucitol ↓, histidine ↓, and inositol ↑	Serum	PDAC vs control	43/42	High sensitivity (86.0%) and specificity (88.1%) for PDAC	[52]
Xylitol ↓, 1,5-anhydro-D-glucitol ↓, histidine ↓, and inositol ↑	Serum	PDAC vs CP vs control	42/23/41	Displayed higher sensitivity (77.8%) in PDAC and lower false discovery rate (17.4%) in CP	[52]
Branched-chain amino acids					
Branched-chain amino acids ↑	Plasma	PDAC vs control	170/340	Increased branched-chain amino acids levels over a period of 10 years associated with increased incidence of PDAC	[55]
Branched-chain amino acids ↑, isoleucine ↑, leucine ↑, and valine ↑	Plasma	PDAC vs control	453/898	Elevated risk was independent of known predisposing factors, with the strongest association observed among subjects with samples collected 2 to 5 years before diagnosis	[54]

(continued)

Table 5.1 (continued)

Metabolites	Sample matrix	Discrimination group	Sample size	Conclusion	References
Choline-containing metabolites					
Glutamate ↓, choline ↓, betaine ↓, methyl-guanidine ↑, and 1,5-anhydro-D-glucitol ↓	Plasma	PDAC vs control	200/200	High sensitivity (97.7%) and specificity (83.1%) (AUC = 0.943, 95%CI = 0.908–0.977). Independent cohort showed satisfactory accuracy (AUC = 0.835; 95%CI = 0.777–0.893)	[60]
Glycolysis-related metabolites					
3-Hydroxybutyrate ↓, 3-hydroxyisovalerate ↓, lactate ↓, and trimethylamine-N-oxide ↓	Serum	PDAC vs control	17/23	Significant higher level of isoleucine, triglyceride, leucine, and creatinine in PDAC	[65]
3-Hydroxybutyrate ↓, 3-hydroxyisovalerate ↓, and lactate ↓	Plasma	PDAC vs CP vs control	19/20/20	Sensitivity of discrimination between PDAC and chronic pancreatitis is 84% with specificity of 90%	[66]

Amino Acids

Cancer cells require certain amino acids for DNA synthesis, building new blood vessels, and duplicating their entire protein content. These proteins work as growth-promoting hormones or tumor growth factors. The increase in the amino acid demand may thus lead to lower availability of plasma free amino acids as detected in cancer patients. Another possibility to explain decreased levels of amino acids is cancer-associated malnutrition. Patients with pancreatic cancer are usually troubled by malnutrition due to exocrine pancreatic insufficiency just to name on one possible explanation [48].

It has been reported that plasma free amino acid (PFAA) concentrations in PDAC, significant decreases arginine levels, regardless of tumor types and stages, weight loss or body mass index are specific features of the presence of a malignant tumor. Concomitantly, a decrease in total amino acids was detected [49]. Fukutake et al. [50] delineated a PFAA index comprising of serine, asparagine, isoleucine, alanine, histidine, and tryptophan as variables to calculate the PDAC risk and successfully discriminate patients with PDAC from control subjects. Several other studies with small sample size [51, 52] reported similar decreases in circulating free amino acid levels in PDAC patients.

Branched-Chain Amino Acids

An accumulating body of evidence demonstrates that branched-chain amino acids (BCAAs), valine, leucine, and isoleucine are essential nutrients for cancer growth and are utilized by tumors in various biosynthetic pathways as a source of energy [9, 53]. It is known that elevated plasma levels of BCAAs are associated with a greater than twofold increased risk of future PDAC diagnosis. This elevated risk was independent of known predisposing factors, with the strongest association observed among subjects with samples collected 2–5 years before diagnosis, when occult disease is probably present [54]. In line, in the Japan Public Health Center-based prospective study, an association between increased plasma BCAA level and increased risk of pancreatic cancer, particularly when an increase in BCAAs was observed at least 10 years before diagnosis, was confirmed [55].

Choline-Containing Metabolites

Aberrant choline metabolism, characterized by increased phosphocholine and total choline-containing metabolites, is a primary cause of choline-containing metabolites due to an overexpression of the choline kinase-α (*CHKA*) and increased expression of choline transporters [56, 57]. PDAC cell lines and pancreatic tumors showed elevated choline-containing metabolites. Total choline-containing metabolites were observed as a single peak in vivo which in turn was resolved in proton spectroscopy to belong to the metabolites phosphocholine, glycerol-phosphocholine, and free choline [57]. However, in an animal study involving rats, choline-containing metabolites were decreased in PDAC [58]. Choline deficiency can also induce severe acute pancreatitis in animal models [59]. Reduced plasma betaine levels enhanced the discrimination of PDAC from control. Because choline is a precursor of betaine, the depletion of both betaine and choline in PDAC may be interrelated [47, 60]. A diagnostic model based on logistic regression incorporating a panel of five metabolites which constitutes choline and betaine (glutamate, choline, betaine, methylguanidine, and 1,5-anhydro-D-glucitol) robustly distinguished PDAC from normal controls [60]. FI-FTICR-MS metabolomic analysis showed significant reductions in serum levels of metabolites belonging to 36-carbon ultra-long-chain fatty acids; multiple choline-related systems including phosphatidylcholines, lysophosphatidylcholines, and sphingomyelins; as well as vinyl ether-containing ethanolamines in PDAC patients if compared to controls [61].

Glycolysis Metabolites

Constitutively active components of the Ras pathway stimulate cellular glucose uptake and metabolic rate, hereby overcoming the capacity of the cell to utilize mainly glucose for its bioenergetic requirements. As a result, tumorigenic cells secrete excess metabolites of the glycolytic pathway in the form of lactic acid. Recent studies have strongly implicated aerobic glycolysis in the malignant etiology of pancreatic tumor cells [62, 63]. The shift to enhanced glucose metabolism in hypoxic pancreatic cancer cells is clearly manifested by the substantial accumulation of the glycolysis end-product lactic acid in the tumor microenvironment. Interestingly, PDAC patients frequently also suffer from diabetes and hyperglycemia, conditions typified by high blood sugar [63, 64]. Serum lactate levels tend to be higher in patients with malignancies [58]. In contrast, serum metabolic analysis revealed significantly lower 3-hydroxybutyrate, 3-hydroxyisovalerate, lactate, and trimethylamine-N-oxide in PDAC compared to that of controls and chronic pancreatitis [65, 66].

Lipid Metabolites

Saturated fatty acids are known to affect insulin secretion and insulin resistance, which might be involved in the carcinogenesis of the pancreas [67]. It has been shown that fatty acids may regulate cancer cells by modulating hypoxia-inducible factor-1 (HIF-1) which encodes for proteins including glucose transporters and growth factors. Several clinical studies demonstrated a significant association between saturated fat intake and pancreatic cancer [68]. Besides, Matters et al. have shown that dietary fat can induce growth and metastasis of pancreatic cancer [69]. Although risk factors in their complexity causing pancreatic cancer are still not fully understood, it is clear that high-fat diet is one of the risk factors associated with PDAC [70].

The two best-studied families of polyunsaturated fatty acids (PUFAs), linoleic acid (n-6) and α-linolenic acid (n-3), are essential fatty acids, and they exert opposite effects on cancer development. n-3 PUFAs can suppress tumor carcinogenesis by giving rise to pro-inflammatory eicosanoids, whereas n-6 PUFAs promote cancer development by giving rise to anti-inflammatory eicosanoids. It has been reported that higher consumption of n-3 PUFAs may protect patients against cancers [71]. Self-reported measures of dietary n-3 PUFAs intake generally derived from food frequency questionnaires (FFQ) are used to assess the n-3 PUFAs intake, but for conformation concentration of serum phospholipid, n-3 LC-PUFAs should be used [72]. Even though growing data, including from epidemiology studies, suggest that n-3 LC-PUFAs may have a protective role on PDAC, the role of n-3 LC-PUFAs as biomarkers and the relationship between these biomarkers and the disease still need to be explored [73]. Lipidomics revealed significant alteration in PDAC for four significant metabolite families, 36-carbon long-chain fatty acid, lysophosphatidyl-choline, phosphatidylcholine, and sphingomyelins [74]. PC-594 is a novel circulating 36-carbon long-chain PUFA that has previously been implicated in Japanese PDAC cohorts. This finding was confirmed in an American cohort with a 86% sensitivity and 91% specificity [75].

Composite Metabolic Signatures

Though metabolomics including lipidomics allowed the identification of clinical metabolite biomarkers, these individual metabolite signatures are far from routine clinical use, partly because of disappointing specificity when challenged to discriminate patients with PDAC from chronic pancreatitis [29, 76]. Also, the performance of these biomarkers may be affected by a significant number of variables, such as age, gender, sample collection method, duration of sample storage, and sample handling. Understanding comorbidities and how they affect the performance of biomarkers are of utmost importance [77]. These conditions may contribute to the heterogeneity in performance of candidate biomarkers [78]. Although some small-scale metabolomic studies have shown promise, the general performance of biomarkers including that of the gold standard cancer antigen 19–9 (CA19–9) in differentiating PDAC from CP is modest, and improvements are needed.

Undoubtedly, one of the greatest biomarker-related challenges in this field is finding biomarkers that accurately distinguish PDAC from other diseases of the pancreas, where overlapping signs and symptoms make differential clinical diagnosis difficult. Recently our own group reported a metabolite-based biomarker signature which distinguishes PDAC from CP with much greater accuracy than achieved by CA19–9 alone [76]. Mayerle et al. reported global analysis of 914 patients analyzed for blood (serum and plasma)-based metabolites including lipids to identify candidate metabolites that distinguish PDAC from CP. Out of 477 metabolites from 10 ontology classes, 29 metabolites were significantly altered between PDAC and CP in serum and plasma of the training set. The Elastic Net algorithm identified 9 metabolites (Table 5.2) plus CA19–9 discriminating PDAC from CP with an AUC of 0.96 [76]. This metabolomic signature was successfully validated in an independent cohort. The study was designed to accurately exclude suspected pancreatic cancer in patients with CP, with an emphasis placed on optimizing the negative predictive value (NPV) [29, 76].

In summary, the only chance of curative treatment for PDAC is based on prompt diagnosis followed by surgical treatment. Unfortunately, routine cancer markers do not seem to be reliable in prediction and detection of early stages of PDAC. Use of metabolomics-based biomarkers points to its potential for the diagnosis of PDAC and indeed for cancer diagnostics in general. The near future probably lies in a carefully selected panel of biomarkers that would allow for earlier diagnosis of PDAC and easier determination of its stage and, ideally, also allow for tailoring of treatment and to provide indicators of prognosis/outcome.

Table 5.2 List of metabolites selected based on the multivariate elastic net analysis comprising the biomarker signature

Metabolites	Ontology class	Fold changes PDAC vs CP Training data	Fold changes PDAC vs CP Test data
CA19–9	Clinical markers	18.36	14.27
Proline	Amino acids	0.69	0.75
Sphingomyelin (d18:2, C17:0)	Complex lipids, fatty acids and related	1.15	1.15
Phosphatidylcholine (C18:0, C22:6)	Complex lipids, fatty acids and related	1.26	1.06
Isocitrate	Energy metabolism and related	1.26	0.99
Sphinganine-1-phosphate (d18:0)	Complex lipids, fatty acids and related	0.79	0.85
Histidine	Amino acid	0.77	0.79
Pyruvate	Energy metabolism and related	0.93	0.97
Ceramide (d18:1, C24:0)	Complex lipids, fatty acids and related	0.79	0.80
Sphingomyelin (d17:1, C18:0)	Complex lipids, fatty acids and related	1.36	1.37

References

1. Griffin JL, Shockcor JP. Metabolic profiles of cancer cells. Nat Rev Cancer. 2004;4(7):551–61.
2. Chakraborty S, Hosen MI, Ahmed M, Shekhar HU. Onco-multi-OMICS approach: a new frontier in cancer research. Biomed Res Int. 2018;2018:1–14.
3. Hager GL, McNally JG, Misteli T. Transcription dynamics. Mol Cell. 2009;35(6):741–53.
4. Hanash SM, Pitteri SJ, Faca VM. Mining the plasma proteome for cancer biomarkers. Nature. 2008;452(7187):571–9.
5. Moffitt RA, Marayati R, Flate EL, Volmar KE, Loeza SGH, Hoadley KA, et al. Virtual microdissection identifies distinct tumor- and stroma-specific subtypes of pancreatic ductal adenocarcinoma. Nat Genet. 2015;47(10):1168–78.
6. Rhodes DR, Yu J, Shanker K, Deshpande N, Varambally R, Ghosh D, et al. Large-scale meta-analysis of cancer microarray data identifies common transcriptional profiles of neoplastic transformation and progression. Proc Natl Acad Sci. 2004;101(25):9309–14.
7. Füzéry AK, Levin J, Chan MM, Chan DW. Translation of proteomic biomarkers into FDA approved cancer diagnostics: issues and challenges. Clin Proteomics. 2013;10(1):13.
8. Collisson EA, Sadanandam A, Olson P, Gibb WJ, Truitt M, Gu S, et al. Subtypes of pancreatic ductal adenocarcinoma and their differing responses to therapy. Nat Med. 2011;17(4):500–3.
9. Mayers JR. Metabolic markers as cancer clues. Science. 2017;358(6368):1265.1–1265.
10. Vander Heiden MG, Cantley LC, Thompson CB. Understanding the Warburg effect: the metabolic requirements of cell proliferation. Science. 2009;324(5930):1029–33.
11. Sullivan LB, Gui DY, Heiden MGV. Altered metabolite levels in cancer: implications for tumor biology and cancer therapy. Nat Rev Cancer. 2016;16(11):680–93.
12. Holmes E, Wilson ID, Nicholson JK. Metabolic phenotyping in health and disease. Cell. 2008;134(5):714–7.
13. Beger R. A review of applications of metabolomics in cancer. Meta. 2013;3(3):552–74.

14. Clayton TA, Lindon JC, Cloarec O, Antti H, Charuel C, Hanton G, et al. Pharmaco-metabonomic phenotyping and personalized drug treatment. Nature. 2006;440(7087):1073–7.
15. Fell DA. Metabolic control analysis: a survey of its theoretical and experimental development. Biochem J. 1992;286(Pt 2):313–30.
16. Cascante M, Boros LG, Comin-Anduix B, de Atauri P, Centelles JJ, Lee PW-N. Metabolic control analysis in drug discovery and disease. Nat Biotechnol. 2002;20(3):243–9.
17. ter Kuile BH, Westerhoff HV. Transcriptome meets metabolome: hierarchical and metabolic regulation of the glycolytic pathway. FEBS Lett. 2001;500(3):169–71.
18. Wenk MR. Lipidomics: new tools and applications. Cell. 2010;143(6):888–95.
19. Stephenson DJ, Hoeferlin LA, Chalfant CE. Lipidomics in translational research and the clinical significance of lipid-based biomarkers. Transl Res J Lab Clin Med. 2017;189:13–29.
20. Griffiths WJ, Koal T, Wang Y, Kohl M, Enot DP, Deigner H-P. Targeted metabolomics for biomarker discovery. Angew Chem Int Ed Engl. 2010;49(32):5426–45.
21. Monteiro MS, Carvalho M, Bastos ML, Guedes de Pinho P. Metabolomics analysis for biomarker discovery: advances and challenges. Curr Med Chem. 2012;20(2):257–71.
22. Goodacre R, Vaidyanathan S, Dunn WB, Harrigan GG, Kell DB. Metabolomics by numbers: acquiring and understanding global metabolite data. Trends Biotechnol. 2004;22(5):245–52.
23. Maitra A, Leach SD. Disputed paternity: the uncertain ancestry of pancreatic ductal neoplasia. Cancer Cell. 2012;22(6):701–3.
24. Louvet C, Philip PA. Accomplishments in 2007 in the treatment of metastatic pancreatic cancer. Gastrointest Cancer Res GCR. 2008;2(3 Suppl):S37–41.
25. Greenhalf W, Ghaneh P, Neoptolemos JP, Palmer DH, Cox TF, Lamb RF, et al. Pancreatic cancer hENT1 expression and survival from gemcitabine in patients from the ESPAC-3 Trial. JNCI J Natl Cancer Inst. 2014;106(1):djt347.
26. Neoptolemos JP, Palmer DH, Ghaneh P, Psarelli EE, Valle JW, Halloran CM, et al. Comparison of adjuvant gemcitabine and capecitabine with gemcitabine monotherapy in patients with resected pancreatic cancer (ESPAC-4): a multicentre, open-label, randomized, phase 3 trial. Lancet Lond Engl. 2017;389(10073):1011–24.
27. Biankin AV, Piantadosi S, Hollingsworth SJ. Patient-centric trials for therapeutic development in precision oncology. Nature. 2015;526(7573):361–70.
28. Costello E, Greenhalf W, Neoptolemos JP. New biomarkers and targets in pancreatic cancer and their application to treatment. Nat Rev Gastroenterol Hepatol. 2012;9(8):435–44.
29. Costello E. A metabolomics-based biomarker signature discriminates pancreatic cancer from chronic pancreatitis. Gut. 2018;67(1):2–3.
30. Armitage EG, Barbas C. Metabolomics in cancer biomarker discovery: current trends and future perspectives. J Pharm Biomed Anal. 2014;87:1–11.
31. Biomarkers Definitions Working Group. Biomarkers and surrogate endpoints: preferred definitions and conceptual framework. Clin Pharmacol Ther. 2001;69(3):89–95.
32. FDA-NIH Biomarker Working Group. BEST (Biomarkers, EndpointS, and other Tools) Resource [Internet]. Silver Spring (MD): Food and Drug Administration (US); 2016 [cited 2018 Dec 19]. Available from: http://www.ncbi.nlm.nih.gov/books/NBK326791/.
33. Bennett MR, Devarajan P. Characteristics of an Ideal Biomarker of Kidney Diseases. In: Biomarkers of Kidney Disease [Internet]. Elsevier; 2017 [cited 2018 Dec 20]. p. 1–20. Available from: https://linkinghub.elsevier.com/retrieve/pii/B9780128030141000017.
34. Davis VW, Bathe OF, Schiller DE, Slupsky CM, Sawyer MB. Metabolomics and surgical oncology: potential role for small molecule biomarkers. J Surg Oncol. 2011;103(5):451–9.
35. Fiehn O, Kristal B, van Ommen B, Sumner LW, Sansone S-A, Taylor C, et al. Establishing reporting standards for metabolomic and metabonomic studies: a call for participation. Omics J Integr Biol. 2006;10(2):158–63.
36. Griffin JL. Metabolic profiles to define the genome: can we hear the phenotypes? Philos Trans R Soc Lond Ser B Biol Sci. 2004;359(1446):857–71.
37. Daemen A, Peterson D, Sahu N, McCord R, Du X, Liu B, et al. Metabolite profiling stratifies pancreatic ductal adenocarcinomas into subtypes with distinct sensitivities to metabolic inhibitors. Proc Natl Acad Sci. 2015 Aug 11;112(32):E4410–7.

38. Daemen A, Liu B, Song K, Kwong M, Gao M, Hong R, et al. Pan-cancer metabolic signature predicts co-dependency on glutaminase and de novo glutathione synthesis linked to a high-mesenchymal cell state. Cell Metab. 2018;28(3):383–99.e9.
39. Jain M, Nilsson R, Sharma S, Madhusudhan N, Kitami T, Souza AL, et al. Metabolite profiling identifies a key role for Glycine in rapid cancer cell proliferation. Science. 2012;336(6084):1040–4.
40. Sreekumar A, Poisson LM, Rajendiran TM, Khan AP, Cao Q, Yu J, et al. Metabolomic profiles delineate potential role for sarcosine in prostate cancer progression. Nature. 2009;457(7231):910–4.
41. Hidalgo M. Pancreatic cancer. N Engl J Med. 2010;362(17):1605–17.
42. Kaur S, Baine MJ, Jain M, Sasson AR, Batra SK. Early diagnosis of pancreatic cancer: challenges and new developments. Biomark Med. 2012;6(5):597–612.
43. Locker GY, Hamilton S, Harris J, Jessup JM, Kemeny N, Macdonald JS, et al. ASCO 2006 update of recommendations for the use of tumor markers in gastrointestinal cancer. J Clin Oncol Off J Am Soc Clin Oncol. 2006;24(33):5313–27.
44. Goggins M. Molecular markers of early pancreatic cancer. J Clin Oncol Off J Am Soc Clin Oncol. 2005;23(20):4524–31.
45. Goonetilleke KS, Siriwardena AK. Systematic review of carbohydrate antigen (CA 19-9) as a biochemical marker in the diagnosis of pancreatic cancer. Eur J Surg Oncol J Eur Soc Surg Oncol Br Assoc Surg Oncol. 2007;33(3):266–70.
46. Kunovsky L, Tesarikova P, Kala Z, Kroupa R, Kysela P, Dolina J, et al. The use of biomarkers in early diagnostics of pancreatic Cancer. Can J Gastroenterol Hepatol. 2018;2018:1–10.
47. Mehta KY, Wu H-J, Menon SS, Fallah Y, Zhong X, Rizk N, et al. Metabolomic biomarkers of pancreatic cancer: a meta-analysis study. Oncotarget [Internet]. 2017 Sep 15 [cited 2018 Dec 18];8(40). Available from: http://www.oncotarget.com/fulltext/20324.
48. Bi X, Henry CJ. Plasma-free amino acid profiles are predictors of cancer and diabetes development. Nutr Diabetes. 2017;7(3):e249.
49. Vissers YL, Dejong CH, Luiking YC, Fearon KC, von Meyenfeldt MF, Deutz NE. Plasma arginine concentrations are reduced in cancer patients: evidence for arginine deficiency? Am J Clin Nutr. 2005;81(5):1142–6.
50. Fukutake N, Ueno M, Hiraoka N, Shimada K, Shiraishi K, Saruki N, et al. A novel multivariate index for pancreatic cancer detection based on the plasma free amino acid profile. PLoS One. 2015;10(7):e0132223.
51. Schrader H, Menge BA, Belyaev O, Uhl W, Schmidt WE, Meier JJ. Amino acid malnutrition in patients with chronic pancreatitis and pancreatic carcinoma. Pancreas. 2009;38(4):416–21.
52. Kobayashi T, Nishiumi S, Ikeda A, Yoshie T, Sakai A, Matsubara A, et al. A novel serum metabolomics-based diagnostic approach to pancreatic cancer. Cancer Epidemiol Biomark Prev. 2013;22(4):571–9.
53. Mayers JR, Torrence ME, Danai LV, Papagiannakopoulos T, Davidson SM, Bauer MR, et al. Tissue of origin dictates branched-chain amino acid metabolism in mutant Kras-driven cancers. Science. 2016;353(6304):1161–5.
54. Mayers JR, Wu C, Clish CB, Kraft P, Torrence ME, Fiske BP, et al. Elevation of circulating branched-chain amino acids is an early event in human pancreatic adenocarcinoma development. Nat Med. 2014;20(10):1193–8.
55. Katagiri R, Goto A, Nakagawa T, Nishiumi S, Kobayashi T, Hidaka A, et al. Increased levels of branched-chain amino acid associated with increased risk of pancreatic cancer in a prospective case-control study of a large cohort. Gastroenterology. 2018;155(5):1474–82.e1.
56. Bagnoli M, Granata A, Nicoletti R, Krishnamachary B, Bhujwalla ZM, Canese R, et al. Choline metabolism alteration: a focus on ovarian cancer. Front Oncol [Internet]. 2016 Jun 22 [cited 2019 Jan 2];6. Available from: http://journal.frontiersin.org/Article/10.3389/fonc.2016.00153/abstract.

57. Penet M-F, Shah T, Bharti S, Krishnamachary B, Artemov D, Mironchik Y, et al. Metabolic imaging of pancreatic ductal adenocarcinoma detects altered choline metabolism. Clin Cancer Res. 2015;21(2):386–95.
58. Fang F, He X, Deng H, Chen Q, Lu J, Spraul M, et al. Discrimination of metabolic profiles of pancreatic cancer from chronic pancreatitis by high-resolution magic angle spinning ^{1}H nuclear magnetic resonance and principal components analysis. Cancer Sci. 2007;98(11):1678–82.
59. Su KH, Cuthbertson C, Christophi C. Review of experimental animal models of acute pancreatitis. HPB. 2006;8(4):264–86.
60. Xie G, Lu L, Qiu Y, Ni Q, Zhang W, Gao Y-T, et al. Plasma metabolite biomarkers for the detection of pancreatic cancer. J Proteome Res. 2015;14(2):1195–202.
61. Ritchie SA, Akita H, Takemasa I, Eguchi H, Pastural E, Nagano H, et al. Metabolic system alterations in pancreatic cancer patient serum: potential for early detection. BMC Cancer [Internet]. 2013 Dec [cited 2019 Jan 2];13(1). Available from: http://bmccancer.biomedcentral.com/articles/10.1186/1471-2407-13-416.
62. Bryant KL, Mancias JD, Kimmelman AC, Der CJ. KRAS: feeding pancreatic cancer proliferation. Trends Biochem Sci. 2014;39(2):91–100.
63. Blum R, Kloog Y. Metabolism addiction in pancreatic cancer. Cell Death Dis. 2014;5(2):e1065.
64. Gapstur SM. Abnormal glucose metabolism and pancreatic cancer mortality. JAMA. 2000;283(19):2552.
65. OuYang D, Xu J, Huang H, Chen Z. Metabolomic profiling of serum from human pancreatic cancer patients using 1H NMR spectroscopy and principal component analysis. Appl Biochem Biotechnol. 2011;165(1):148–54.
66. Zhang L, Jin H, Guo X, Yang Z, Zhao L, Tang S, et al. Distinguishing pancreatic cancer from chronic pancreatitis and healthy individuals by 1H nuclear magnetic resonance-based metabonomic profiles. Clin Biochem. 2012;45(13–14):1064–9.
67. Sievenpiper JL, Jenkins AL, Whitham DL, Vuksan V. Insulin resistance: concepts, controversies, and the role of nutrition. Can J Diet Pract Res Publ Diet Can Rev Can Prat Rech En Diet Une Publ Diet Can. 2002;63(1):20–32.
68. Weisbeck A, Jansen RJ. Nutrients and the pancreas: an epigenetic perspective. Nutrients. 2017 Mar;15:9(3).
69. Matters GL, Cooper TK, McGovern CO, Gilius EL, Liao J, Barth BM, et al. Cholecystokinin mediates progression and metastasis of pancreatic cancer associated with dietary fat. Dig Dis Sci. 2014;59(6):1180–91.
70. Iovanna J, Mallmann MC, Gonçalves A, Turrini O, Dagorn J-C. Current knowledge on pancreatic cancer. Front Oncol. 2012;2:6.
71. Saini RK, Keum Y-S. Omega-3 and omega-6 polyunsaturated fatty acids: dietary sources, metabolism, and significance — a review. Life Sci. 2018;203:255–67.
72. Brunvoll SH, Thune I, Frydenberg H, Flote VG, Bertheussen GF, Schlichting E, et al. Validation of repeated self-reported n-3 PUFA intake using serum phospholipid fatty acids as a biomarker in breast cancer patients during treatment. Nutr J. 2018;17(1):94.
73. Colomer R, Moreno-Nogueira JM, García-Luna PP, García-Peris P, García-de-Lorenzo A, Zarazaga A, et al. N-3 fatty acids, cancer and cachexia: a systematic review of the literature. Br J Nutr. 2007;97(5):823–31.
74. Akita H, Ritchie SA, Takemasa I, Eguchi H, Pastural E, Jin W, et al. Serum metabolite profiling for the detection of pancreatic cancer: results of a large independent validation study. Pancreas. 2016;45(10):1418–23.
75. Ritchie SA. Pancreatic cancer serum biomarker PC-594: diagnostic performance and comparison to CA19-9. World J Gastroenterol. 2015;21(21):6604.
76. Mayerle J, Kalthoff H, Reszka R, Kamlage B, Peter E, Schniewind B, et al. Metabolic biomarker signature to differentiate pancreatic ductal adenocarcinoma from chronic pancreatitis. Gut. 2018;67(1):128–37.

77. Pannala R, Leirness JB, Bamlet WR, Basu A, Petersen GM, Chari ST. Prevalence and clinical profile of pancreatic cancer–associated diabetes mellitus. Gastroenterology. 2008;134(4):981–7.
78. Jenkinson C, Elliott VL, Evans A, Oldfield L, Jenkins RE, O'Brien DP, et al. Decreased serum Thrombospondin-1 levels in pancreatic cancer patients up to 24 months prior to clinical diagnosis: association with diabetes mellitus. Clin Cancer Res. 2016;22(7):1734–43.

Chapter 6
Blood-Based Circulating RNAs as Preventive, Diagnostic, Prognostic and Druggable Biomarkers for Pancreatic Ductal Adenocarcinoma

Bo Kong and Helmut Friess

Despite enormous advances in understanding pancreatic cancer biology, the prognosis of patients diagnosed with pancreatic ductal adenocarcinoma (PDAC) remains poor. This also holds for patients who undergo surgical resections [1]. Here, metastasis is the primary reason leading to cancer-related death in that 70% of patients die eventually from remote metastasis. In particular, a portion of them dies from widespread metastasis within 2 years following curative-aimed surgery [2]. Although the surgical resection is the only "curative" option for PDAC patients, the majority of patients (ca. 80% of patients) are diagnosed at the advanced and often unresectable stage. This is because PDAC with its aggressive tumour biology develops in general without specific symptoms. Thus, it is essential to develop biomarkers, which enable a risk stratification for PDAC in the general population, and eventually contributes to earlier detection. Recent studies have uncovered a stable presence of circulating RNAs in blood, which may serve as the promising biomarkers for PDAC prevention, diagnosis, prognosis and targeted therapy.

B. Kong (✉)
Department of Surgery, Klinikum rechts der Isar, School of Medicine,
Technical University of Munich (TUM), Munich, Germany

Department of Gastroenterology, Affiliated Drum Tower Hospital of Nanjing University,
Medical School, Nanjing, China

H. Friess
Department of Surgery, Klinikum rechts der Isar, School of Medicine,
Technical University of Munich (TUM), Munich, Germany

© Springer Nature Switzerland AG 2020
C. W. Michalski et al. (eds.), *Translational Pancreatic Cancer Research*,
Molecular and Translational Medicine,
https://doi.org/10.1007/978-3-030-49476-6_6

Blood-Based Circulating RNAs

Circulating mRNA in PDAC

Blood-based circulating RNAs consist of two major categories: mRNAs (messenger RNAs) and ncRNAs (noncoding RNAs, Fig. 6.1) [3, 4]. In blood, mRNAs exist either in a cell-free or in a cellular form. Due to the abundance of RNases, cell-free mRNA can only be detected at a very low concentration in blood, and it is thought to be incorporated into exosomes or microvesicles [5]. Here, Kang and co-author reported that the serum level of type IV collagen (COL6A3) mRNA constituted potentially a diagnostic biomarker for PDAC with high sensitivity (0.91), but low specificity (0.46). As for cellular mRNA, it is mainly used as a surrogate marker for circulating tumour cells (CTCs). In 1996, Funaki and co-authors first reported the detection of carcinoembryonic antigen (CEA) mRNA in the whole blood of PDAC patients using classic RT-PCR methods [6]. Two years later, the same group reported a quantitative analysis of CEA mRNA using portal blood; they successfully detected high levels of CEA mRNAs in PDAC preoperatively, which declined significantly after tumour resection [7]. These initial data suggested that CEA mRNA in blood could be used to monitor the disease progression. Indeed, this hypothesis was tested in a study published in 2004 [8]. As such, Mataki and co-authors investigated the CEA mRNA expression in 53 patients in whole blood samples after surgical resection of biliary-pancreatic cancers. Among these 53 patients, 16 of them developed recurrence. The detection rate of blood CEA mRNA in these 16 patients was significantly higher than those without recurrence (75% vs. 5.4%, $p < 0.001$). In their analysis, the sensitivity and specificity of blood CEA mRNA were 75% and 94.6%, respectively, which is superior to conventional biomarkers such as CA19–9. More recently, the detection of cancer cell-specific blood mRNA markers such as CK20 (keratin 20) and alpha-1,4-N-acetylglucosaminyltransferase (a4GnT) was also reported [9, 10]. However, these methods were not further analysed in larger PDAC cohorts.

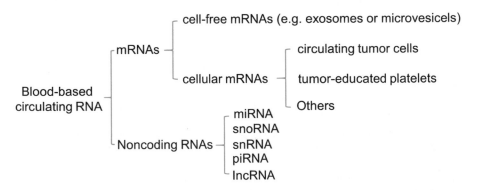

Fig. 6.1 Classification of blood RNAs

Apart from CTCs, mRNA profiles of tumour-educated platelets (TEPs) have the potential to function as diagnostic biomarkers for PDAC [11]. Taking advantage of next-generation sequencing techniques, Best and co-authors performed mRNA sequencing in 283 platelets samples including 35 PDAC patients. A panel of mRNA classifier was identified to distinguish cancer patients from healthy individuals with 96% accuracy.

Circulating ncRNAs in PDAC

It is now known that only a small part of human genomic DNAs code proteins and a large part of them are transcribed into ncRNAs [12]. ncRNAs contain miRNAs (microRNAs), small ncRNAs (nucleolar RNA (snoRNA), nuclear RNA (snRNA) and piwi-interacting RNA (piRNA)) and long ncRNAs (lncRNA). Initially, the function of these ncRNAs was thought to be merely a signal intermediate transferring genetic information from DNA to proteins. However, it became recently clear that they also played crucial roles in many cellular processes including pancreatic carcinogenesis [13].

Among these ncRNAs, miRNA is presently the most characterized one. miRNAs contain 18–22 nucleotides. They control cell proliferation, differentiation and cell death by regulating the post-transcriptional expression of genes [14]. In 2008, Mitchell and co-authors first demonstrated that miRNAs were detected in blood in a remarkably stable form protected from endogenous RNase activity [15]. Later studies revealed that circulating miRNAs are either packaged into exosome vesicles or bound to proteins in serum/plasma. Hence, they are protected from the degradation of endogenous RNase activity [16, 17]. This stable feature of miRNA in blood together with improved detection methods opens up a novel research field focusing on their potentials as noninvasive tumour diagnostic biomarkers in blood. As for PDAC, many studies have revealed that blood miRNAs might be useful for PDAC prevention, diagnosis, prognosis and therapy (Table 6.1). Also, lncRNA and snRNA were also found to be promising diagnostic biomarkers.

Table 6.1 Circulating ncRNAs as biomarkers of PDAC

	Preventive	Diagnostic	Prognostic	Druggable
Blood RNAs	miRNA	miRNA lncRNA snRNA	miRNA	miRNA
Other blood markers	BCAAs FBG	CA19–9	CA19–9	None

BCAAs branched-chain amino acids, FBG fasting blood glucose

Circulating ncRNAs as Preventive/Predictive Biomarkers of PDAC

Previous Blood Preventive/Predictive Biomarkers for PDAC

As for the preventive/predictive markers of PDAC, previous studies mainly focus on diabetes mellitus, which has a bi-directional connection with PDAC, with diabetes being both a risk factor and in some cases an early sign of the disease (Table 6.2) [18]. In a well-designed case-control study, fasting blood glucose (FBG) levels were increased (>126 mg/dL) in PDAC patients for a mean period of 36 to 30 months before cancer diagnosis [19]. Similarly, increased plasma levels of branched-chain amino acids (BCAAs), a marker for insulin resistance, were associated with the development of PDAC. The strongest association (risk) was observed among samples collected 24 to 60 months before cancer diagnosis [20].

Blood miRNA: "Late" Preventive/Predictive Biomarkers

As for blood miRNAs, Duell and co-authors recently published a prospective cohort study involving 225 healthy controls and 225 PDAC patients (Table 6.2) [21]. A panel of eight miRNAs (miR-10a, miR-10b, miR-21-3p, miR-21-5p, miR-30c, miR-106b, miR-155 and miR-212) was screened for their expressions in plasma samples taken before PDAC diagnosis. Four of these eight miRNAs (miR-10b, miR-21-5p, miR-30c and miR-106b) were significantly higher in PDAC plasma samples collected within 24 months before cancer diagnosis compared to healthy controls. However, compared to other preventive/predictive markers, alterations of blood miRNAs seem to take place late in the disease course of PDAC. This notion was confirmed by a recent case-control study published by Franklin and co-authors [22]. In this study, 15 miRNAs were investigated in 67 plasma samples sequentially collected before PDAC diagnosis, and their expressions were compared with 132 matched controls. However, none of these 15 miRNAs was significantly altered in prediagnostic plasma samples. In comparison, CA19–9 levels were already significantly increased in plasma samples collected less than 5 years before diagnosis. Collectively, these data suggest that alterations in blood miRNAs tend to occur late in the disease course of PDAC and blood miRNAs, as preventive/predictive early biomarkers for PDAC, are in general inferior to classical biomarkers. Thus, the current evidence does not support the notion to use blood miRNA as preventive/ predictive biomarkers for patient selection in a PDAC surveillance programme.

Table 6.2 Preventive/predictive blood biomarkers of PDAC

Biomarkers	Study design	Patient number	Time before diagnosis	Year/reference
FBG	Case-control	526 PDAC	36–30 months	2018/ [19]
BCAAs	Case-control	454 PDAC 908 controls	24–60 months	2014/ [20]
miRNAs	Case-control	225 PDAC 225 controls	<24 months	2017/ [21]

Circulating ncRNAs as Diagnostic Biomarkers of PDAC

Despite its limitations, CA19–9 is the only blood biomarker that is routinely used for PDAC diagnosis [23]. Thus, it is essential to develop further blood-based bio-markers with better sensitivity and specificity especially in early tumour stage. Upon the discovery of miRNA stable presence in blood in 2008 [15], the first study exploring the diagnostic potentials of plasma miRNAs was published in 2009 [24]. In this study, 4 miRNAs, miR-21, miR-210, miR-155 and miR-196, were investigated for their expressions in 49 PDAC and 36 control plasma samples using real-time PCR. This analysis revealed that this panel of four miRNAs discriminated PDAC patients from healthy controls with a sensitivity of 64% and a specificity of 89%, respectively. However, no comparison to CA19–9 was performed in this study. Moreover, as the first "proof of principle" study, it opened a door for the clinical translation of blood miRNAs as diagnostic markers for PDAC. In the last decade, numerous studies have been published on this topic (Table 6.3). Regarding diagnostic performance, blood miRNAs tend to have comparable sensitivity, but consistently a lower specificity as compared to serum CA19–9. For instance, blood

Table 6.3 Diagnostic performance of CA19–9 and ncRNAs in PDAC

Biomarkers	Source	Patient number	AUC	Sensitivity	Specificity	Year/ reference
miR panel miR-16 miR-196a vs. CA19–9	Plasma	140 PDAC 68 controls	0.89 vs. 0.90	87% vs. 81%	73% vs. 100%	2012/ [29]
miR-1290 vs. CA19–9	Serum	41 PDAC 19 controls	0.96 vs. 0.86	88% vs. 71%	84% vs. 90%	2013/ [25]
miR panel (miR-885-5p, 22-3p,642b-3p) vs. CA19–9	Plasma	11 PDAC 11 controls	0.97 vs. Unclear	91% vs. 73%	91% vs. 100%	2014/ [27]
miR panels Panel 1 Panel 2 vs. CA19–9	Whole blood	409 PDAC 312 controls	0.80 0.91 vs. 0.81	77% 80% vs. 74%	66% 82% vs. 99%	2014/ [28]
miR-483-3p miR-21 vs. CA19–9	Plasma	32 PDAC 30 controls	0.74 0.73 vs. 0.86	Undefined	Undefined	2015/ [30]
Linc-pint vs. CA 19–9	Plasma	59 PDAC 35 controls	0.78 vs. 0.87	87% Vs. 54%	77% Vs. 82%	2016/ [32]
miR-1290 vs. CA19–9	Plasma	267 PDAC 167 controls	0.73 vs. 0.91	56.3% Vs. 85%	89.5% Vs. 95.9%	2018/ [26]

miR-1290 was found to have a sensitivity of 88% and a specificity of 84% in a small cohort consisting of 41 PDAC patients and 19 controls [25]. In this cohort, serum CA19–9 differentiated PDAC patients from controls with a sensitivity of 71% and a specificity of 90%. This trend was seen in another large series containing 267 PDAC patients and 167 controls [26]. Here, blood miR-1290 distinguished PDAC patients from healthy controls with a sensitivity of 56.3% and a specificity of 89.5%, respectively. However, this was significantly lower than a sensitivity of 85% and a specificity of 95.9% for serum CA19–9 in the same cohort. This limited specificity was also observed when panels of blood miRNAs were tested [27–29]. For example, Schultz and co-authors identified two panels of whole blood miRNAs diagnosing PDAC with a specificity of 66% and 82% in a cohort of 409 PDAC patients and 312 controls, which was also lower than 99% for CA19–9 [28]. Similarly, Liu and co-authors compared the diagnostic accuracy of a panel of plasma miRNAs (miR-16 and miR-196a) and serum CA19–9 in a cohort of 140 PDAC patients and 68 controls [30]. As compared to serum CA19–9, this panel of plasma miRNAs had a similar sensitivity (87% vs. 81%), but a lower specificity (73% vs. 100%) in differentiating PDAC patients from healthy controls. Taken together, blood miRNAs have similar sensitivity, but unfavourable specificity in detecting PDAC as compared to the routinely used serum marker CA19–9.

Apart from blood miRNAs, other blood ncRNAs such as lncRNA and snRNA were also reported to be potential diagnostic biomarkers for PDAC [31, 32]. Here, Baraniskin et al. identified fragments of circulating U2 snRNAs as a novel diagnostic marker for PDAC in a retrospective cohort [31]. Recently, Linc-pint (p53-induced transcript) was identified as a potential diagnostic lncRNA in plasma for PDAC patients [32]. Certainly, these data need to be validated by further studies with large patient numbers (e.g. prospective studies).

Circulating ncRNAs as Prognostic Biomarkers of PDAC

As earlier demonstrated, serum CA19–9 is a well-validated diagnostic marker for PDAC. Recent studies revealed that it also constituted a prognostic biomarker for PDAC patients [33, 34]. However, the cut-off value of CA19–9 as a prognostic biomarker is not routinely used "37 U/ml", but much higher values. For instance, Dong et al. analysed the serum CA19–9 levels in a cohort of 120 PDAC patients and their prognostic impact. This analysis revealed that PDAC patients with serum CA19–9 levels less than 338 U/ml had a significantly longer median overall survival than those with serum CA19–9 above 338 U/ml (24.9 vs. 11.9 months, p = 0.009). The same principle also applies to blood miRNAs: many of the above-mentioned blood miRNAs with diagnostic potentials are also prognostic biomarkers when an appropriate cut-off value is applied (Table 6.4). Also, some blood miRNAs were found to be associated with other clinical factors of PDAC. For example, miR-744 is associated with the tumour size (T) [35]; miR-744 and miR-107 mainly are linked with the lymphatic status(N) [35, 36]; miR-221, miR-1290, miR-21 and miR-107 are

Table 6.4   ncRNAs as prognostic biomarkers for PDAC

Biomarkers	Patient number	Survival	Tumour size (T)	Lymphatic status (N)	Metastatic status (M)	Recurrence	Year/reference
miR-1290 miR-486-3p	n = 41	+ +	–	–	–	–	2013/ [25]
miR-221	n = 47	–	–	–	+	–	2014/ [37]
miR-744	n = 94	+	+	+	–	+	2015/ [35]
miR-21	n = 32	+	–	–	+	–	2015/ [30]
miR-107	n = 74	+	–	+	+	+	2017/ [36]
miR-1290	n = 167	+	–	–	+	–	2018/ [26]

related to the metastatic status (M, Table 6.4); miR-744 and miR-107 are associated with tumour recurrence (Table 6.4) [37]. Thus, blood miRNAs not only affect PDAC prognosis but also are associated with multiple clinical parameters of PDAC.

Circulating ncRNAs as Druggable Targets of PDAC

Recently, miRNA-based therapy has been developed [38, 39]. For instance, miravirsen (also known as SPC3649) is a potent miR-122 inhibitor, which is currently tested for treating hepatitis C infection in humans. As for PDAC, Immaura and co-authors identified plasma miR-107 as a potentially druggable target [36]. Firstly, they observed that miR-107 was significantly down-regulated in plasmas from PDAC patients compared to healthy controls. In a xenograft mouse model of PDAC, the restoration and maintenance of plasma miR-107 using miRNA mimics significantly inhibited tumour growth. These data provided first evidence defining plasma miR-107 as a potentially druggable target in PDAC patients.

Conclusion and Outlook

Hereby, we summarized the potential utility of blood-based circulating RNAs as preventive, diagnostic, prognostic and druggable biomarkers for PDAC. Due to the abundance of RNases, the reliable detection of cell-free mRNA in blood may not be easy to realize in clinical practice, thus compromising its future application. For the cellular form of mRNAs in blood, the exact dissection of blood mRNA composition (e.g. CTCs or TEPs) is crucial for future clinical translation. As for ncRNAs, blood miRNA is the most promising candidate. However, the alteration in blood miRNAs tends to take place late in the disease course of PDAC, arguing against its role as a preventive/predictive biomarker. Despite a lower specificity, blood miRNAs, as diagnostic biomarkers, are generally as useful as serum CA19–9 in diagnosing PDAC. The poor specificity of blood miRNAs might be improved by selectively using exosomal levels of miRNAs [40]. Furthermore, by applying appropriate cut-off values, many blood miRNAs might also serve as prognostic biomarkers useful for preoperative patient stratification. Finally, a few blood miRNAs are currently explored as druggable biomarkers at the preclinical stage.

References

1. Salman B, Zhou D, Jaffee EM, Edil BH, Zheng LJO. Vaccine therapy for pancreatic cancer. Oncoimmunology. 2013;2:e26662.
2. Iacobuzio-Donahue CA, Fu B, Yachida S, et al. DPC4 gene status of the primary carcinoma correlates with patterns of failure in patients with pancreatic cancer. J Clin Oncol. 2009;27:1806.
3. Okajima W, Komatsu S, Ichikawa D, et al. Liquid biopsy in patients with hepatocellular carcinoma: circulating tumor cells and cell-free nucleic acids. World J Gastroenterol. 2017;23:5650.
4. Kishikawa T, Otsuka M, Ohno M, Yoshikawa T, Takata A, Koike K. Circulating RNAs as new biomarkers for detecting pancreatic cancer. World J Gastroenterol. 2015;21:8527.
5. Kang CY, Wang J, Axell-House D, et al. Clinical significance of serum COL6A3 in pancreatic ductal adenocarcinoma. J Gastrointest Surg. 2014;18:7–15.
6. Funaki NO, Tanaka J, Kasamatsu T, et al. Identification of carcinoembryonic antigen mRNA in circulating peripheral blood of pancreatic carcinoma and gastric carcinoma patients. Life Sci. 1996;59:2187–99.
7. Funaki NO, Tanaka J, Hosotani R, Kogire M, Suwa H, Imamura M. Quantitative analysis of carcinoembryonic antigen messenger RNA in peripheral venous blood and portal blood of patients with pancreatic ductal adenocarcinoma. Clin Cancer Res. 1998;4:855–60.
8. Mataki Y, Takao S, Maemura K, et al. Carcinoembryonic antigen messenger RNA expression using nested reverse transcription-PCR in the peripheral blood during follow-up period of patients who underwent curative surgery for biliary-pancreatic cancer: longitudinal analyses. Clin Cancer Res. 2004;10:3807–14.
9. Zhang Y-L, Feng J-G, Gou J-M, Zhou L-X, Wang P. Detection of CK20mRNA in peripheral blood of pancreatic cancer and its clinical significance. World J Gastroenterol. 2005;11:1023.
10. Ishizone S, Yamauchi K, Kawa S, et al. Clinical utility of quantitative RT-PCR targeted to α1, 4-N-acetylglucosaminyltransferase mRNA for detection of pancreatic cancer. Cancer Sci. 2006;97:119–26.
11. Best MG, Sol N, Kooi I, et al. RNA-Seq of tumor-educated platelets enables blood-based pan-cancer, multiclass, and molecular pathway cancer diagnostics. Cancer Cell. 2015;28:666–76.
12. Nature IHGSCJ. Initial sequencing and analysis of the human genome. Nature 2001;409:860.
13. Szymanski M, Barciszewska MZ, Erdmann VA, Barciszewski J. A new frontier for molecular medicine: noncoding RNAs. Biochim Biophys Acta. 1756;2005:65–75.
14. Brennecke J, Stark A, Russell RB, Cohen SM. Principles of microRNA–target recognition. PLoS Biol. 2005;3:e85.
15. Mitchell PS, Parkin RK, Kroh EM, et al. Circulating microRNAs as stable blood-based markers for cancer detection. Proc Natl Acad Sci U S A. 2008;105:10513–8.
16. Kosaka N, Iguchi H, Yoshioka Y, Takeshita F, Matsuki Y, Ochiya T. Secretory mechanisms and intercellular transfer of microRNAs in living cells. J Biol Chem. 2010;285(23):17442–52.

17. Arroyo JD, Chevillet JR, Kroh EM, et al. Argonaute2 complexes carry a population of circulating microRNAs independent of vesicles in human plasma. Proc Natl Acad Sci U S A. 2011;108:5003–8.
18. Bosetti C, Rosato V, Li D, et al. Diabetes, antidiabetic medications, and pancreatic cancer risk: an analysis from the International Pancreatic Cancer Case-Control Consortium. Ann Oncol. 2014;25:2065–72.
19. Sharma A, Smyrk TC, Levy MJ, Topazian MA, Chari ST. Fasting blood glucose levels provide estimate of duration and progression of pancreatic cancer before diagnosis. Gastroenterology. 2018. 155(2):490–500.e2.
20. Mayers JR, Wu C, Clish CB, et al. Elevation of circulating branched-chain amino acids is an early event in human pancreatic adenocarcinoma development. Nat Med. 2014;20:1193.
21. Duell EJ, Lujan-Barroso L, Sala N, et al. Plasma microRNAs as biomarkers of pancreatic cancer risk in a prospective cohort study. Int J Cancer. 2017;141:905–15.
22. Franklin O, Jonsson P, Billing O, et al. Plasma micro-RNA alterations appear late in pancreatic cancer. Ann Surg. 2018;267:775.
23. Ballehaninna UK, Chamberlain RS. Serum CA 19–9 as a biomarker for pancreatic cancer—a comprehensive review. Indian J Surg Oncol. 2011;2:88–100.
24. Wang J, Chen J, Chang P, et al. MicroRNAs in plasma of pancreatic ductal adenocarcinoma patients as novel blood-based biomarkers of disease. Cancer Prev Res (Phila). 2009;2(9):807–13. CAPR-09-0094.
25. Ang L, Jun Y, Haeryoung K, et al. MicroRNA array analysis finds elevated serum miR-1290 accurately distinguishes patients with low-stage pancreatic cancer from healthy and disease controls. Clin Cancer Res. 2013;19:3600–10.
26. Tavano F, Gioffreda D, Valvano MR, et al. Droplet digital PCR quantification of miR-1290 as a circulating biomarker for pancreatic cancer. Scientific Reports 06 November 2018.
27. Ganepola Ap G, Rutledge JR, Paritosh S, Anusak Y, Chang DH. Novel blood-based microRNA biomarker panel for early diagnosis of pancreatic cancer. World J Gastrointest Oncol. 2014;6:22.
28. Schultz NA, Christian D, Jensen BV, et al. MicroRNA biomarkers in whole blood for detection of pancreatic cancer. JAMA. 2014;311:392.
29. Liu J, Gao J, Du Y, et al. Combination of plasma microRNAs with serum CA19–9 for early detection of pancreatic cancer. Int J Cancer. 2012;131:683–91.
30. Makoto A, Misa Y, Rie S, et al. Circulating miR-483-3p and miR-21 is highly expressed in plasma of pancreatic cancer. Int J Oncol. 2015;46:539–47.
31. Alexander B, Stefanie NPD, Maike A, et al. Circulating U2 small nuclear RNA fragments as a novel diagnostic biomarker for pancreatic and colorectal adenocarcinoma. Int J Cancer. 2013;132:E48–57.
32. Li L, Zhang GQ, Chen H, et al. Plasma and tumor levels of Linc-pint are diagnostic and prognostic biomarkers for pancreatic cancer. Oncotarget. 2016;7:71773–81.
33. Xu HX, Liu L, Xiang JF, et al. Postoperative serum CEA and CA125 levels are supplementary to perioperative CA19–9 levels in predicting operative outcomes of pancreatic ductal adenocarcinoma. Surgery. 2017;161:373–84.
34. Dong Q, Yang XH, Zhang Y, et al. Elevated serum CA19–9 level is a promising predictor for poor prognosis in patients with resectable pancreatic ductal adenocarcinoma: a pilot study. World J Surg Oncol. 2014;12:1–8.
35. Mahito M, Shuhei K, Daisuke I, et al. Plasma microRNA profiles: identification of miR-744 as a novel diagnostic and prognostic biomarker in pancreatic cancer. Br J Cancer. 2015;113:1467–76.
36. Imamura T, Komatsu S, Ichikawa D, et al. Depleted tumor suppressor miR-107 in plasma relates to tumor progression and is a novel therapeutic target in pancreatic cancer. Sci Rep. 2017;7:e120.
37. Kawaguchi T, Komatsu S, Ichikawa D, et al. Clinical impact of circulating miR-221 in plasma of patients with pancreatic cancer. Br J Cancer. 2013;108:361–9.

38. Gebert LFR, Rebhan MAE, Crivelli SEM, Rémy D, Markus S, Jonathan H. Miravirsen (SPC3649) can inhibit the biogenesis of miR-122. Nucleic Acids Res. 2014;42:609–21.
39. Lanford RE, Hildebrandt-Eriksen ES, Andreas P, et al. Therapeutic silencing of microRNA-122 in primates with chronic hepatitis C virus infection. Science. 2010;327(5962):198–201.
40. Lai X, Wang M, Mcelyea SD, Sherman S, House M, Korc M. A microRNA signature in circulating exosomes is superior to exosomal glypican-1 levels for diagnosing pancreatic cancer. Cancer Lett. 2017;393:86.

Chapter 7
Circulating Tumor DNA as a Novel Biomarker for Pancreatic Cancer

Andreas W. Berger and Alexander Kleger

Models to Derive Biomarkers

The pancreas functions as both an endocrine and an exocrine organ, with crucial roles in digestion of food and maintenance of blood glucose levels. Obstruction of pancreatic endocrine function contributes to the development of *diabetes mellitus* (DM). Alternatively, exocrine dysfunction, frequently due to *chronic pancreatitis,* causes malnutrition, and oncogene activation can lead to *pancreatic cancer.* Pancreatic ductal adenocarcinoma (PDAC) is the most common type of pancreatic cancer and has a devastating prognosis despite intensive efforts in basic and translational research. PDAC has an overall 5-year survival rate of only 4%. According to recent predictions, pancreatic cancer will surpass colorectal and breast cancer to rank as the second most common cause of cancer-related deaths in Germany by 2030 [1]. The only potentially curative treatment is surgery, but only 15–20% of PDAC patients are eligible, and after surgery still just 25–30% survive. The genetic complexity and inter−/intratumoral heterogeneity of PDAC prevent the development of tailored therapies. Further, there are no predictive biomarkers that take individual tumor characteristics into account [1, 2]. The most promising way to diagnose PDAC in its curable phase would be identification of tumors at a premalignant stage, as we do with colon adenomas in the prevention of colorectal cancer [3]. The progression of PDAC begins with acinar-to-ductal metaplasia (ADM) and further development into more advanced precursor lesions called pancreatic intraepithelial

A. W. Berger
Department of Gastroenterology, Gastrointestinal Oncology and Interventional Endoscopy, Vivantes Klinikum Im Friedrichshain, Berlin, Germany

Department of Internal Medicine I, Ulm University, Ulm, Germany

A. Kleger (✉)
Department of Internal Medicine I, Ulm University, Ulm, Germany
e-mail: alexander.kleger@uniklinik-ulm.de

© Springer Nature Switzerland AG 2020
C. W. Michalski et al. (eds.), *Translational Pancreatic Cancer Research,*
Molecular and Translational Medicine,
https://doi.org/10.1007/978-3-030-49476-6_7

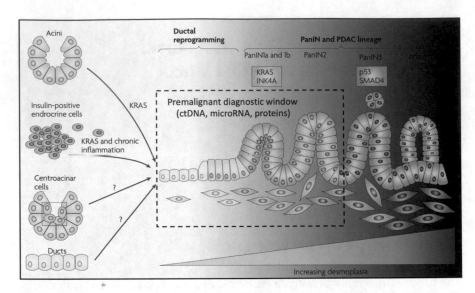

Fig. 7.1 Illustration of the sequential steps in pancreatic cancer development and the from secreted cargo arising premalignant diagnostic window. (Modified from Morris et al. [7], with permission)

neoplasia (PanIN). Hence, a biomarker to sense the development of PanIN lesions would be desirable [4]. Currently, PDAC models are limited to genetically engineered mouse models, 2D culture systems, patient-derived xenografts, and most recently pancreatic organoid cultures. The lattermost can be derived from primary cancer specimens and have been shown to be a superior model for PDAC; however, they only allow analysis of the static endpoint once the stage of early diagnosis has already passed [5]. Most biomarkers were discovered in these advanced-stage PDAC model systems that are not representative of earlier stages, when detection would be most relevant [6]. We reason that cargo such as ctDNA, proteins, or microRNA derived from precursor lesions, such as PanINs or cystic pancreatic tumors progressing to PDAC, might provide an innovative and effective opportunity to discover diagnostic biomarkers. Currently, however, there are no genetically clean, purified, and human in vitro pancreas organ culture systems, which allow spatiotemporal resolution of the secreted cargo of the developing precursor lesions of PDAC (Fig. 7.1).

ctDNA Biomarkers in the Bloodstream: Different Approaches and Technical Issues

Nowadays it is well established that cancer-specific genetic signatures are depicted in the bloodstream of cancer patients and can assist for non-invasive diagnosis, treatment monitoring under real-time conditions, and estimation of patients' prognosis of pancreatic cancer patients. Various origins of these blood-based genetic biomarkers in pancreatic ductal adenocarcinoma (PDAC) were reported. Circulating tumor DNA (ctDNA) is considered to be the most intensively studied target for this purpose. ctDNA is released into the bloodstream in the context of active-spontaneous [8, 9] and passive secretion (apoptosis, necrosis, insufficient clearance) [10–13]. Molecular characterization of ctDNA allows non-invasive tumor-specific genotyping in malignancy [14, 15]. The exquisite biological specificity qualifies ctDNA as a promising biomarker in oncology. ctDNA is defined by the presence of (tumor-specific) mutations and is detectable in a variety of malignancies. The individual ctDNA concentrations are disease stage-dependent [16, 17]. The hype in cfDNA/ctDNA analytics is also explained by massive investments and developments in the technology sector. New digital technologies and sequencing approaches are meanwhile delivering ever higher sensitivities. Single point mutations are detectable as well as amplifications, rearrangements, and aneuploidy [18]. However, all ctDNA approaches, also the detection of minimal residual disease, require a certain degree of analytical sensitivity. Some authors demonstrated that gender, chronic inflammation, age, or tumor heterogeneity could influence the level of ctDNA [19]. The challenges can be summarized as follows:

1. The discrimination of ctDNA and physiologically occurring cfDNA in a cost-effective manner
2. The handling of extremely low concentrations of ctDNA
3. The exact quantification of the number of mutated fragments
4. Handling technical artifacts (errors) introduced during sequencing [20–23].

Recently it was reasoned that a specific enrichment of methylated DNA fragments from cfDNA could overcome the abovementioned limitations or challenges. A sensitive, immunoprecipitation-based protocol was recently published to analyze the methylome of small quantities of cfDNA. The authors even demonstrate the ability to classify early-stage cancers based on plasma cfDNA methylation patterns [24].

Furthermore, microvesicles or even exosomes, which are present in the blood of every human being, contain DNA cargo. Specifically, exosomes contain proteins and nucleic acids derived from their cell of origin. Exosomes can be isolated from blood plasma and, in addition to other markers, can be identified as tumor-specific by Glypican-1 on their surface [25]. Generally, the DNA contained in exosomes (exoDNA) is present in larger fragments of more than 10 kKB and is protected against degradation [26, 27]. Recently, it was shown that treatment with engineered exosomes (called iExosomes) facilitates for direct and specific targeting of oncogenic *KRAS* in pancreatic tumors and subsequently can delay tumor growth [28]. Thus, both types of DNA, ctDNA and exoDNA, can provide access to the molecular signature of the respective tumor by means of a simple blood sample; although the technical requirements for both approaches are very different, both demand a minutely developed methodological setup.

Recent work on material from patients with different types of tumors has shown that ctDNA maps the mutational makeup of a given tumor and may therefore be used to reconstruct the latter and subsequently to monitor tumor evolution during therapy [16, 29, 30]. However, most of these works only show the feasibility based on a single analytical time point. For example, in cystic premalignant lesions of the pancreas, it was demonstrated that a diagnosis can be made by molecular character-ization of ctDNA from blood plasma using highly sensitive methods (digital PCR) [4]. Based on this, mutational signatures in ctDNA were investigated in the course of therapy. Studies showed that in patients with colon cancer, the detection of *KRAS* mutation status in ctDNA and the determination of allelic frequencies in the further course allow non-invasive imaging of tumor burden and disease progression. In subgroups, a correlation of cfDNA amount under treatment with the duration of progression-free survival (PFS) could be presented [31]. Other work has shown that the seven most frequently mutated genes in PDAC are depicted in ctDNA, assessed by targeted deep sequencing, delivering comparable results with tissue-derived DNA. Such panel or digital PCR-based approaches operate generally fast, are effi-cient, and are rather easy to be elaborated; however, despite these promising results, small gene panels are overall not insufficient to map the entire heterogeneity. In addition, the complexity of biological processes such as clonal evolution of pancre-atic carcinoma, in all cases, to completely trace the clinical course [32]. However, this is essential if therapeutic decisions based on molecular ctDNA characterization should be made. Here, whole-exome sequencing from ctDNA samples can step in but deliver the appropriate results at expensive of feasibility and pricing.

ctDNA as Biomarker for Premalignant Pancreatic Cystic Tumors and Early PDAC Progression

Earlier detection is the key to reduce cancer-related deaths. Based on published results, it appears realistic that early detection can become possible by simple blood tests [33] operating on ctDNA analytical basis [34]. PDAC is the most common malignant tumor of the pancreas and the fourth leading cause of cancer deaths in the western world with an increasing incidence [35]. Overall, PDAC has a very poor prognosis despite intensive treatment regimens [36, 37]. Therefore, all efforts for prevention and for early detection of pancreatic malignancy must be made. A prom-ising approach in this regard is the non-invasive monitoring of PDAC precursor lesions using liquid biopsy approaches, to avoid the malignant transformation of precursor lesions. In that sense, it is necessary to define high-risk lesions in the pancreas, which are known to develop into PDAC. These include primarily cystic pancreatic neoplasms, such as mucinous cystic neoplasms (MCN) or intraductal papillary-mucinous cystic neoplasm (IPMN) [38, 39]. Consequently, correct man-agement of cystic pancreatic tumors may prevent progression to PDAC while mini-mizing the need for lifelong screening and related costs [40]. The diagnosis and monitoring of these lesions has so far invariably been based on instrumental examinations. In a retrospective analysis, it was shown that the genetic profile of cystic pancreatic tumors is depicted in the blood and is usable for, e.g., diagnostics in the form of a liquid biopsy. Indeed, *GNAS* and *KRAS* mutations in ctDNA significantly discriminated patients with strictly benign pancreatic lesions (serous cystadenomas) from others with borderline cysts (IPMN) or pancreatic cancer [40].

Obviously, proteins released from precursor lesions during tumor progression such as pancreatic intraepithelial neoplasia (PanIN) might serve also as innovative and effective diagnostic biomarkers. In turn, a future path to succeed in early diagnosis of PDAC might be the combination and complementary use of established markers such as CA19-9 together with novel protein and cfDNA-based approaches. Thrombospondin-2 (THBS2) is a disulfide-linked homotrimer glycoprotein that mediates cell-to-cell and cell-to-matrix interactions. THBS2 probably inhibits angiogenesis, and depletion of the THBS2 gene in a mouse model increases the susceptibility to cancer [41]. THBS2 is secreted or released from human precursor PanIN organoids and may hence serve as a biomarker for early PDAC [41, 42]. Preclinical data were recently validated in a large cohort with PDAC patients at various disease stages compared to healthy controls and patients with cystic tumors or chronic pancreatitis. Normal pancreatic cells express the THBS2 antigen, but under physiological conditions, the plasma concentration is low. In contrary, it is highly expressed by PDAC tumor cells, and the plasma of PDAC patients shows elevated THBS2 levels. The concentration of THBS2 in plasma is reported to allow the discrimination between resectable PDAC stage I cancer and advanced stage III/IV. However, the mechanism of THBS2 release into the bloodstream remains elusive [43]. The value of THBS2 by complementing with cfDNA measurements and CA19-9 in a large cohort of PDAC patients prior to intended curative surgery was evaluated and compared to strictly benign IPMN patients and healthy controls. The authors reported that the combination of CA19-9 and THBS2 showed a promising c-statistics of 0.87 and could be further increased to 0.94 when combining CA19-9, THBS2, and total cfDNA quantification. This marker combination performed best for all PDAC stages, especially in the group of stage I PDAC (c-statistics of 0.90 for the three-marker combination) [44].

Recent studies have shown that dynamic changes in the global DNA methylation and gene expression patterns play key roles in the PDAC development, which was supported by integrated genomic analysis of hundreds of PDAC cases which allows to define distinct molecular subtype of PDAC [45]. Differential methylation is observed in genes associated, for example, with pancreatic development and pancreatic cancer core signaling pathways [46]. First data are now available that epigenetic targeting might be a new therapeutic option in PDAC [47]. The sensitivity of ctDNA mutagenome analyzing methods may be low among patients with early-stage cancer given the limited number of recurrent mutations [33, 34, 48, 49]. Shen SY et al. assumed that large-scale epigenetic alterations potentially have greater ability to detect and classify cancers in patients with early-stage disease and developed a sensitive blood test by using plasma cfDNA methylomes [24].

Prognostic Relevance of ctDNA Signatures During Treatment of Resectable PDAC

Liquid biopsy approaches also were studied in the context of resectable PDAC as a prognostic biomarker. A French study by Pietrasz D et al. could show that patients, resected from PDAC, with undetectable ctDNA after surgery had a longer disease-free survival (17.6 vs. 4.6 months; log-rank $P = 0.03$) and a longer overall survival (32.2 vs. 19.3; $P = 0.027$) than those with detectable ctDNA, based on genotyping of ctDNA for frequent mutations such as in *CDKN2A*, *SMAD4*, *TP53*, or *KRAS* [50]. In patients with advanced PDACs, ctDNA was also an independent prognostic biomarker for survival (HR = 1.94; $P = 0.007$). Chen and colleagues have previously described the prognostic value of ctDNA as a biomarker in PDAC [51]. In their series, the presence of *KRAS* mutation in plasma was correlated with poor OS (3.9 vs. 10.2 months; $P < 0.001$) in nonresectable patients. More recently, Sausen and colleagues reported that, in resectable patients, ctDNA was a prognostic factor of early tumor relapse if detected before surgery (log-rank $P = 0.015$). In this study, in a subgroup of 20 patients collected after surgical resection, detectable ctDNA was also a prognostic biomarker of DFS (9.9 months vs. median not reached; log-rank $P = 0.02$). Taken together, the detection of ctDNA after resection predicts clinical relapse and poor outcome, with recurrence by ctDNA detected 6.5 months earlier than with CT imaging. These observations provide genetic predictors of outcome in pancreatic cancer and have implications for new avenues of therapeutic intervention [52]. Hadano and colleagues reported that among 105 PDAC cases, ctDNA was detected in 33 (31%) plasma samples. The median OS durations were 13.6 months for patients with ctDNA (ctDNA+) and 27.6 months for patients without ctDNA. Patients who were ctDNA+ had a significantly poorer prognosis with respect to OS ($P < 0.0001$) [53]. The combination of ctDNA and exoDNA analyses in PDAC was recently published. Bernard and colleagues performed a prospective cohort study and collected liquid biopsy samples 34 resectable PDAC patients. Droplet digital polymerase chain reaction was used to determine *KRAS* mutant allele fraction (MAF) from ctDNA and exoDNA purified from plasma and was correlated with prognostic and predictive outcomes [54]. Interestingly, an increase in exoDNA level after neoadjuvant therapy was significantly associated with disease progression ($P = 0.003$), whereas ctDNA did not show correlations with outcomes [54].

ctDNA in Metastatic PDAC: Prognostics and Real-Time Treatment Guidance

The first studies on ctDNA in PDAC focused on *KRAS* mutations that are present in the majority of PDACs [52, 55, 56]. But for treatment-associated tumor evolution, more genomic alterations are likely to play a role. Currently, there are only limited data available from ctDNA analyses over and above *KRAS* profiling [50, 57]. Pietrasz and colleagues reported that 64.7% of the patients with metastatic PDAC had detectable ctDNA in comparison with only 16.6% with locally advanced disease ($P < 0.001$ [50]). In the group of metastatic patients, no significant correlation was found between the presence of ctDNA and the number of metastatic sites ($P = 0.13$). The presence of ctDNA was strongly correlated with poor OS (6.5 vs. 19.0 months; log-rank $P < 0.001$) in patients with advanced pancreatic adenocarcinoma. Patients with higher MAF had the worst OS. The OS decreased from 18.9, 7.8, and 4.9 months (log-rank $P < 0.001$) for the lowest, middle, and highest MAF tertiles, respectively [50].

In addition, a recently published study applied a targeted next-generation sequencing approach of ctDNA, combined with droplet digital PCR, (i) to examine ctDNA as a tool for non-invasive diagnosis and (ii) to inform on therapy-induced tumor evolution in metastatic PDAC during different lines of systemic treatment [32]. All therapy-naïve patients presented with detectable ctDNA at baseline. The combined mutational allele frequency (CMAF) of *KRAS* and *TP53* was reported to reflect the amount of ctDNA. The median CMAF level significantly decreased during treatment ($P = 0.0027$) and increased at progression ($P = 0.0104$). CA19-9 tumor marker analyses did not show significant differences. In treatment-naïve patients, the CMAF levels during therapy significantly correlated with progression-free survival (Spearman, $r = -0.8609$, $P = 0.0013$) [32].

Kruger and colleagues stated in a previously published study that repeated ctDNA measurements on mutated *KRAS* alleles represent a novel and promising tool for early response prediction and therapy monitoring in advanced pancreatic cancer [58]. The authors reported that mut*KRAS* ctDNA was present in a majority of advanced PDAC patients (67%). The presence of mut*KRAS* ctDNA was significantly correlated to an adverse overall survival. A decrease in mut*KRAS* ctDNA levels during therapy was an early indicator of response to therapy, while there was no significant correlation between kinetics of CA19-9 tumor marker [58].

Summary and Conclusion

ctDNA-based measurements have the capacity to relaunch the biomarker debate in pancreatic cancer. The reason for this ascent is multilayered but primarily links a novel grade of specificity due to the opportunity to detect tumor-specific alterations with an unreached sensitivity resulting from technological progress in this field. The latter can be particularly interesting when a PDAC needs to be differentiated from its yet benign precursor lesions or to risk stratify a cystic tumor in the pancreas. A further additive value is given by complementary action with established biomarkers such as CA19-9. Besides the diagnostic value of ctDNA measures, the most important strength lies in its capacity to mimic the entire mutational makeup and thus PDAC's heterogeneity plus the opportunity to quantitatively follow the mutational load to track and trace chemotherapy-driven tumor evolution. In that light, a therapeutic blueprint based on repetitive ctDNA genotyping can be envisioned to specifically tailor patients' therapy. Still, clinical grade standards and future validation of this novel tool need to developed, and economical hurdles to bring this method to a broader range have to be negotiated.

References

1. Kleger A, Perkhofer L, Seufferlein T. Smarter drugs emerging in pancreatic cancer therapy. Ann Oncol. 2014;25:1260–70.
2. Waddell N, Pajic M, Patch AM, et al. Whole genomes redefine the mutational landscape of pancreatic cancer. Nature. 2015;518:495–501.
3. Tomasello G, Petrelli F, Barni S. Risk of primary tumor sidedness as a criterion for screening, diagnostic colonoscopy, and surveillance intervals-reply. JAMA Oncol. 2017;3(10):1427.
4. Berger AW, Schwerdel D, Costa IG, et al. Detection of hot-spot mutations in circulating cell-free DNA from patients with intraductal papillary mucinous neoplasms of the pancreas. Gastroenterology. 2016;151:267–70.
5. Boj SF, Hwang CI, Baker LA, et al. Organoid models of human and mouse ductal pancreatic cancer. Cell. 2015;160:324–38.
6. Costello E, Greenhalf W, Neoptolemos JP. New biomarkers and targets in pancreatic cancer and their application to treatment. Nat Rev Gastroenterol Hepatol. 2012;9:435–44.
7. Morris JP, Wang SC, Hebrok M. KRAS, Hedgehog, Wnt and the twisted developmental biology of pancreatic ductal adenocarcinoma. Nat Rev Cancer. 2010;10:683–95.
8. Schwarzenbach H, Hoon DS, Pantel K. Cell-free nucleic acids as biomarkers in cancer patients. Nat Rev Cancer. 2011;11:426–37.
9. Pisetsky DS, Fairhurst AM. The origin of extracellular DNA during the clearance of dead and dying cells. Autoimmunity. 2007;40:281–4.
10. Anker P, Stroun M, Maurice PA. Spontaneous release of DNA by human blood lymphocytes as shown in an in vitro system. Cancer Res. 1975;35:2375–82.
11. Rogers JC, Boldt D, Kornfeld S, et al. Excretion of deoxyribonucleic acid by lymphocytes stimulated with phytohemagglutinin or antigen. Proc Natl Acad Sci U S A. 1972;69:1685–9.
12. Stroun M, Anker P. Nucleic acids spontaneously released by living frog auricles. Biochem J. 1972;128:100P–1P.
13. Stroun M, Lyautey J, Lederrey C, et al. About the possible origin and mechanism of circulating DNA apoptosis and active DNA release. Clin Chim Acta. 2001;313:139–42.
14. Murtaza M, Dawson SJ, Tsui DW, et al. Non-invasive analysis of acquired resistance to cancer therapy by sequencing of plasma DNA. Nature. 2013;497:108–12.
15. Pantel K, Diaz LA Jr, Polyak K. Tracking tumor resistance using 'liquid biopsies'. Nat Med. 2013;19:676–7.
16. Bettegowda C, Sausen M, Leary RJ, et al. Detection of circulating tumor DNA in early- and late-stage human malignancies. Sci Transl Med. 2014;6:224ra224.
17. Speicher MR, Pantel K. Tumor signatures in the blood. Nat Biotechnol. 2014;32:441–3.
18. Diaz LA Jr, Bardelli A. Liquid biopsies: genotyping circulating tumor DNA. J Clin Oncol. 2014;32:579–86.
19. Gall TM, Frampton AE, Krell J, et al. Circulating molecular markers in pancreatic cancer: ready for clinical use? Future Oncol. 2013;9:141–4.
20. Diehl F, Li M, Dressman D, et al. Detection and quantification of mutations in the plasma of patients with colorectal tumors. Proc Natl Acad Sci U S A. 2005;102:16368–73.
21. Diehl F, Schmidt K, Choti MA, et al. Circulating mutant DNA to assess tumor dynamics. Nat Med. 2008;14:985–90.

22. Holdhoff M, Schmidt K, Donehower R, Diaz LA Jr. Analysis of circulating tumor DNA to confirm somatic KRAS mutations. J Natl Cancer Inst. 2009;101:1284–5.
23. Spindler KG, Boysen AK, Pallisgard N, et al. Cell-free DNA in metastatic colorectal cancer: a systematic review and meta-analysis. Oncologist. 2017;22:1049–55.
24. Shen SY, Singhania R, Fehringer G, et al. Sensitive tumour detection and classification using plasma cell-free DNA methylomes. Nature. 2018;563:579–83.
25. Melo SA, Luecke LB, Kahlert C, et al. Glypican-1 identifies cancer exosomes and detects early pancreatic cancer. Nature. 2015;523:177–82.
26. Kahlert C, Melo SA, Protopopov A, et al. Identification of double-stranded genomic DNA spanning all chromosomes with mutated KRAS and p53 DNA in the serum exosomes of patients with pancreatic cancer. J Biol Chem. 2014;289:3869–75.
27. Nuzhat Z, Kinhal V, Sharma S, et al. Tumour-derived exosomes as a signature of pancreatic cancer – liquid biopsies as indicators of tumour progression. Oncotarget. 2017;8:17279–91.
28. Kamerkar S, LeBleu VS, Sugimoto H, et al. Exosomes facilitate therapeutic targeting of onco-genic KRAS in pancreatic cancer. Nature. 2017;546:498–503.
29. Oellerich M, Schutz E, Beck J, et al. Using circulating cell-free DNA to monitor personalized cancer therapy. Crit Rev Clin Lab Sci. 2017;54:205–18.
30. Riva F, Dronov OI, Khomenko DI, et al. Clinical applications of circulating tumor DNA and circulating tumor cells in pancreatic cancer. Mol Oncol. 2016;10:481–93.
31. Berger AW, Schwerdel D, Welz H, et al. Treatment monitoring in metastatic colorectal cancer patients by quantification and KRAS genotyping of circulating cell-free DNA. PLoS One. 2017;12:e0174308.
32. Berger AW, Schwerdel D, Ettrich TJ, et al. Targeted deep sequencing of circulating tumor DNA in metastatic pancreatic cancer. Oncotarget. 2018;9:2076–85.
33. Cohen JD, Li L, Wang Y, et al. Detection and localization of surgically resectable cancers with a multi-analyte blood test. Science. 2018;359:926–30.
34. Phallen J, Sausen M, Adleff V, et al. Direct detection of early-stage cancers using circulating tumor DNA. Sci Transl Med. 2017;9(403):eaan2415.
35. Rahib L, Smith BD, Aizenberg R, et al. Projecting cancer incidence and deaths to 2030: the unexpected burden of thyroid, liver, and pancreas cancers in the United States. Cancer Res. 2014;74:2913–21.
36. Conroy T, Hammel P, Hebbar M, et al. FOLFIRINOX or gemcitabine as adjuvant therapy for pancreatic cancer. N Engl J Med. 2018;379:2395–406.
37. Neoptolemos JP, Palmer DH, Ghaneh P, et al. Comparison of adjuvant gemcitabine and capecitabine with gemcitabine monotherapy in patients with resected pancreatic cancer (ESPAC-4): a multicentre, open-label, randomised, phase 3 trial. Lancet. 2017;389:1011–24.
38. European Study Group on Cystic Tumours of the P. European evidence-based guidelines on pancreatic cystic neoplasms. Gut. 2018;67:789–804.
39. Tanaka M, Fernandez-Del Castillo C, Kamisawa T, et al. Revisions of international con-sensus Fukuoka guidelines for the management of IPMN of the pancreas. Pancreatology. 2017;17:738–53.
40. Del Chiaro M, Segersvard R, Lohr M, Verbeke C. Early detection and prevention of pancreatic cancer: is it really possible today? World J Gastroenterol. 2014;20:12118–31.
41. Hawighorst T, Velasco P, Streit M, et al. Thrombospondin 2 plays a protective role in multistep carcinogenesis: a novel host anti-tumor defense mechanism. EMBO J. 2001;20:2631–40.
42. Kim J, Hoffman JP, Alpaugh RK, et al. An iPSC line from human pancreatic ductal adeno-carcinoma undergoes early to invasive stages of pancreatic cancer progression. Cell Rep. 2013;3:2088–99.
43. Kim J, Bamlet WR, Oberg AL, et al. Detection of early pancreatic ductal adenocarcinoma with thrombospondin-2 and CA19-9 blood markers. Sci Transl Med. 2017;9(398):eaah5583.
44. Berger AW, Schwerdel D, Reinacher-Schick A, et al. A blood-based multi marker assay supports the differential diagnosis of early-stage pancreatic cancer. Theranostics. 2019;9(5):1280–7.

45. Bailey P, Chang DK, Nones K, et al. Genomic analyses identify molecular subtypes of pancreatic cancer. Nature. 2016;531:47–52.
46. Mishra NK, Guda C. Genome-wide DNA methylation analysis reveals molecular subtypes of pancreatic cancer. Oncotarget. 2017;8:28990–9012.
47. Huang MH, Chou YW, Li MH, et al. Epigenetic targeting DNMT1 of pancreatic ductal adenocarcinoma using interstitial control release biodegrading polymer reduced tumor growth through hedgehog pathway inhibition. Pharmacol Res. 2018;139:50–61.
48. Aravanis AM, Lee M, Klausner RD. Next-generation sequencing of circulating tumor DNA for early cancer detection. Cell. 2017;168:571–4.
49. Newman AM, Bratman SV, To J, et al. An ultrasensitive method for quantitating circulating tumor DNA with broad patient coverage. Nat Med. 2014;20:548–54.
50. Pietrasz D, Pecuchet N, Garlan F, et al. Plasma circulating tumor DNA in pancreatic cancer patients is a prognostic marker. Clin Cancer Res. 2017;23:116–23.
51. Chen H, Tu H, Meng ZQ, et al. K-ras mutational status predicts poor prognosis in unresectable pancreatic cancer. Eur J Surg Oncol. 2010;36:657–62.
52. Sausen M, Phallen J, Adleff V, et al. Clinical implications of genomic alterations in the tumour and circulation of pancreatic cancer patients. Nat Commun. 2015;6:7686.
53. Hadano N, Murakami Y, Uemura K, et al. Prognostic value of circulating tumour DNA in patients undergoing curative resection for pancreatic cancer. Br J Cancer. 2016;115:59–65.
54. Bernard V, Kim DU, San Lucas FA, et al. Circulating nucleic acids are associated with outcomes of patients with pancreatic cancer. Gastroenterology. 2019;156:108–18.. e104
55. Kinde I, Wu J, Papadopoulos N, et al. Detection and quantification of rare mutations with massively parallel sequencing. Proc Natl Acad Sci U S A. 2011;108:9530–5.
56. Takai E, Totoki Y, Nakamura H, et al. Clinical utility of circulating tumor DNA for molecular assessment and precision medicine in pancreatic cancer. Adv Exp Med Biol. 2016;924:13–7.
57. Zill OA, Greene C, Sebisanovic D, et al. Cell-free DNA next-generation sequencing in pancreatobiliary carcinomas. Cancer Discov. 2015;5:1040–8.
58. Kruger S, Heinemann V, Ross C, et al. Repeated mutKRAS ctDNA measurements represent a novel and promising tool for early response prediction and therapy monitoring in advanced pancreatic cancer. Ann Oncol. 2018;29:2348–55.

Chapter 8
PDAC Subtypes/Stratification

Holly Brunton, Giuseppina Caligiuri, Gareth J. Inman, and Peter Bailey

Large-scale sequencing analyses have transformed our understanding of pancreatic ductal adenocarcinoma (PDAC) and have defined several molecular taxonomies that now guide pre-clinical and clinical therapeutic development. The identification of molecularly defined subgroups of patients with distinct biological underpinnings and potential therapeutic vulnerabilities promises a step change in clinical practice. However, the ability of these molecular taxonomies to guide therapy and ultimately improve patient outcomes remains to be established. This review examines the current status of molecular subtyping in PDAC and explores subtype-specific biology, potential subtype-specific vulnerabilities and their potential relevance to clinical practice.

H. Brunton
Cancer Research UK Beatson Institute, Glasgow, UK

G. Caligiuri
Cold Spring Harbor Laboratory, Cold Spring Harbor, NY, USA

G. J. Inman
Cancer Research UK Beatson Institute, Glasgow, UK and Institute of Cancer Sciences, University of Glasgow, Glasgow, UK

P. Bailey (✉)
Cancer Research UK Beatson Institute, Glasgow, UK and Institute of Cancer Sciences, University of Glasgow, Glasgow, UK

Department of General Surgery, University of Heidelberg, Heidelberg, Germany
e-mail: Peter.Bailey.2@glasgow.ac.uk

© Springer Nature Switzerland AG 2020
C. W. Michalski et al. (eds.), *Translational Pancreatic Cancer Research*,
Molecular and Translational Medicine,
https://doi.org/10.1007/978-3-030-49476-6_8

From Single Genetic Aberrations to Actionable Genomic Subtypes

International sequencing consortia have molecularly profiled over 25,000 genomes [1, 2]. At the outset, these studies promised to transform clinical decision-making by identifying genetic aberrations or actionable mutations in individual patients, such as recurrent hot-spot mutations in oncogenes, that are susceptible to therapeutic intervention. To date, however, this promise has only been realised in a relatively small number of cancer types with recurrent BCR-ABL gene fusions in chronic myeloid leukaemia (CML) being a prime example of a recurrent actionable mutation (targetable by tyrosine kinase inhibitors) that has transformed clinical practice and patient outcomes [3, 4].

PDAC is one cancer type where the utility of patient selection, based on the presence of a single actionable mutation, is severely challenged by a paucity of recurrent clinically actionable events [5–12]. The PDAC mutational landscape is dominated by recurrent, predominantly overlapping mutations in KRAS, TP53, SMAD4 and CDKN2A (>50%) with a subset of additional genes including KDM6A, MLL3, ARID1A, TGFBR2, RBM10 and BCORL1 recurrently mutated in 5–10% of patient samples [6, 10]. The mutational landscape of PDAC is, however, complex with a long tail of low prevalence mutations contributing to significant intra-tumour heterogeneity. The majority of single gene aberrations occur at low prevalence (<2%) with genetic biomarkers of drug response such as ERBB2 amplification, BRAF gene fusions/mutations and BRCA1/2 falling within this long tail of low prevalence mutations [6, 13, 14]. Despite the obvious relevance of these predictive biomarkers to clinical practice, their low prevalence in PDAC patient populations has limited their uptake as economically viable therapeutic targets.

Notwithstanding the inherent challenges in defining patient groups using single genetic biomarkers of therapeutic response, other readouts of genomic abnormality including structural variation (SV) and mutational signatures have defined larger patient subgroups with potential clinical utility [6, 15]. SVs including deletions, amplifications, duplications and translocations can be grouped on the basis of frequency and distribution to define four genomic SV subtypes, namely, stable (<50 structural variations per genome); scattered (50–200 structural variants per genome); locally rearranged (>200 structural variants clustered on less than 3 chromosomes); or unstable (>200 structural variants distributed across the genome). Of these, the unstable SV subtype is significantly associated with subgroups of patients having mutations in DNA damage repair pathway (DDR) genes including BRCA1, BRCA2 and PALB2 [6]. Six mutational signatures, which define specific mutational processes active in tumour cells, have been identified in PDAC. Four of these mutational signatures are associated with known mutational processes and include a BRCA mutational signature, an age-related signature, a DNA mismatch repair (MMR) deficiency signature and an APOBEC signature (APOBEC family of cytidine deaminases) [6, 15].

The identification of subgroups of patients harbouring genomic abnormalities that are associated with defects in DNA damage repair and/or MMR highlights the potential utility of these genomic readouts for clinical decision-making. A hallmark of cancers with defective DDR is their vulnerability to specific DNA damaging agents such as platinum and PARP inhibitors. Platinum-based therapies are widely used in other cancer settings, and there is growing evidence for their efficacy in PDAC [6, 16]. Exceptional responders to platinum therapy are well documented in small subsets of PDAC patients, and BRCA1 and BRCA2 germline carriers show significant responses to both platinum and PARP inhibitors [6]. Although germline and somatic mutations in DDR pathway genes such as BRCA1/2 occur at low prevalence, the integration of orthogonal genomic readouts of DDR deficiency suggests that platinum therapy and/or novel drugs targeting similar mechanisms (such as PARP inhibitors) may be effective in a large subset of PDAC patients [6]. It has been calculated that 24% of all PDAC tumours harbour either an unstable genomes (>200 structural variants per genome); somatic and germline mutations in BRCA pathway genes; a BRCA mutational signature; or combinations thereof [6]. Importantly, the classification of PDAC patients using a combination of these orthogonal measures can predict response to platinum therapy [6].

Microsatellite instability (MSI) occurs in 1–2% of resectable PDAC and is a hallmark of DNA mismatch repair deficiency which is commonly associated with mutations in the MMR genes MSH2 and MLH1 [7]. MSI is reliably detectable using immunohistochemical assays for MSH1, PMS2, MLH1 and MSH6 expression [7] or NGS (single gene mutations and MMR mutational signature) [6, 17] and is a predictive biomarker of response to immune checkpoint inhibitors [18]. Pembrolizumab, which selectively targets the lymphocyte programmed cell death 1 receptor (PD-1), has recently been approved as a first-line treatment for solid tumours with MSI [19]. Recent evidence also suggests that ARID1A plays a role in DNA mismatch repair with deleterious mutations in ARID1A associated with increased immune infiltrates and significant antitumor response to immune checkpoint inhibitors [20]. These findings suggest that the combination of both MSI and deleterious ARID1A mutations may define a larger group of PDAC patients responsive to immune checkpoint inhibitors but this remains to be determined. In addition, ARID1A mutations have been shown to induce an increased reliance on ATR as a consequence of topoisomerase 2A and cell cycle defects and are consequently more sensitive to ATR inhibitors [21]. This study highlights the potential of using ARID1A mutational status as a readout for ATR targeting and provides further evidence that ARID1A mutational status may be an important biomarker of therapeutic response in PDAC.

A key challenge in deploying mutational profiling in the clinic is defining which genomic events in a given tumour are "actionable" [22]. In particular, although platforms and methodologies to detect mutations and/or genomic abnormalities are proceeding at pace, our ability to understand the relevance of these aberrations with respect to clinical decision-making remains a significant challenge. Further, despite some success in defining DDR deficiency as a large actionable segment in PDAC (approx. <= 24% of patient cohorts), additional biomarkers of therapeutic response are urgently required. In this regard, the transcriptomic profiling of PDAC has defined additional patient subgroups with potential therapeutic vulnerabilities and is helping to redefine our understanding of PDAC tumour biology [10, 12, 23–26].

Transcriptomic Subtypes of PDAC

The identification of intrinsic subtypes using gene expression data has been successfully employed in a number of different cancer settings to define broad and potentially actionable subgroups of patients. As an exemplar, the classification of colorectal cancer by gene expression profiling has identified robust and reproducible subtypes that show promise in clinical practice [27–30]. mRNA profiling of PDAC by several different groups has defined *at least* four intrinsic molecular subtypes and produced three major classification schemes with differing nomenclature [10, 12, 23–26]. A comparison of these schemes highlights several important similarities and dichotomies and underlines the need to align efforts to generate a new consensus classification for PDAC that better defines patient subgroups and clinical decision-making.

Three major studies, in particular, have shaped debate concerning the classification of PDAC using gene expression profiles. The first of these, performed by *Collisson and Sadanandam* et al., used primary resected PDAC (micro-dissected to remove stromal contamination) to define three subtypes referred to as exocrine-like, classical and quasi-mesenchymal [23]. Genes associated with exocrine function (digestive enzyme genes), markers of epithelial adhesion and terminal differentiation (e.g. GATA6) and gain in mesenchymal function were specifically expressed in either the exocrine-like, classical or quasi-mesenchymal subtypes, respectively. In addition, the quasi-mesenchymal subtype was correlated with high tumour grade and poor patient outcomes.

The second major study performed by Moffit et al. used a supervised classification approach to informatically segregate tumour cell *intrinsic* gene expression signatures from "contaminating" gene expression signatures commonly associated with terminally differentiated normal pancreas (exocrine and endocrine genes signatures) and stromal cell populations (pancreatic stellate gene signatures) [24]. This analysis identified two major PDAC tumour cell *intrinsic* subtypes named classical and basal-like and additional tumour cell *extrinsic* or stromal subtypes referred to as normal and activated. Importantly, this study was the first to model the complex interplay between tumour cell intrinsic subtypes and specific stromal cell signals with combinations of tumour-specific and stromal subtypes associated with different patient survival.

The third major classification scheme proposed by Bailey et al. used primary resectable PDAC with >40% cellularity to define four subtypes referred to as aberrantly differentiated endocrine exocrine (ADEX), pancreatic progenitor, immunogenic and squamous [31]. These subtypes overlapped directly with the Collisson classification Scheme [23] with the exception of the immunogenic subtype which was defined by the significant enrichment of genes associated with specific immune cell populations, including T cells and B cells. Although gene expression values defining the immunogenic subtype most certainly originate from immune infiltrates resident in the tumour stroma, an underlying pancreatic progenitor-like gene expression profile was clearly evident in tumours falling within this subtype. In addition, the quasi-mesenchymal subtype of Collisson was renamed squamous due to the significant enrichment of several pan-squamous characteristics, including mutations in KDM6A, enrichment of the ΔNTP63 isoform of p63 and a significant association with adenosquamous PDAC histology. This study also demonstrated for the first time that squamous tumours undergo a profound epigenetic shift, with changes in DNA methylation orchestrating the downregulation of pancreatic specific transcription factors (PDX1, GATA6, HNF1A), which control pancreatic cell fate determination, and the activation of multigene programmes regulated by ΔNTP63 and c-MYC that drive squamous-like differentiation. Supporting a role for epigenetic dysregulation in the genesis of PDAC subtypes, the squamous subtype was found to be enriched for mutations in COMPASS (COMplex of Proteins Associated with Set1-like) complex members KDM6A, MLL2 and MLL3 that function as chromatin-modifying enzymes.

Recent studies performed by Puleo et al. [26] and Maurer et al. [32] have started to refine our understanding of these established classification schemes and in particular describe in greater detail how different stromal cell populations exist in concert with tumour cell intrinsic subtypes. Puleo et al. transcriptomically profiled 309 resected PDAC tumours to define 5 subtypes using both tumour cell intrinsic and microenvironment-derived expression signatures. This work identified two subtypes with low stromal content referred to as pure basal-like and pure classical and three additional subtypes with high stromal content referred to as stroma activated, desmoplastic and immune classical. In a complementary study, Maurer et al. performed laser capture microdissection on resected PDAC to transcriptomically profile pure epithelial or stromal cell populations. This analysis identified two major stromal subtypes, an extracellular matrix-rich (ECM-rich) and immune-rich subtype, with basal-like tumours exhibiting an ECM profile having the worst overall survival. Importantly, both Puleo et al. and Maurer et al. provide evidence that the previously proposed exocrine-like/ADEX subtype is not a genuine PDAC subtype but rather a consequence of normal pancreatic contamination in profiled tumour samples.

Towards a Consensus Transcriptomic Classification of PDAC

The transcriptomic classification of PDAC by several different groups has generated a number of interesting contrasts and ultimately divided opinion. A major point of difference concerns the inclusion of the exocrine-like/ADEX subtype as a bona fide subtype of disease. The weight of current opinion is now favouring the exclusion of this subtype on the basis that it represents normal pancreatic contamination [12, 24, 26, 32]; however, the identification of exocrine-like/ADEX gene expression in patient-derived xenografts and cell lines suggests that further study is required [8, 33, 34]. A second point of contention concerns the inclusion of a separate immunogenic subtype. Bailey et al. demonstrate that the immunogenic subtype is a complex admixture of gene expression comprising both pancreatic progenitor-like and immune gene expression (predominantly associated with T cells and B cells) [10]. The separation of the pancreatic progenitor signature into immune high (Immunogenic) and immune low (pancreatic progenitor) suggests that signals from the underlying epithelium (immunogenic subset) may drive tumour cell immunogenicity. Recent studies, however, argue that immune infiltrates are enriched across all tumour intrinsic subtypes and their prevalence is primarily driven by tumour cellularity of sequenced samples [12]. In addition, these studies advocate the use of integrated classification schemes that apply both tumour cell intrinsic and stromal subtype signatures to optimally define prognostic PDAC subtypes [26, 32].

Despite differences in nomenclature and interpretation, a direct "side-by-side" comparison of the established classification schemes demonstrates considerable overlap and several common themes. In particular, strong alignment exists between the classical-pancreatic progenitor and quasi-mesenchymal/basal-like/squamous subtypes. Together these overlapping subtypes define two broad prognostic classes (referred to herein as classical-pancreatic and squamous) with squamous tumours associated with significantly poorer outcomes. These classes are delineated by the differential expression of pancreatic specific transcription factors, such as GATA6, PDX1 and HNF1A, that act to specify and maintain pancreatic identity and which are lost in squamous tumours. Importantly, the dynamic changes in gene expression observed between the classical-pancreatic and squamous classes are driven by an underlying shift in the epigenome. Multiple studies have now established that the squamous subtype is defined by changes in DNA methylation that ultimately repress pancreatic identity and activate multigene programmes that drive squamous-like differentiation [12, 26, 35]. Further, despite different approaches in modelling stromal infiltrate and the ever-growing number of stromal subtypes, there is a clear consensus that signals from the stroma play an important role in disease progression. An outstanding question in this regard is whether tumour cell intrinsic subtypes contribute to the levels and/or composition of stromal (fibroblasts and immune cell) infiltrate. Additional refinement and integration of tumour cell intrinsic and stromal subtype signatures will help to drive a greater understanding of tumour-stroma crosstalk and ultimately inform better prognostic models of disease.

Pre-clinical Models, Transcriptomic Subtypes and Subtype Plasticity

The LSL-Kras$^{G12D/+}$, LSL-Trp53$^{R172H/+}$, Pdx-1-Cre (KPC) genetically engineered mouse model (GEMM) is the standard model for understanding PDAC and recapitulates many of the key characteristics of human disease including the formation of precursor lesions (PanINs) leading to frank PDAC and the development of metastatic lesions within distant organs including the liver [36, 37]. The comprehensive interrogation of KPC GEMMs has identified distinct cellular populations important for disease progression and in particular has highlighted an important role for stromal cells including cancer-associated fibroblasts (CAFs) and immune cells in this process [38, 39]. Importantly, recent work has demonstrated that epithelial-derived cells isolated from KPC tumours recapitulate the transcriptionally defined subtypes of human PDAC [40]. Consistent with human disease, murine tumours having squamous transcriptional profiles are associated with high-grade poorly differentiated histologies, whereas tumours having classical-progenitor gene expression profiles are associated with low-grade well-differentiated histologies. This work also demonstrates that these histological and transcriptionally distinguishable PDAC subtypes exhibit distinct modes of migration.

Recent evidence demonstrates that stromal cues play an important role in modulating tumour cell intrinsic subtypes [39, 41, 42]. Extensive desmoplasia is a hallmark of PDAC and is characterised by a dense fibrotic stroma comprising CAFs and immune cells. A complex cocktail of tumour cell intrinsic and stromal cues help to shape this tumour microenvironment (TME) with signals from both CAFs and specific immune cell populations directing the differentiation state of PC tumour cells. In particular, PDAC exhibits substantial immune cell heterogeneity, and there is now a growing appreciation that tumour cell intrinsic factors shape the immune TME [10, 39, 42, 43]. PDAC subtypes are associated with distinct immune cell populations with tumours exhibiting a classical-pancreatic subtype enriched for transcripts associated with B cells, CD4+ and CD8+ tumour-infiltrating lymphocytes (TILs) and tumours falling within the squamous subtype characterised by myeloid cell gene enrichment and a general absence of B-cell and T-cell transcripts [10]. Remarkably, targeted ablation of myeloid cells in KPC GEMMs by the selective inhibition of CSF1R produces a profound shift in subtype from predominantly squamous-like to classical-pancreatic [42]. Inhibition of CSF1R causes a profound reprogramming of the tumour cell intrinsic pathways underpinning PDAC subtypes, including the re-activation of transcriptional networks controlled by transcription factors that act as master regulators of exocrine or endocrine pancreatic identity. Further underpinning an important paracrine role for the stroma in PC, signalling cues originating from CAFs have also been shown to modulate tumour cell intrinsic pathways [41]. Specifically, stromal cues have been shown to drive distinct changes in tumour cell metabolic pathways and to re-programme the tumour epigenome [41].

Recent evidence also demonstrates that the two major transcriptomic subtypes of PDAC are defined by distinct epigenetic landscapes that are largely shaped by specific subsets of TFs that orchestrate subtype-specific multigene programmes [10, 35, 44]. Using a collection of 23 PDAC patient-derived tumour xenografts, Lomberk et al. used chromatin states to epigenetically classify PDAC subtypes [35]. Three major epigenetic states were established described as cluster 1 (composed of enhancers active in most squamous samples), cluster 2 (enhancers active in classical-pancreatic samples) and cluster 3 (active promoters in classical-pancreatic samples). TFs associated with super-enhancers in the classical-pancreatic subtype included GATA6, FOS, FOXP1, FOXP4, KLF4, ELF3 and CUX1. Squamous-specific super-enhancer regulation was associated with the hepatocyte growth factor receptor MET. Interestingly, MET siRNA-mediated knockdown in squamous samples induced a transcriptional switch towards classical-pancreatic associated gene programmes, in particular those driven by GATA6. This evidence implicates super-enhancers as critical regulatory hubs that both maintain pancreatic identity and control the activation of genes that drive squamous differentiation. Additionally, this data demonstrates that certain subtype-specific gene programmes maintain a degree of plasticity that can be manipulated therapeutically.

Dysregulation of super-enhancer activity by inactivation of key chromatin modifiers including KDM6A may lead to a loss of both pancreatic identity and the activation of squamous gene programmes. Consistent with this hypothesis, squamous tumours are enriched for mutations in COMPASS-like complex members KDM6A, MLL2 and MLL3. These findings suggest that mutations in key chromatin effectors may rewire the regulatory landscape of PDAC and subvert cell fate decisions to favour squamous-like cell states. In support of this notion, GEMMs of PDAC with targeted deletion of Kdm6a in the context of oncogenic Kras develop squamous-like metastatic pancreatic cancer that phenocopies the progression and histological features of human disease [45]. Mechanistically, deregulation of the COMPASS complex by Kdm6a deletion induces the aberrant activation of super-enhancers regulating the expression of ΔNTP63, MYC and RUNX3 that in turn subvert pancreatic identity and induce squamous differentiation. In a complementary study, the overexpression of ΔNTP63 was shown to drive a classical-pancreatic to squamous transcriptional reprogramming in human classical-pancreatic PDAC cells [46]. As found in the mouse Kdm6a GEMM, squamous identity was associated with profound alterations in enhancer landscape.

The plasticity exhibited by PDAC cells has important implications for disease progression, drug resistance and the development of subtype-specific therapies. Deciphering the transcriptional regulatory networks underpinning subtype plasticity will provide important mechanistic insights into disease progression and highlight potential therapeutic vulnerabilities.

PDAC Subtyping and Translational Protocols

The translation of molecular subtypes into clinical practice is in its infancy; however, several groups have made significant gains in applying genomic and/or transcriptomic subtyping to inform patient selection for targeted therapy. To bridge the translational gap between molecular subtyping and clinical decision-making, the PancSeq protocol was developed which enables rapid turnaround genomic analysis of metastatic or locally advanced PDAC [47]. Mutational signature analysis of WES data identified four main mutational signatures described as COSMIC 1 (C > T transitions at CpG dinucleotides, Aging), COSMIC2 and 13 (APOBEC), COSMIC3 (HRD and BRCA deficient) and COSMIC17 (unknown) which converged on at least two well-established subtypes of PDAC including a classical-pancreatic subtype and a squamous subtype. Interestingly integrated analysis which included normal tissue gene expression as well as that of tumours was able to identify not only samples by subtype but also site of biopsy, suggesting that different tumour locations have differing tumour biology. In this cohort of 71 patients, 37% harboured germline or somatic mutations in DDR genes, 9 of whom were characterised as having an enrichment for the HRD/COSMIC3 signature. A further 7% of patients also had enrichment for the HRD/COSMIC3 signature but no apparent HR gene mutations. Two of these patients could be explained by downregulation of the mRNA of the HR repair protein RAD51C, highlighting the importance of using multiple methods of omics characterisation to obtain the full spectrum of potential therapeutic candidates. Furthermore, integration of the unstable SV subtype with the HRD/COSMIC3 mutation signature and DDR gene mutations could further identify potential responders to DDR therapy.

Using genomics-driven precision medicine, Aung et al. demonstrate the feasibility of using whole genome and RNA sequencing within a clinically relevant timeframe to direct clinical decision-making and identify individuals predicted to be sensitive to chemotherapy [48]. The COMPASS (Comprehensive Molecular Characterization of Advanced Pancreatic Ductal Adenocarcinoma for Better Treatment Selection) trial identified that PDAC patients with stage III/IV and transcriptionally subtyped as classical-pancreatic responded better to first-line chemotherapy compared to squamous tumours, demonstrating that better or exceptional responders could be identified using subtyping methodology.

Recent success to map clinical response with transcriptomic subtypes has been observed using a pancreatic cancer patient-derived organoid (PDO) library [49]. The PDO library is composed of 66 PDO cultures obtained from primary tumours and metastases that recapitulates the transcriptional classical-pancreatic and squamous subtypes and the mutational landscape of primary pancreatic cancer. Within the library, 57 of these organoids were isolated from 55 treatment-naïve patients, which offers a unique research tool to establish the transcriptional landscape before neoadjuvant therapy that typically occurs before surgical resection. Tiriac and colleagues demonstrate that within a clinically meaningful timeframe, drug-sensitivity profiles can be generated that reflect a patient's response to therapy. Therapeutic profiling which was termed "pharmacotyping" was performed on the PDAC PDOs using commonly used chemotherapeutics used to treat PDAC, and for each chemotherapeutic agent, the PDO library was subtyped into three groups: the least responsive, the most responsive and those exhibiting intermediate response. Gene expression signatures were further refined to include genes whose expression correlated with drug sensitivity. When the gemcitabine-specific PDO-sensitive signature was applied to a subgroup of patients who received gemcitabine monotherapy, patients with significantly better PFS were found to be enriched for the gemcitabine-sensitive signature. Importantly, the same analysis on treatment-naïve patients failed to identify individuals with improved PFS or OS suggesting that this signature is treatment dependent and may be clinically relevant for predicting response to and ultimately selection of patients for gemcitabine treatment.

Conclusions

Pancreatic cancer is associated with dismal patient outcomes. Most patients are unsuitable for surgical resection, and current treatment regimens have not required routine molecular profiling. Consequently, most patients receive non-targeted and unselected combination chemotherapy. Recent comprehensive molecular landscaping studies on samples obtained from fine needle biopsies, surgical biopsy and autopsy coupled with profiling of patient-derived cell lines and organoids are beginning to reveal a potentially brighter future for PC management. Integrated genomic and transcriptomic analyses have enabled the generation of molecular signatures that reveal the underlying biology of PC, identify potential therapeutic vulnerabilities and may predict patient response to chemotherapy. The robustness of these signatures will only increase with the inclusion of more samples, the development of sequencing methodologies and integration of pre-clinical, clinical and clinical trial-associated datasets. Increasing the breadth and depth of our datasets will enable the use of artificial intelligence and deep learning approaches to generate more clinically meaningful classifiers. Ultimately, we hope that these studies will enable the development of molecularly based and cost-effective companion diagnostics that inform clinical decisions that result in improved patient outcomes.

References

1. Cancer Genome Atlas Research N. Comprehensive genomic characterization defines human glioblastoma genes and core pathways. Nature. 2008;455(7216):1061–8.
2. International Cancer Genome C, Hudson TJ, Anderson W, Artez A, Barker AD, Bell C, et al. International network of cancer genome projects. Nature. 2010;464(7291):993–8.
3. Druker BJ, Tamura S, Buchdunger E, Ohno S, Segal GM, Fanning S, et al. Effects of a selective inhibitor of the Abl tyrosine kinase on the growth of Bcr-Abl positive cells. Nat Med. 1996;2(5):561–6.
4. Nicolini FE, Basak GW, Kim DW, Olavarria E, Pinilla-Ibarz J, Apperley JF, et al. Overall survival with ponatinib versus allogeneic stem cell transplantation in Philadelphia chromosome-positive leukemias with the T315I mutation. Cancer. 2017;123(15):2875–80.
5. Biankin AV, Waddell N, Kassahn KS, Gingras MC, Muthuswamy LB, Johns AL, et al. Pancreatic cancer genomes reveal aberrations in axon guidance pathway genes. Nature. 2012;491(7424):399–405.
6. Waddell N, Pajic M, Patch AM, Chang DK, Kassahn KS, Bailey P, et al. Whole genomes redefine the mutational landscape of pancreatic cancer. Nature. 2015;518(7540):495–501.
7. Humphris JL, Patch AM, Nones K, Bailey PJ, Johns AL, McKay S, et al. Hypermutation in pancreatic cancer. Gastroenterology. 2017;152(1):68–74.. e2
8. Smit VT, Boot AJ, Smits AM, Fleuren GJ, Cornelisse CJ, Bos JL. KRAS codon 12 mutations occur very frequently in pancreatic adenocarcinomas. Nucleic Acids Res. 1988;16(16):7773–82.
9. Jones S, Zhang X, Parsons DW, Lin JC, Leary RJ, Angenendt P, et al. Core signaling pathways in human pancreatic cancers revealed by global genomic analyses. Science. 2008;321(5897):1801–6.
10. Bailey P, Chang DK, Nones K, Johns AL, Patch AM, Gingras MC, et al. Genomic analyses identify molecular subtypes of pancreatic cancer. Nature. 2016;531(7592):47–52.

11. Witkiewicz AK, McMillan EA, Balaji U, Baek G, Lin WC, Mansour J, et al. Whole-exome sequencing of pancreatic cancer defines genetic diversity and therapeutic targets. Nat Commun. 2015;6:6744.

12. Cancer Genome Atlas Research Network. Electronic address aadhe, Cancer Genome Atlas Research N. Integrated genomic characterization of pancreatic ductal adenocarcinoma. Cancer Cell. 2017;32(2):185–203 e13.

13. Chou A, Waddell N, Cowley MJ, Gill AJ, Chang DK, Patch AM, et al. Clinical and molecular characterization of HER2 amplified-pancreatic cancer. Genome Med. 2013;5(8):78.

14. Chmielecki J, Hutchinson KE, Frampton GM, Chalmers ZR, Johnson A, Shi C, et al. Comprehensive genomic profiling of pancreatic acinar cell carcinomas identifies recurrent RAF fusions and frequent inactivation of DNA repair genes. Cancer Discov. 2014;4(12):1398–405.

15. Alexandrov LB, Nik-Zainal S, Wedge DC, Aparicio SA, Behjati S, Biankin AV, et al. Signatures of mutational processes in human cancer. Nature. 2013;500(7463):415–21.

16. Pishvaian MJ, Biankin AV, Bailey P, Chang DK, Laheru D, Wolfgang CL, et al. BRCA2 secondary mutation-mediated resistance to platinum and PARP inhibitor-based therapy in pancreatic cancer. Br J Cancer. 2017;116(8):1021–6.

17. Niu B, Ye K, Zhang Q, Lu C, Xie M, McLellan MD, et al. MSIsensor: microsatellite instability detection using paired tumor-normal sequence data. Bioinformatics. 2014;30(7):1015–6.

18. Le DT, Uram JN, Wang H, Bartlett BR, Kemberling H, Eyring AD, et al. PD-1 blockade in tumors with mismatch-repair deficiency. N Engl J Med. 2015;372(26):2509–20.

19. Le DT, Durham JN, Smith KN, Wang H, Bartlett BR, Aulakh LK, et al. Mismatch repair deficiency predicts response of solid tumors to PD-1 blockade. Science. 2017;357(6349):409–13.

20. Shen J, Ju Z, Zhao W, Wang L, Peng Y, Ge Z, et al. ARID1A deficiency promotes mutability and potentiates therapeutic antitumor immunity unleashed by immune checkpoint blockade. Nat Med. 2018;24(5):556–62.

21. Williamson CT, Miller R, Pemberton HN, Jones SE, Campbell J, Konde A, et al. ATR inhibitors as a synthetic lethal therapy for tumours deficient in ARID1A. Nat Commun. 2016;7:13837.

22. Carr TH, McEwen R, Dougherty B, Johnson JH, Dry JR, Lai Z, et al. Defining actionable mutations for oncology therapeutic development. Nat Rev Cancer. 2016;16(5):319–29.

23. Collisson EA, Sadanandam A, Olson P, Gibb WJ, Truitt M, Gu S, et al. Subtypes of pancreatic ductal adenocarcinoma and their differing responses to therapy. Nat Med. 2011;17(4):500–3.

24. Moffitt RA, Marayati R, Flate EL, Volmar KE, Loeza SG, Hoadley KA, et al. Virtual microdissection identifies distinct tumor- and stroma-specific subtypes of pancreatic ductal adenocarcinoma. Nat Genet. 2015;47(10):1168–78.

25. Cancer Genome Atlas Research N. Comprehensive molecular profiling of lung adenocarcinoma. Nature. 2014;511(7511):543–50.

26. Puleo F, Nicolle R, Blum Y, Cros J, Marisa L, Demetter P, et al. Stratification of pancreatic ductal adenocarcinomas based on tumor and microenvironment features. Gastroenterology. 2018;155(6):1999–2013.. e3

27. Sadanandam A, Lyssiotis CA, Homicsko K, Collisson EA, Gibb WJ, Wullschleger S, et al. A colorectal cancer classification system that associates cellular phenotype and responses to therapy. Nat Med. 2013;19(5):619–25.

28. De Sousa EMF, Wang X, Jansen M, Fessler E, Trinh A, de Rooij LP, et al. Poor-prognosis colon cancer is defined by a molecularly distinct subtype and develops from serrated precursor lesions. Nat Med. 2013;19(5):614–8.

29. Marisa L, de Reynies A, Duval A, Selves J, Gaub MP, Vescovo L, et al. Gene expression classification of colon cancer into molecular subtypes: characterization, validation, and prognostic value. PLoS Med. 2013;10(5):e1001453.

30. Guinney J, Dienstmann R, Wang X, de Reynies A, Schlicker A, Soneson C, et al. The consensus molecular subtypes of colorectal cancer. Nat Med. 2015;21(11):1350–6.

31. Bailey P, Chang DK, Forget MA, Lucas FA, Alvarez HA, Haymaker C, et al. Exploiting the neoantigen landscape for immunotherapy of pancreatic ductal adenocarcinoma. Sci Rep. 2016;6:35848.

32. Maurer C, Holmstrom SR, He J, Laise P, Su T, Ahmed A, et al. Experimental microdissection enables functional harmonisation of pancreatic cancer subtypes. Gut. 2019;68(6):1034–43.
33. Noll EM, Eisen C, Stenzinger A, Espinet E, Muckenhuber A, Klein C, et al. CYP3A5 mediates basal and acquired therapy resistance in different subtypes of pancreatic ductal adenocarcinoma. Nat Med. 2016;22(3):278–87.
34. Knudsen ES, Balaji U, Mannakee B, Vail P, Eslinger C, Moxom C, et al. Pancreatic cancer cell lines as patient-derived avatars: genetic characterisation and functional utility. Gut. 2018;67(3):508–20.
35. Lomberk G, Blum Y, Nicolle R, Nair A, Gaonkar KS, Marisa L, et al. Distinct epigenetic landscapes underlie the pathobiology of pancreatic cancer subtypes. Nat Commun. 2018;9(1):1978.
36. Hingorani SR, Wang L, Multani AS, Combs C, Deramaudt TB, Hruban RH, et al. Trp53R172H and KrasG12D cooperate to promote chromosomal instability and widely metastatic pancreatic ductal adenocarcinoma in mice. Cancer Cell. 2005;7(5):469–83.
37. Gopinathan A, Morton JP, Jodrell DI, Sansom OJ. GEMMs as preclinical models for testing pancreatic cancer therapies. Dis Model Mech. 2015;8(10):1185–200.
38. Ohlund D, Handly-Santana A, Biffi G, Elyada E, Almeida AS, Ponz-Sarvise M, et al. Distinct populations of inflammatory fibroblasts and myofibroblasts in pancreatic cancer. J Exp Med. 2017;214(3):579–96.
39. Steele CW, Karim SA, Leach JDG, Bailey P, Upstill-Goddard R, Rishi L, et al. CXCR2 inhibition profoundly suppresses metastases and augments immunotherapy in pancreatic ductal adenocarcinoma. Cancer Cell. 2016;29(6):832–45.
40. Aiello NM, Maddipati R, Norgard RJ, Balli D, Li J, Yuan S, et al. EMT subtype influences epithelial plasticity and mode of cell migration. Dev Cell. 2018;45(6):681–95.. e4
41. Sherman MH, Yu RT, Tseng TW, Sousa CM, Liu S, Truitt ML, et al. Stromal cues regulate the pancreatic cancer epigenome and metabolome. Proc Natl Acad Sci U S A. 2017;114(5):1129–34.
42. Candido JB, Morton JP, Bailey P, Campbell AD, Karim SA, Jamieson T, et al. CSF1R(+) macrophages sustain pancreatic tumor growth through T cell suppression and maintenance of key gene programs that define the squamous subtype. Cell Rep. 2018;23(5):1448–60.
43. Li J, Byrne KT, Yan F, Yamazoe T, Chen Z, Baslan T, et al. Tumor cell-intrinsic factors underlie heterogeneity of immune cell infiltration and response to immunotherapy. Immunity. 2018;49(1):178–93.. e7
44. Sivakumar S, de Santiago I, Chlon L, Markowetz F. Master regulators of oncogenic KRAS response in pancreatic cancer: an integrative network biology analysis. PLoS Med. 2017;14(1):e1002223.
45. Andricovich J, Perkail S, Kai Y, Casasanta N, Peng W, Tzatsos A. Loss of KDM6A activates super-enhancers to induce gender-specific squamous-like pancreatic cancer and confers sensitivity to BET inhibitors. Cancer Cell. 2018;33(3):512–26.. e8
46. Somerville TDD, Xu Y, Miyabayashi K, Tiriac H, Cleary CR, Maia-Silva D, et al. TP63-mediated enhancer reprogramming drives the squamous subtype of pancreatic ductal adenocarcinoma. Cell Rep. 2018;25(7):1741–55.. e7
47. Aguirre AJ, Nowak JA, Camarda ND, Moffitt RA, Ghazani AA, Hazar-Rethinam M, et al. Real-time genomic characterization of advanced pancreatic cancer to enable precision medicine. Cancer Discov. 2018;8(9):1096–111.
48. Aung KL, Fischer SE, Denroche RE, Jang GH, Dodd A, Creighton S, et al. Genomics-driven precision medicine for advanced pancreatic cancer – early results from the COMPASS trial. Clin Cancer Res. 2017;24(6):1344–54.
49. Tiriac H, Belleau P, Engle DD, Plenker D, Deschenes A, Somerville TDD, et al. Organoid profiling identifies common responders to chemotherapy in pancreatic cancer. Cancer Discov. 2018;8(9):1112–29.

Chapter 9
Circulating Tumor Cells as Biomarkers in Pancreatic Cancer

Alina Hasanain and Christopher L. Wolfgang

Pancreatic cancer is highly lethal; the majority of patients present with metastatic disease at diagnosis, precluding surgical resection, which remains the only possibility for a cure in most cases [1]. Moreover, in those patients with clinically localized disease who undergo potentially curative surgical resection and systemic therapy, nearly 80% will have a metastatic relapse [2]. In recent years, there have been significant advances in understanding the biology of pancreatic cancer at the molecular level, including the characterization of the pancreatic cancer genome [3], global expression profiling [4–8], and proteomic analysis [9, 10]. In addition, it has been shown that the dense stroma associated with pancreatic cancer is important in tumor progression and metastasis [11, 12]. Extensive work in this area has demonstrated details of the interaction of supporting cells and cancer cells and of the role of the stroma in creating a barrier to chemotherapy and immunotherapy [13, 14]. This work has provided insight into how more efficacious treatments might be developed in the future. For example, the molecular analysis supports the clinical observation that pancreatic cancer is comprised of different subtypes, each with unique behaviors and responses to therapy. Thus, more effective therapy will need to be developed using a tailored approach that has become known as precision medicine.

One necessary step in the development of a precision approach to pancreatic cancer will require the identification of clinically useful biomarkers. A biomarker is defined as a characteristic that can be objectively measured and evaluated as an indicator of some biological process. An ideal biomarker must demonstrate the ability to accurately function as a surrogate of the biological feature in question. In this

A. Hasanain
Division of Surgical Oncology, Johns Hopkins Medical Institution, Baltimore, MD, USA

C. L. Wolfgang (✉)
Division of Surgical Oncology, Department of Surgery, Pathology and Oncology,
Johns Hopkins Medical Institution, Baltimore, MD, USA
e-mail: cwolfga2@jhmi.edu

© Springer Nature Switzerland AG 2020
C. W. Michalski et al. (eds.), *Translational Pancreatic Cancer Research*,
Molecular and Translational Medicine,
https://doi.org/10.1007/978-3-030-49476-6_9

sense, biomarkers can be derived from pathological specimens or non-pathologic tissues and fluids. The most commonly used biomarkers for the management of cancers are molecular measurements. Examples include tailored therapy for HER2/neu-positive lung cancers [15] or estrogen/progesterone-receptor-positive breast cancers [16].

In the case of pancreatic cancer, very few clinical biomarkers exist. Commonly, carbohydrate antigen 19-9 (CA19-9) is used as an adjunct in diagnosis and as marker of disease course, but has numerous limitations, which are described below. Other markers, such as SMAD4 status or GATA6 upregulation, currently require a tissue biopsy acquired through invasive means. Recently, the concept of blood-based liquid biopsy has been tested and been found useful in assessing cancer biomarkers [17]. Circulating tumor DNA (ctDNA), microsomes, and CTCs, among other factors, can all be identified in a blood sample. In particular, ctDNA and CTCs have shown promise in the search for biomarkers for pancreatic cancer.

The majority of published reports on liquid biopsy for pancreatic cancer have focused on ctDNA [18–20]. However, recent work on CTCs has demonstrated their utility as a possible biomarker, and for some applications, CTCs have advantages over ctDNA [21–24].

First described in the peripheral circulation of a woman with metastatic breast cancer in 1869 by Australian physician Thomas Ashworth [25], CTCs are rare, with 1 CTC per billion normal blood cells per milliliter of blood [26]. Their movement to and persistence in circulation indicates an ability to both migrate away from and survive after detachment from established tumor deposits and suggests that they are an important step in the metastasis of cancer. However, it has been shown that a very small percentage of CTCs contribute to metastatic lesions [27].

CTCs can express both epithelial and mesenchymal characteristics [28–30] and can exist as single cells or clusters of tumor microemboli, which appear to have increased metastatic potential [31]. Their half-life is extremely short, ranging from estimates of 25–30 minutes for single cells and 6–10 minutes for clusters [31] to 1–2.4 hours on average [32]. Thus, CTCs are an opportunity to view the behavior of a tumor in real time, from a single peripheral blood draw, and could possibly be used to both monitor the entire course of disease and more closely explore the dynamics of cancer biology and metastasis.

The purpose of this chapter is to review the current status of CTCs as a biomarker in pancreatic cancer and to additionally discuss the advantages and disadvantages of CTCs as a liquid biopsy.

Liquid Biopsy

A traditional biopsy has been the workhorse of cancer care in terms of establishing a diagnosis and assessment of biomarkers. Unfortunately, traditional biopsies have several limitations. They are a one-time measurement in an entire treatment course; serial sampling throughout the administration of surgical or medical therapy would be necessary to provide accurate and timely information about changing tumor biology. However, traditional biopsies are invasive, as they require resection or instrumentation of the tumor, meaning it is neither feasible nor practical to perform serial biopsies to guide treatment in real time.

Most tumors, including pancreatic cancer, consist of multiple cellular clones, and each has the potential for a unique biological behavior [33]. This creates a challenge in the choice and monitoring of therapy, as an effective treatment might be introduced early, with a significant initial response, and then fail to maintain results as resistant clones survive and multiply. Tumor heterogeneity also increases the probability of sampling error with the use of traditional biopsy. The inability to detect aggressive clones, which drive outcome, among all subclones has clinical implications in terms of guiding management in a precision approach.

As such, there has been recent interest in the development of biomarkers from bodily fluids – in particular, blood. A liquid biopsy can overcome the limitations of traditional biopsy, as it provides the opportunity to gain access to biomarkers through a minimally invasive method such as a blood draw, with little discomfort and virtually no risks. This advantage goes beyond patient comfort and safety, as a liquid biopsy is amenable to real-time analysis with multiple samples over time to monitor tumor progression and response to therapy. Finally, a liquid biopsy potentially represents the biomarkers of all clones of the primary tumor, metastatic deposits, and subclinical disease. The utility of liquid biopsies has been reported extensively in literature [19, 20, 34].

Currently, no blood-borne biomarker exists for pancreatic cancer that can be used to guide therapy or develop a true liquid biopsy. The most extensively used blood test for pancreatic cancer is CA19-9, which has been shown to be helpful in establishing a diagnosis and in determining recurrence or progression of disease following therapeutic interventions. Beyond these features, CA19-9 is limited in its capacity as a biomarker. Approximately 10% of Caucasians and 22% of African Americans are Lewis antigen negative, rendering this test useless in this population [35–37]. Moreover, CA19-9 is not specific for pancreatic cancer and can be elevated in other cancers as well as in benign conditions such as biliary obstruction, a common concomitant feature in pancreatic cancer [36].

The ideal liquid biopsy for the detection of pancreatic cancer biomarkers would be obtained through a blood draw, represent known intra- and inter-tumor heterogeneity, and give real-time information about the disease course and response to therapy. The ability to perform liquid biopsies for the management of cancer is based on the principle that either cells or molecular markers unique to the tumor are found in the plasma. These include intact cells, free DNA, RNA, and proteins.

The best studied forms of liquid biopsy are ctDNA and CTCs. One method is not superior to the other, and both have shown promise as clinically useful biomarkers in the treatment of pancreatic cancer. The information provided by ctDNA and CTCs is complementary; the isolation and analysis of both provides both the opportunity for a more accurate and extensive understanding of both tumor biology in general, possibly leading to novel therapeutic options, and the ability to predict outcomes in individual patients [34, 38].

While ctDNA, which consists of short DNA fragments released from dying or apoptotic primary tumor or metastatic lesions into blood, is a representation of the genome of all clones of the primary tumor and metastatic sites, CTCs, cells shed from all tumor deposits into circulation, provide not only DNA but also RNA and proteins for analysis. Unlike ctDNA, CTCs have the ability to represent each unique clone present within the tumor and are, as such, not an "average" of the entire disease burden. These cells are the probable source of metastatic lesions; hence, they provide the potential for direct analysis of tumor biology. Moreover, as a manifestation of disease relapse, their analysis may provide a real-time assessment of treatment failure [39–41]. Compared to ctDNA, however, CTCs are less prevalent in plasma, rendering them less sensitive as both a screening marker and for tracking the evolution of disease.

General Methods of CTC Detection

To comprehend the role of CTCs as a biomarker and to interpret literature on the subject, it is important to have a basic understanding of the methods of CTC isolation. Large discrepancies are noted in the data on this subject; much of the variability stems from the abundance of methods used to isolate and identify CTCs. Thus, enumeration and characterization of CTCs taken from the same patient at the same time point can differ depending on the method of isolation utilized.

A number of isolation techniques exist for CTC enrichment, including affinity-based methods relying on antibody-antigen interactions; size-based systems taking advantage of the differences in size between CTCs and other cells in the circulation, such as epithelial tumor cells; negative and positive selection-based approaches, such as flow cytometry; and electric-field-based systems, which separate CTCs by their dielectric properties. Additionally, microfluidic devices work to separate CTCs using laminar flow and allow for detection of multiple properties, such as cell size, deformability, and affinity [42–47].

As CTCs are rare and heterogeneous, isolation can be a challenge. More invasive experimental approaches, such as leukapheresis [48], may heighten the probability of capturing greater numbers of CTCs, but these methods are not ideally suited for clinical use. The type of collection tube, storage and transport conditions, time to analysis, and processing techniques can also impact CTC capture and are especially important when mRNA transcript identification is required or when attempts are being made to culture these cells [49].

Isolation of CTCs presents the additional limitation of possibly excluding cells with certain phenotypes, as current systems designed for this purpose all exploit a specific property of these cells (e.g., surface markers or size). For example, the Veridex CellSearch system (Janssen Diagnostics, Raritan, NJ), approved by the Food and Drug Administration (FDA) in 2004 for CTC detection in breast, prostate, and colorectal tumors, relies on surface EpCAM expression to immunomagnetically capture CTCs, which are further identified as CD45 negative and cytokeratin

(CK) 8-, 18-, or 19-positive cells [50]. However, this system will have limited success in isolating cells with low EpCAM expression. Contrastingly, size-based systems (e.g., ISET, or isolation by size of epithelial tumor cells – Rarecells, Paris, France) [43], while capable of greater sensitivity than platforms such as CellSearch [51, 52], will fail to detect cells smaller than the determined cutoff.

Once a pool of CTCs has been isolated, not only the cell itself but also its DNA, RNA, and proteins are available for analysis for relevant mutations and molecules that might become targets of therapeutic agents. Genomic analysis follows the same principles as for ctDNA with the added need for the extraction of genetic material. RNA and protein characterization allow for a more functional profiling of tumor cells.

CTCs as a Biomarker in Pancreatic Cancer

The prospects for the development of CTC-based biomarkers are immense, and this field is currently in its initial stages. Possibilities include simple enumeration, detailing of subclasses, mutational profiling, and expression profiling of these cells, to name a few. It should be noted that similar work is being done in other cancers – a worse prognosis has been linked to the presence of CTCs in breast cancer [21, 53–58], small cell lung cancer [59, 60], non-small cell lung cancer (NSCLC) [61, 62], cholangiocarcinoma [63], colorectal cancer [64–68], melanoma [69], and prostate cancer [70, 71]. Though CTC research in other cancer types is more well established, a growing body of evidence has demonstrated the predictive value of CTCs in pancreatic cancer. For example, de Albuquerque et al. reported a shorter progression-free survival in patients with CTCs in peripheral blood than in those without CTCs [41]. Similarly, Zhang et al. demonstrated a correlation between CTC positivity and both the development of metastases and worse survival in a cohort that was followed for 18 months [72].

Two meta-analysis reports, each comprising more than 600 patients with pancreatic cancer, have demonstrated a clear correlation between CTC positivity and worse outcomes. One of these studies drew associations between CTC positivity and poorer overall survival (HR = 1.64, 95% CI 1.39–1.94, $p < 0.00001$) and progression-free survival/recurrence-free survival (PFS/RFS) (HR = 2.36, 95% CI 1.41–3.96, $p < 0.00001$), concluding that CTCs can be predictive of pancreatic cancer disease course. CTCs predicted unfavorable outcomes at all time points throughout treatment (before, during, and posttreatment); CTCs were most predictive at the posttreatment time point (PFS/RFS HR = 8.36, 95% CI 3.22–21.67, $p < 0.0001$) [73]. Similarly, a separate meta-analysis, including 623 patients, concluded that CTC-positive patients have worse PFS (HR = 1.89, 95% CI 1.25–4.00, $p < 0.001$) and OS (HR = 1.23, 95% CI 0.88–2.08, $p < 0.001$) [74].

Circulating tumor cells within a given patient exhibit phenotypic heterogeneity, and not all types correlate with outcome. In a series of 50 patients with localized pancreatic cancer who underwent resection, Poruk et al. identified CTCs in 78% of

patients using ISET, followed by negative exclusion of leukocytes using immunofluorescence. In this study, two subpopulations of CTCs were identified – those
expressing cytokeratin alone (epithelial-type) and those expressing both cytokeratin
and vimentin (mesenchymal-type). On multivariate analysis with typical predictive
pathological features and CTC subtypes, there was no correlation between total
CTCs or epithelial-type CTCs with recurrence. Interestingly, there was a strong correlation between the mesenchymal-type CTCs and recurrence (HR 2.78 95% CI
1.3–5.9; $p = 0.01$) [29].

These results were further investigated by our group in a longitudinal study
called the CLUSTER trial (NCT2974764), where 200 patients undergoing surgical
resection of pancreatic cancer were enrolled and CTC concentrations in the patient
peripheral blood were measured at fixed intervals, starting prior to surgical resection, at 4 and 6 postoperative days, and every 2–3 months after this time point. In the
initial report on the subset of 136 patients who achieved a 12-month median follow-
up, CTCs were isolated based on size (>8 microns) and then stratified into epithelial
or epithelial-mesenchymal types (Fig. 9.1). Circulating tumor cells were identified
in the blood of 131 (96%) patients. The 58% of patients who had received no chemotherapy prior to surgery had significantly higher CTC numbers before resection
compared to patients who were post-neoadjuvant therapy (42%). There was a statis-
tically significant decrease in the number of CTCs counted in both the treated and
untreated patient populations after surgery; those with early recurrence, defined as
recurrence within 1 year of surgery, had significantly higher pre- and postoperative
CTC counts and a higher proportion of mixed epithelial-mesenchymal phenotype
CTCs. These findings appear to indicate that cells with this epithelial-mesenchymal
or transitional phenotype have a more aggressive biology, demonstrating the heterogeneity of CTCs [30]. The epithelial-mesenchymal transition (EMT) is defined as a

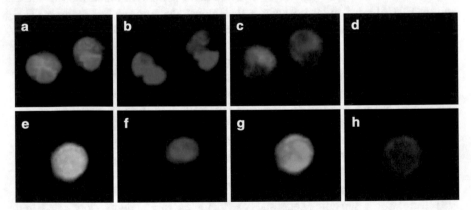

Fig. 9.1 Circulating tumor cells from pancreatic cancer patients. Immunofluorescence micros-
copy (at 20× magnification) here demonstrating epithelial-like (**a–d**) and epithelial-mesenchymal,
or transitional (**e–h**) circulating tumor cells in patients with pancreatic ductal adenocarcinoma. (**a**)
Pan-cytokeratin-positive, vimentin-negative CTC (merged), (**b**) DAPI (blue), (**c**) pan-cytokeratin
(green), (**d**) absence of vimentin (red); (**e**) pan-cytokeratin-positive and vimentin-positive CTC
(merge), (**f**) DAPI (blue), (**g**) pan-cytokeratin (green), and (**h**) vimentin (red)

reversible phenotypic change where a cancer cell with epithelial characteristics becomes more mesenchymal and invasive in phenotype, distinguished by a downregulation of E-cadherin, increased expression of mesenchymal markers such as N-cadherin and vimentin, and a loss of its ability to adhere to adjacent cells [75–79]. Prior work in pancreatic cancer has similarly linked EMT to disease dissemination and poorer prognosis [78, 80], and previous studies in other cancer types, such as breast, prostate, and lung carcinoma, have also connected EMT with metastatic disease [28, 81–83].

It is presumed that CTCs are directly responsible for mediating the dissemination of cancer. In order to accomplish this end, these cells must be capable of long periods of quiescence, self-renewal, and differentiation to form a tumor similar to the parent tumor. These are all features of cancer stem cells (Fig. 9.2) [84], also called tumor-initiating cells. Tumor-initiating cells are thought to constitute a small percentage of all cells within cancer (<0.01), but are necessary for driving growth [85]. In animal studies, cancer stem cells are able to establish tumors with as few as 100 cells; to compare, millions of cells from bulk tumor are required to produce the same results. A cancer stem cell from pancreatic cancer expresses CD133, CD44, and aldehyde dehydrogenase (ALDH) [86].

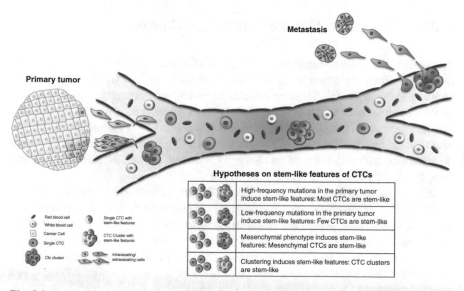

Fig. 9.2 Steps of cancer metastasis. This figure demonstrates what are proposed to be the steps required for the generation of cancer stem cells (tumor-initiating cells) and metastasis. A small percentage of cancer cells within the primary tumor undergo a phenotypic change to become more mesenchymal-like. This change is called an epithelial-mesenchymal transition (EMT) and is associated with cells developing the ability to grow in the absence of contact with the basement membrane, migrate into the circulatory system, and survive the harsh environment of circulation. These cells, now called CTCs, leave circulation through a poorly understood process and take up residence in the stroma of distant organs. A small subset acquire stemlike features; different possible mechanisms of this change are enumerated in the figure. (From Gkountela and Aceto [84], with permission)

Based on the finding of the importance of epithelial-mesenchymal-type CTCs and their correlation with outcome, the hypothesis that a subclass of CTCs would have a stem-cell phenotype was tested by our group. In a cohort of patients undergoing surgical resection, we reported the presence of a CK+/ALDH+ phenotype in 77% of all patients with CTCs at the time of resection. This phenotype predicted worse overall and disease-free survival (HR 3.4, 95% CI 1.2–9.8; $p = 0.03$). In further stratification of this cohort, patients with CTCs that were "triple-positive" for CK/CD133/CD44 had a much higher risk of recurrence compared to those with CK+/CD133+/CD44- cells (6.45, HR 6.45; 95% CI 2.1–19.7).

These results support the idea that at least a subset of CTCs have tumor-initiating cell properties, but there is currently no direct evidence that CTCs from pancreatic cancer are able to form metastases. To show that this is possible, it will be necessary to establish that these cells can be cultured. Attempts to culture CTCs from pancreatic cancer have not yet been successful, but CTC cultures have been reported for some other tumor types, such as colorectal and breast cancers [87–89], and co-culture of CTCs from early stage lung cancer patients using cancer-associated fibroblasts as a template on the CTC-Chip platform has also been reported [46].

Future Potential of CTCs in Pancreatic Cancer

The current literature demonstrates a role for CTCs as a biomarker to predict patient outcomes. However, much work still needs to be done, and the full potential of research in the field of CTCs in pancreatic cancer has not yet been reached. A wealth of information exists in the detailed evaluation of phenotype, expression profiling, and genetic data. Genome analysis of viable and intact CTCs indirectly reflects the tumor of origin. Studies show that sequencing CTC genomes is possible, and high concordance with a clonal relation between CTCs and the corresponding tumor has been found [22, 90].

In 2013, a group from Graz, Austria, was the first to outline a complete genomic profile of CTCs from patients with colorectal cancer through the implementation of array CGH and next-generation sequencing; they compared their findings with a broad panel of 68 known colorectal cancer-related genes and found matching mutations of cancer driver genes (KRAS, APC, PIK3CA) in the primary tumor, in metastatic deposits, and in the corresponding CTCs of the same patients [91]. Other studies confirmed these findings: exome sequencing on patients with lung cancer found that CTCs and tumor metastases had the same mutations [92], and the same held true for prostate cancer [90]. Ni et al. studied the copy number variations (CNVs) of CTCs in patients with lung adenocarcinoma and SCLC and concluded both that CNVs are specific to the type of cancer and that this pattern did not vary with therapy. However, it was also observed that chemotherapy did result in insertions/deletions and single nucleotide variations and that CTCs harbored tumor-related genes, including ones linked to resistance [92]. Therapy can halt cancer growth; nonetheless, it alters the clonal distribution of cancer and confers a selective advantage to certain cells, coupling the progression of disease with chemoresistance [93].

Similar work is now being reported in the field of pancreatic cancer. For example, RNA expression analysis of pancreatic cancer CTCs in a mouse model identified alterations in the expression of the gene Wnt2, which has been implicated in increasing the metastatic tendency of this cancer [23]. Court et al. analyzed CTCs for KRAS, an oncogene known to be involved at early stages in 95% of pancreatic cancers, and they were able to detect the mutation in 92% of the samples. However, due to difficulties in sequencing and accidental allele dropout during amplification, they were not able to identify KRAS in all the cells and concluded that at least ten CTCs were needed to consistently determine KRAS status due to decreased sensitivity below this threshold number [94]. Another study aimed to examine KRAS in CTCs and interestingly found that patients with detectable KRAS mutations in CTCs had a better survival compared to those with wild-type KRAS in CTCs (19.4 vs. 7.4 months, $p = 0.015$) [95].

The ability to directly evaluate tumor cell phenotype with molecular profiling at diagnosis will be an important and necessary feature for a biomarker for pancreatic cancer to possess. Circulating tumor cells can be assessed at the time of diagnosis and throughout the course of treatment. Since the half-life of CTCs is estimated to be on the order of minutes and as they can be obtained with a simple blood draw, they may prove useful to track subclinical responses to therapy. In this regard, a drop in CTCs has been reported in as few as 4 days following resection [30] and in response to neoadjuvant therapy. In addition, it is possible that the development of chemoresistance could be measured in real time and that patients could be spared months of therapy that will later be found to be ineffective by clinical assessment.

However, the significance of CTCs extends beyond their use as a simple biomarker in that a better understanding of their disease biology may directly improve therapy. Unlike ctDNA, CTCs are a part of the disease process and can essentially be considered as a liquid phase of the tumor. In fact, since the majority of patients with pancreatic cancer die from metastatic disease, CTCs may represent the most clinically important part of the tumor. In patients who undergo surgical resection, the majority of recurrence results from metastases, which are presumed to originate from micrometastatic disease, also called disseminated tumor cells, seeded by CTCs. A better understanding of these cells may help identify unique vulnerabilities that contrast with those of the primary tumor and could result in targeted therapies.

Summary

In the application of precision medicine to pancreatic cancer, novel biomarkers will be necessary to guide therapy. Biomarkers obtained from a traditional biopsy of the primary tumor will be limited in terms of their ability to deliver real-time feedback and to represent and predict tumor behavior as a result of tumor heterogeneity.

Liquid biopsy has the ability to overcome many of these limitations. The use of CTCs as a biomarker in pancreatic cancer has shown initial promise. However, the science regarding CTCs is immature, and to better understand the potential role of CTCs, it is essential to perform further molecular investigations with broader and longer-term studies. More sensitive, advanced, and automated techniques are required to analyze cells from a genetic and molecular perspective and to retrieve a greater number of viable CTCs such that culturing these cells from pancreatic cancer becomes a possibility.

References

1. Noone AM, Cronin KA, Altekruse SF, et al. Cancer incidence and survival trends by subtype using data from the surveillance epidemiology and end results program, 1992-2013. Cancer Epidemiol Biomark Prev. 2017;26(4):632–41. https://doi.org/10.1158/1055-9965. EPI-16-0520.
2. Groot VP, Rezaee N, Wu W, et al. Patterns, timing, and predictors of recurrence following pancreatectomy for pancreatic ductal adenocarcinoma. Ann Surg. 2018;267(5):936–45. https://doi.org/10.1097/SLA.0000000000002234.
3. Jones S, Zhang X, Parsons DW, et al. Core signaling pathways in human pancreatic cancers revealed by global genomic analyses. Science. 2008;321(5897):1801–7.
4. Bailey P, Chang DK, Nones K, et al. Genomic analyses identify molecular subtypes of pancreatic cancer. Nature. 2016;531(7592):47–52. https://doi.org/10.1038/nature16965.
5. Waddell N, Pajic M, Patch AM, et al. Whole genomes redefine the mutational landscape of pancreatic cancer. Nature. 2015;518(7540):495–501. https://doi.org/10.1038/nature14169.
6. Collisson EA, Sadanandam A, Olson P, et al. Subtypes of pancreatic ductal adenocarcinoma and their differing responses to therapy. Nat Med. 2011;17(4):500–3. https://doi.org/10.1038/ nm.2344.
7. Iacobuzio-Donahue CA, Maitra A, Olsen M, et al. Exploration of global gene expression patterns in pancreatic adenocarcinoma using cDNA microarrays. Am J Pathol. 2003;162(4):1151–62. https://doi.org/10.1016/S0002-9440(10)63911-9.
8. Moffitt RA, Marayati R, Flate EL, et al. Virtual microdissection identifies distinct tumor- and stroma-specific subtypes of pancreatic ductal adenocarcinoma. Nat Genet. 2015;47(10):1168–78. https://doi.org/10.1038/ng.3398.
9. Pan S, Brentnall TA, Kelly K, Chen R. Tissue proteomics in pancreatic cancer study: discovery, emerging technologies, and challenges. Proteomics. 2013;13:710–21. https://doi.org/10.1002/ pmic.201200319.
10. Cohen JD, Javed AA, Thoburn C, et al. Combined circulating tumor DNA and protein biomarker-based liquid biopsy for the earlier detection of pancreatic cancers. Proc Natl Acad Sci U S A. 2017;114(38):10202–7. https://doi.org/10.1073/PNAS.1704961114.
11. Iacobuzio-Donahue CA, Ryu B, Hruban RH, Kern SE. Exploring the host desmoplastic response to pancreatic carcinoma: gene expression of stromal and neoplastic cells at the site of primary invasion. Am J Pathol. 2002;160(1):91–9. https://doi.org/10.1016/S0002-9440(10)64353-2.
12. Laklai H, Miroshnikova YA, Pickup MW, et al. Genotype tunes pancreatic ductal adenocarcinoma tissue tension to induce matricellular fibrosis and tumor progression. Nat Med. 2016;22(5):497–505. https://doi.org/10.1038/nm.4082.
13. Olive KP, Jacobetz MA, Davidson CJ, et al. Inhibition of Hedgehog signaling enhances delivery of chemotherapy in a mouse model of pancreatic cancer. Science. 2009;324(5933):1457–61. https://doi.org/10.1126/science.1171362.

14. Beatty GL, Eghbali S, Kim R. Deploying immunotherapy in pancreatic cancer: defining mechanisms of response and resistance. Am Soc Clin Oncol Educ Book. 2017;37:267–78. https://doi.org/10.14694/edbk_175232.
15. Hirsch FR, Franklin WA, Veve R, Varella-Garcia M, Bunn PA. HER2/neu expression in malignant lung tumors. Semin Oncol. 2002;29(1 Suppl 4):51–8.
16. Chand P, Anubha G, Singla V, Rani N. Evaluation of immunohistochemical profile of breast cancer for prognostics and therapeutic use. Niger J Surg. 2018;24(2):100. https://doi.org/10.4103/njs.NJS_2_18.
17. Cohen JD, Li L, Wang Y, et al. Detection and localization of surgically resectable cancers with a multi-analyte blood test. Science. 2018;359(6378):926–30. https://doi.org/10.1126/science.aar3247.
18. Cristofanilli M, Fortina P. Circulating tumor DNA to monitor metastatic breast cancer. N Engl J Med. 2013;369(1):93–4. https://doi.org/10.1056/NEJMc1306040.
19. Perets R, Greenberg O, Shentzer T, et al. Mutant KRAS circulating tumor DNA is an accurate tool for pancreatic cancer monitoring. Oncologist. 2018;23(5):566–72. https://doi.org/10.1634/theoncologist.2017-0467.
20. Heitzer E, Haque IS, Roberts CES, Speicher MR. Current and future perspectives of liquid biopsies in genomics-driven oncology. Nat Rev Genet. 2019;20:71–88. https://doi.org/10.1038/s41576-018-0071-5.
21. Dong X, Alpaugh KR, Cristofanilli M. Circulating tumor cells (CTCs) in breast cancer: a diagnostic tool for prognosis and molecular analysis. Chin J Cancer Res. 2012;24(4):388–98. https://doi.org/10.3978/j.issn.1000-9604.2012.11.03.
22. Buim ME, Fanelli MF, Souza VS, et al. Detection of KRAS mutations in circulating tumor cells from patients with metastatic colorectal cancer. Cancer Biol Ther. 2015;16(9):1289–95. https://doi.org/10.1080/15384047.2015.1070991.
23. Yu M, Ting DT, Stott SL, et al. RNA sequencing of pancreatic circulating tumour cells implicates WNT signalling in metastasis. Nature. 2012;487(7408):510–3. https://doi.org/10.1038/nature11217.
24. Woo D, Yu M. Circulating tumor cells as "liquid biopsies" to understand cancer metastasis. Transl Res. 2018;201:128–35. https://doi.org/10.1016/j.trsl.2018.07.003.
25. Ashworth TR. A case of cancer in which cells similar to those in the tumours were seen in the blood after death. Australas Med J. 1869;14:146–9. http://ci.nii.ac.jp/naid/10029590080/en/. Accessed 28 Dec 2018.
26. DiPardo BJ, Winograd P, Court CM, Tomlinson JS. Pancreatic cancer circulating tumor cells: applications for personalized oncology. Expert Rev Mol Diagn. 2018;18(9):809–20. https://doi.org/10.1080/14737159.2018.1511429.
27. Massagué J, Obenauf AC. Metastatic colonization by circulating tumour cells. Nature. 2016;529(7586):298–306. https://doi.org/10.1038/nature17038.
28. Yu M, Bardia A, Wittner BS, et al. Circulating breast tumor cells exhibit dynamic changes in epithelial and mesenchymal composition. Science. 2013;339(6119):580–4. https://doi.org/10.1126/science.1228522.
29. Poruk KE, Valero V 3rd, Saunders T, et al. Circulating tumor cell phenotype predicts recurrence and survival in pancreatic adenocarcinoma. Ann Surg. 2016;264(6):1073–81. https://doi.org/10.1097/SLA.0000000000001600.
30. Gemenetzis G, Groot VP, Yu J, et al. Circulating tumor cells dynamics in pancreatic adenocarcinoma correlate with disease status: results of the prospective CLUSTER study. Ann Surg. 2018;268(3):408–20. https://doi.org/10.1097/SLA.0000000000002925.
31. Aceto N, Bardia A, Miyamoto DT, et al. Circulating tumor cell clusters are oligoclonal precursors of breast cancer metastasis. Cell. 2014;158(5):1110–22. https://doi.org/10.1016/j.cell.2014.07.013.
32. Meng S, Tripathy D, Frenkel EP, et al. Circulating tumor cells in patients with breast cancer dormancy. Clin Cancer Res. 2004;10(24):8152–62. https://doi.org/10.1158/1078-0432.CCR-04-1110.

33. Makohon-Moore A, Iacobuzio-Donahue CA. Pancreatic cancer biology and genetics from an evolutionary perspective. Nat Rev Cancer. 2016;16(9):553–65. https://doi.org/10.1038/nrc.2016.66.
34. Pantel K, Alix-Panabières C. Liquid biopsy and minimal residual disease – latest advances and implications for cure. Nat Rev Clin Oncol. 2019;16(7):409–24. https://doi.org/10.1038/s41571-019-0187-3.
35. Tempero MA, Uchida E, Takasaki H, Burnett DA, Steplewski Z, Pour PM. Relationship of carbohydrate antigen 19-9 and Lewis antigens in pancreatic cancer. Cancer Res. 1987;47(20):5501–3.
36. Poruk KE, Gay DZ, Brown K, et al. The clinical utility of CA 19-9 in pancreatic adenocarcinoma: diagnostic and prognostic updates. Curr Mol Med. 2013;13(3):340–51. https://doi.org/10.2174/1566524011313030003.
37. Goonetilleke KS, Siriwardena AK. Systematic review of carbohydrate antigen (CA 19-9) as a biochemical marker in the diagnosis of pancreatic cancer. Eur J Surg Oncol. 2007;33(3):266–70. https://doi.org/10.1016/j.ejso.2006.10.004.
38. Pantel K, Speicher MR. The biology of circulating tumor cells. Oncogene. 2016;35(10):1216–24. https://doi.org/10.1038/onc.2015.192.
39. Bidard FC, Huguet F, Louvet C, et al. Circulating tumor cells in locally advanced pancreatic adenocarcinoma: the ancillary CirCe 07 study to the LAP 07 trial. Ann Oncol. 2013;24(8):2057–61. https://doi.org/10.1093/annonc/mdt176.
40. Kurihara T, Itoi T, Sofuni A, et al. Detection of circulating tumor cells in patients with pancreatic cancer: a preliminary result. J Hepato-Biliary-Pancreat Surg. 2008;15(2):189–95. https://doi.org/10.1007/s00534-007-1250-5.
41. de Albuquerque A, Kubisch I, Breier G, et al. Multimarker gene analysis of circulating tumor cells in pancreatic cancer patients: a feasibility study. Oncology. 2012;82(1):3–10. https://doi.org/10.1159/000335479.
42. Bhagwat N, Dulmage K, Pletcher CH, et al. An integrated flow cytometry-based platform for isolation and molecular characterization of circulating tumor single cells and clusters. Sci Rep. 2018;8:5035. https://doi.org/10.1038/s41598-018-23217-5.
43. Vona G, Sabile A, Louha M, et al. Isolation by size of epithelial tumor cells. Am J Pathol. 2000;156(1):57–63.
44. Pimienta M, Edderkaoui M, Wang R, Pandol S. The potential for circulating tumor cells in pancreatic cancer management. Front Physiol. 2017;8:1–13. https://doi.org/10.3389/fphys.2017.00381.
45. Alix-Panabières C, Pantel K. Challenges in circulating tumour cell research. Nat Rev Cancer. 2014;14(9):623–31. https://doi.org/10.1038/nrc3820.
46. Zhang Z, Shiratsuchi H, Lin J, et al. Expansion of CTCs from early stage lung cancer patients using a microfluidic co-culture model. Oncotarget. 2014;5(23):12383–97. https://doi.org/10.18632/oncotarget.2592.
47. Nagrath S, Sequist LV, Maheswaran S, et al. Isolation of rare circulating tumour cells in cancer patients by microchip technology. Nature. 2007;450(7173):1235–9. https://doi.org/10.1038/nature06385.
48. Rox JM, Stoecklein NH, Kasprowicz NS, et al. Diagnostic leukapheresis enables reliable detection of circulating tumor cells of nonmetastatic cancer patients. Proc Natl Acad Sci U S A. 2013;110(41):16580–5. https://doi.org/10.1073/pnas.1313594110.
49. Luk AWS, Ma Y, Ding PN, et al. CTC-mRNA (AR-V7) analysis from blood samples – impact of blood collection tube and storage time. Int J Mol Sci. 2017;18(5):1047. https://doi.org/10.3390/ijms18051047.
50. Riethdorf S, Fritsche H, Müller V, et al. Detection of circulating tumor cells in peripheral blood of patients with metastatic breast cancer: a validation study of the cell search system. Clin Cancer Res. 2007;13(3):920–8. https://doi.org/10.1158/1078-0432.CCR-06-1695.
51. Hofman V, Ilie MI, Long E, et al. Detection of circulating tumor cells as a prognostic factor in patients undergoing radical surgery for non-small-cell lung carcinoma: comparison of the

efficacy of the CellSearch Assay™ and the isolation by size of epithelial tumor cell method. Int J Cancer. 2011;129(7):1651–60. https://doi.org/10.1002/ijc.25819.

52. Hou JM, Krebs M, Ward T, et al. Circulating tumor cells as a window on metastasis biology in lung cancer. Am J Pathol. 2011;178(3):989–96. https://doi.org/10.1016/j.ajpath.2010.12.003.

53. Zhang L, Riethdorf S, Wu G, et al. Meta-analysis of the prognostic value of circulating tumor cells in breast cancer. Clin Cancer Res. 2012;18(20):5701–10. https://doi.org/10.1158/1078-0432.CCR-12-1587.

54. Helissey C, Berger F, Cottu P, et al. Circulating tumor cell thresholds and survival scores in advanced metastatic breast cancer: the observational step of the CirCe01 phase III trial. Cancer Lett. 2015;360(2):213–8. https://doi.org/10.1016/j.canlet.2015.02.010.

55. Lucci A, Hall CS, Lodhi AK, et al. Circulating tumour cells in non-metastatic breast cancer: a prospective study. Lancet Oncol. 2012;13(7):688–95. https://doi.org/10.1016/S1470-2045(12)70209-7.

56. Cristofanilli M, Budd GT, Ellis MJ, et al. Circulating tumor cells, disease progression, and survival in metastatic breast cancer. N Engl J Med. 2004;351(8):781–91. https://doi.org/10.1056/NEJMoa040766.

57. Tarhan MO, Gonel A, Kucukzeybek Y, et al. Prognostic significance of circulating tumor cells and serum CA15-3 levels in metastatic breast cancer, single center experience, preliminary results. Asian Pac J Cancer Prev. 2013;14(3):1725–9.

58. Smerage JB, Barlow WE, Hortobagyi GN, et al. Circulating tumor cells and response to chemotherapy in metastatic breast cancer: SWOG S0500. J Clin Oncol. 2014;32(31):1–8. https://doi.org/10.1200/JCO.2014.56.2561.

59. Hiltermann TJN, Pore MM, van den Berg A, et al. Circulating tumor cells in small-cell lung cancer: a predictive and prognostic factor. Ann Oncol. 2012;23(11):2937–42. https://doi.org/10.1093/annonc/mds138.

60. Hou J-M, Krebs MG, Lancashire L, et al. Clinical significance and molecular characteristics of circulating tumor cells and circulating tumor microemboli in patients with small-cell lung cancer. J Clin Oncol. 2012;30(5):525–32. https://doi.org/10.1200/jco.2010.33.3716.

61. Hofman V, Bonnetaud C, Ilie MI, et al. Preoperative circulating tumor cell detection using the isolation by size of epithelial tumor cell method for patients with lung cancer is a new prognostic biomarker. Clin Cancer Res. 2011;17(4):827–35. https://doi.org/10.1158/1078-0432.CCR-10-0445.

62. Maheswaran S, Sequist LV, Nagrath S, et al. Detection of mutations in *EGFR* in circulating lung-cancer cells. N Engl J Med. 2008;359(4):366–77. https://doi.org/10.1056/NEJMoa0800668.

63. Yang JD, Campion MB, Liu MC, et al. Circulating tumor cells are associated with poor overall survival in patients with cholangiocarcinoma. Hepatology. 2016;63(1):148–58. https://doi.org/10.1002/hep.27944.

64. Cohen SJ, Punt CJA, Iannotti N, et al. Relationship of circulating tumor cells to tumor response, progression-free survival, and overall survival in patients with metastatic colorectal cancer. J Clin Oncol. 2008;26(19):3213–21. https://doi.org/10.1200/JCO.2007.15.8923.

65. Uen Y-H, Lu C-Y, Tsai H-L, et al. Persistent presence of postoperative circulating tumor cells is a poor prognostic factor for patients with stage I-III colorectal cancer after curative resection. Ann Surg Oncol. 2008;15(8):2120–8. https://doi.org/10.1245/s10434-008-9961-7.

66. Aggarwal C, Meropol NJ, Punt CJ, et al. Relationship among circulating tumor cells, CEA and overall survival in patients with metastatic colorectal cancer. Ann Oncol. 2013;24(2):420–8. https://doi.org/10.1093/annonc/mds336.

67. van Dalum G, Stam GJ, Scholten LF, et al. Importance of circulating tumor cells in newly diagnosed colorectal cancer. Int J Oncol. 2015;46(3):1361–8. https://doi.org/10.3892/ijo.2015.2824.

68. Kaifi JT, Kunkel M, Das A, et al. Circulating tumor cell isolation during resection of colorectal cancer lung and liver metastases: a prospective trial with different detection techniques. Cancer Biol Ther. 2015;16(5):699–708. https://doi.org/10.1080/15384047.2015.1030556.

69. Mazzini C, Pinzani P, Salvianti F, et al. Circulating tumor cells detection and counting in uveal melanomas by a filtration-based method. Cancers (Basel). 2014;6(1):323–32. https://doi.org/10.3390/cancers6010323.

70. Goodman OB, Symanowski JT, Loudyi A, Fink LM, Ward DC, Vogelzang NJ. Circulating tumor cells as a predictive biomarker in patients with hormone-sensitive prostate cancer. Clin Genitourin Cancer. 2011;9(1):31–8. https://doi.org/10.1016/j.clgc.2011.04.001.

71. Wang F-B, Yang XQ, Yang S, Wang BC, Feng MH, Tu JC. A higher number of circulating tumor cells (CTC) in peripheral blood indicates poor prognosis in prostate cancer patients – a meta-analysis. Asian Pac J Cancer Prev. 2011;12(10):2629–35.

72. Zhang Y, Wang F, Ning N, et al. Patterns of circulating tumor cells identified by CEP8, CK and CD45 in pancreatic cancer. Int J Cancer. 2015;136(5):1228–33. https://doi.org/10.1002/ijc.29070.

73. Ma XL, Li YY, Zhang J, et al. Prognostic role of circulating tumor cells in patients with pancreatic cancer: a meta-analysis. Asian Pac J Cancer Prev. 2014;15(15):6015–20. https://www.ncbi.nlm.nih.gov/pubmed/25124566.

74. Han L, Chen W, Zhao Q. Prognostic value of circulating tumor cells in patients with pancreatic cancer: a meta-analysis. Tumour Biol. 2014;35(3):2473–80. https://doi.org/10.1007/s13277-013-1327-5.

75. Brabletz T, Jung A, Spaderna S, Hlubek F, Kirchner T. Opinion: migrating cancer stem cells – an integrated concept of malignant tumour progression. Nat Rev Cancer. 2005;5(9):744–9. https://doi.org/10.1038/nrc1694.

76. Mani SA, Guo W, Liao MJ, et al. The epithelial-mesenchymal transition generates cells with properties of stem cells. Cell. 2008;133(4):704–15. https://doi.org/10.1016/j.cell.2008.03.027.

77. Morel AP, Lievre M, Thomas C, Hinkal G, Ansieau S, Puisieux A. Generation of breast cancer stem cells through epithelial-mesenchymal transition. PLoS One. 2008;3(8):e2888. https://doi.org/10.1371/journal.pone.0002888.

78. Rhim AD, Mirek ET, Aiello NM, et al. EMT and dissemination precede pancreatic tumor formation. Cell. 2012;148(1–2):349–61. https://doi.org/10.1016/j.cell.2011.11.025.

79. Thiery JP, Acloque H, Huang RY, Nieto MA. Epithelial-mesenchymal transitions in development and disease. Cell. 2009;139(5):871–90. https://doi.org/10.1016/j.cell.2009.11.007.

80. Handra-Luca A, Hong SM, Walter K, Wolfgang C, Hruban R, Goggins M. Tumour epithelial vimentin expression and outcome of pancreatic ductal adenocarcinomas. Br J Cancer. 2011;104(8):1296–302. https://doi.org/10.1038/bjc.2011.93.

81. Kallergi G, Papadaki MA, Politaki E, Mavroudis D, Georgoulias V, Agelaki S. Epithelial to mesenchymal transition markers expressed in circulating tumour cells of early and metastatic breast cancer patients. Breast Cancer Res. 2011;13(3):R59. https://doi.org/10.1186/bcr2896.

82. Planchard D, Farace F, Soria JC, Vielh P, Perez-Moreno P, Lecharpentier A. Detection of circulating tumour cells with a hybrid (epithelial/mesenchymal) phenotype in patients with metastatic non-small cell lung cancer. Br J Cancer. 2011;105(9):1338–41. https://doi.org/10.1038/bjc.2011.405.

83. Armstrong AJ, Marengo MS, Oltean S, et al. Circulating tumor cells from patients with advanced prostate and breast cancer display both epithelial and mesenchymal markers. Mol Cancer Res. 2012;9(8):997–1007. https://doi.org/10.1158/1541-7786.MCR-10-0490. Circulating.

84. Gkountela S, Aceto N. Stem-like features of cancer cells on their way to metastasis. Biol Direct. 2016;11:1–14. https://doi.org/10.1186/s13062-016-0135-4.

85. Kreso A, Dick JE. Evolution of the cancer stem cell model. Cell Stem Cell. 2014;14(3):275–91. https://doi.org/10.1016/j.stem.2014.02.006.

86. Lee CJ, Dosch J, Simeone DM. Pancreatic cancer stem cells. J Clin Oncol. 2008;26(17):2806–12. https://doi.org/10.1200/JCO.2008.16.6702.

87. Cauley CE, Pitman MB, Zhou J, et al. Circulating epithelial cells in patients with pancreatic lesions: clinical and pathologic findings. J Am Coll Surg. 2015;221(3):699–707. https://doi.org/10.1016/j.jamcollsurg.2015.05.014.

88. Franken B, de Groot MR, Mastboom WJ, et al. Circulating tumor cells, disease recurrence and survival in newly diagnosed breast cancer. Breast Cancer Res. 2012;14(5):R133. https://doi.org/10.1186/bcr3333.

89. Pantel K, Deneve E, Nocca D, et al. Circulating epithelial cells in patients with benign colon diseases. Clin Chem. 2012;58(5):936–40. https://doi.org/10.1373/clinchem.2011.175570.

90. Lohr JG, Adalsteinsson VA, Cibulskis K, et al. Whole-exome sequencing of circulating tumor cells provides a window into metastatic prostate cancer. Nat Biotechnol. 2014;32(5):479–84. https://doi.org/10.1038/nbt.2892.

91. Heitzer E, Auer M, Gasch C, et al. Complex tumor genomes inferred from single circulating tumor cells by array-CGH and next-generation sequencing. Cancer Res. 2013;73(10):2965–75. https://doi.org/10.1158/0008-5472.CAN-12-4140.

92. Ni X, Zhuo M, Su Z, et al. Reproducible copy number variation patterns among single circulating tumor cells of lung cancer patients. Proc Natl Acad Sci U S A. 2013;110(52):21083–8. https://doi.org/10.1073/pnas.1320659110.

93. Vanharanta S, Massagué J. Origins of metastatic traits. Cancer Cell. 2013;24(4):410–21. https://doi.org/10.1016/j.ccr.2013.09.007.

94. Court CM, Ankeny JS, Sho S, et al. Reality of single circulating tumor cell sequencing for molecular diagnostics in pancreatic cancer. J Mol Diagn. 2016;18(5):688–96. https://doi.org/10.1016/j.jmoldx.2016.03.006.

95. Kulemann B, Liss AS, Warshaw AL, et al. KRAS mutations in pancreatic circulating tumor cells: a pilot study. Tumor Biol. 2016;37(6):7547–54. https://doi.org/10.1007/s13277-015-4589-2.

Part IV
Personalized Treatment Approaches

Chapter 10
Personalized Models of Human PDAC

Hanna Heikenwälder and Susanne Roth

Most patients with PDAC are diagnosed with advanced, unresectable disease, and even highly selected patients with initially limited disease who underwent potential curative resection finally succumb from recurrent disease, while long-term survival remains rare. Although significant progress has been achieved in PDAC patient care, such as neoadjuvant treatment strategies, or more effective combined adjuvant and palliative chemotherapeutic regimens [1, 2], the overall beneficial effect on prognosis has been marginal in unselected patient populations. Currently, chemotherapeutic regimens in pancreatic cancer are still mostly limited by a "one-size-fits-all" approach, meaning that therapeutic decisions are mainly based on the clinical tumour stage and ignoring the patient's individual cancer biology. Recently, high-throughput sequencing technologies have revealed a complex mutational landscape in pancreatic cancer with multiple mutated genes at low prevalence and significant intertumoural heterogeneity [3–8]. Due to the diverse genetic landscape, tumour biology and thus responses to antitumour therapies vary substantially. Although several signature-based mutational and transcriptional subtypes have been proposed in PDAC, so far no reliable biomarker for predicting the effectiveness of antitumour therapies is currently available [2]. Many antitumour therapies are highly toxic and associated with serious side effects. Therefore, it is of central importance to identify those individuals that would benefit from specific antitumour therapies, matching the right treatment to the right patient. Such a personalized treatment strategy could improve prognosis for patients with this devastating disease and also reduce therapy-associated toxicity. Yet, response prediction to antitumour drugs remains a major challenge in cancer treatment. Prediction based solely on cancer genome sequencing is limited, and recent evidence indicates that intratumoural heterogeneity and the tumour

---

H. Heikenwälder · S. Roth (✉)
Department of General, Visceral and Transplantation Surgery,
Heidelberg University Hospital, Heidelberg, Germany
e-mail: susanne.roth@med.uni-heidelberg.de

© Springer Nature Switzerland AG 2020
C. W. Michalski et al. (eds.), *Translational Pancreatic Cancer Research*,
Molecular and Translational Medicine,
https://doi.org/10.1007/978-3-030-49476-6_10

microenvironment can restrict biomarker-guided strategies for therapy selection. This limitation could be addressed by direct functional response testing of live patient tumour tissues exposed to potential therapies. Several functional assays assessing antitumour activity of drugs have been developed, such as stable tumour cell lines, organoids, or xenograft models from individual patients [9], which possess unique drug sensitivity profiles that could not be predicted using genetic analyses [10]. Personalized models of PDAC should recapitulate the genetic complexity and heterogeneity of the disease and prevent the process of adaption to in vitro growth conditions that leads to significant changes in the biology of cancer cells. Those models might help to choose the right therapy in a clinically relevant time frame, enabling more effective individualized treatment options to improve outcomes for patients with pancreatic cancer and prevent the unnecessary use of chemotherapeutics to which patients are resistant, thereby reducing toxicity. In this chapter, we provide a brief overview of the most promising personalized models of human PDAC, including patient-derived xenograft models, cell lines, organoids, tumour tissue slice cultures and circulating tumour cells, as well as potential future applications (Fig. 10.1).

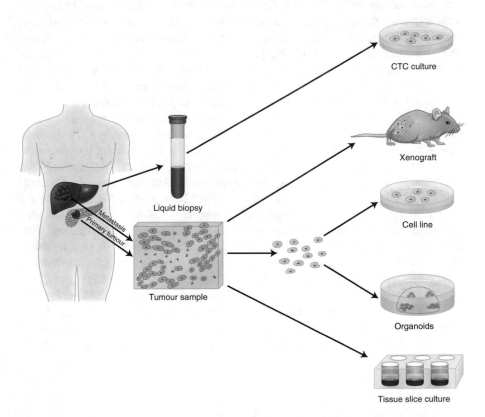

Fig. 10.1 Personalized models of human PDAC. Tumour specimen and liquid biopsies from PDAC patients can be used to generate individualized tumour models, including xenografts, patient-derived cell lines, 3D organoids, tissue slice cultures and cultures of circulating tumour cells, respectively. In-depth molecular and functional characterizations of these models help to select most effective therapies in each individual patient

Xenograft Models

Xenograft models have been used for decades in preclinical research as a valuable tool to study tumour biology and for drug screening. Xenografts can be generated from small pieces of primary human tumours and metastases collected by surgery or even from biopsy samples. These small tissue pieces are then transplanted either subcutaneously or orthotopically into immunodeficient mouse strains such as athymic nude or NOD-SCID mice. Orthotopic transplantation refers to transplantation of the original tumour tissue into the corresponding anatomical location in the mouse, e.g., primary human PDAC tissue into the murine pancreas. Although the orthotopic approach would most accurately mimic the natural tumour microenvironment, subcutaneous transplantation into the dorsal flank of immunodeficient mice is the standard procedure. This is mainly due to practical reasons, as orthotopic transplantation does not only require advanced surgical skills and is more time-consuming but also makes it much more difficult to monitor the engraftment success and tumour growth. Patient-derived xenograft models are a suitable tool for personalized treatment approaches in PDAC, as they allow studying tumour cells in their highly heterogeneous environment, composed of a dense extracellular matrix and other cell types that typically reside within these tumours. However, studies have shown that the non-malignant cell types of patient-derived xenografts are substituted over time by murine cells [11]. The cells that infiltrate the xenograft have been shown to be overall the murine counterparts of the original stroma and even produce comparable extracellular matrix components [12–14]. Nonetheless, the substitution of human by murine stroma might interfere with the original interaction of tumour cells with their microenvironment and impose a selective pressure on cancer cells towards an adaption to the new environment. In addition, xenograft models require the use of immunocompromised mice, which prevents the analysis of tumour interactions with the immune system that plays a pivotal role in PDAC development. Human PDAC displays an immune cell signature that is commonly highly immunosuppressive and is thought to be a major contributor to its poor prognosis [1]. Furthermore, the immunocompromised background of mouse strains employed for xenograft generation renders it difficult to test immunotherapies such as checkpoint inhibitors. A potential solution to this problem might be the generation of humanized mice that are irradiated prior to xenograft transplantation and reconstituted with bone marrow containing haematopoietic stem cells from the individual human xenograft donor [15, 16].

Despite these apparent drawbacks, patient-derived xenograft models show gene-expression profiles that are similar to the original tumour [13], and chemotherapy response rates are comparable between patient-derived xenografts and clinical data [13]. Notwithstanding, patient-derived xenograft models have considerable limitations for the use of personalized treatment approaches such as chemosensitivity testing. Especially the low engraftment rates and time required for growth in the recipient mouse remain an unsolved problem. Some approaches tried to increase engraftment rates by transplanting tissue pieces coated with Matrigel or additional cell types such as human fibroblasts or mesenchymal stem cells. Interestingly, patient-derived xenograft engraftment rates in PDAC showed to be similarly low for subcutaneous or orthotopic transplantation protocols in nude mice with 61% and 62%, respectively [17, 18]. Generally, metastases were found to have higher engraftment rates than primary tumours [13], and successful engraftment was shown to be associated with worse recurrence-free and overall survival in PDAC [19]. These engraftment rates are definitely too low to allow for reliable individualized drug testing or co-clinical trials analysing the underlying mechanisms of treatment responses. Another major problem is the long engraftment time of 4–8 months before drug testing and analyses can be performed [20]. Especially in PDAC, this time gap between initial surgery and start of adjuvant therapy is unacceptable [2].

Patient-Derived Cell Lines

Patient-derived tumour cell lines are generated from human PDAC specimen by tissue dissociation producing single cell suspensions. Once isolated from the fresh tumour sample, the cells first need to adapt to growth in serum containing media in tissue culture dishes, which is the main critical step in the generation of tumour cell lines. Patient-derived cell lines are usually established only from more aggressive tumours and hence are not representative of the full clinical spectrum of PDAC in humans [13]. For PDAC, the efficiency to generate cell lines from a resected primary tumour is even lower than the efficiency of generating 3D cultures such as organoids [21]. In most cases this excludes the generation of cell lines from patients that are diagnosed with early disease. Thus, at the moment being patient-derived cell lines seem to be a rather insufficient strategy for personalized treatment applications [13]. Once patient-derived tumour cells have successfully adapted to their new in vitro environment, they are easy to culture, passage, cryopreserve and manipulate chemically and genetically [11]. Yet, this adaption also represents a major disadvantage, as it induces fundamental changes in cell physiology such as altered gene expression. Newly developed pancreatic cancer cell lines seem to harbour strong genetic conservation with the primary tumour, but this conservation is diminishing with increasing numbers of passages [22]. Thus, low passage cell lines could be used to dissect therapeutic vulnerabilities based on genetic features of individual PDAC samples. Furthermore, the development of various cell lines derived from distinct subclones of the same primary tumour specimen would allow to study tumour heterogeneity. Still, those monolayer forming cell lines fail to recapitulate many key features of the primary tumour, such as 3D organization, interactions with fibroblasts, immune cells and the ECM [11]. Despite these apparent disadvantages, patient-derived cell lines still hold some benefits over other personalized models of human PDAC. The development of patient-derived cell lines is relatively cost-effective, easy to handle and feasible within a time frame that allows the employment of the obtained information for treatment choices, however with the exclusion of those patients, whose tumour cells do not adapt to growth under culture conditions.

Organoids

The limitations of monolayer cell cultures have inspired the development of more physiological organoid cultures, in which cells grow in 3D structures inside or on top of matrices that compensate for the primary ECM. 3D culture methods prevent cells from attaching to the cell culture dish, enable PDAC cells to develop polarity and organize into ductlike structures resembling the original PDAC architecture. Yet, those organoids have been missing stroma components. Recently, more complex organotypic cultures of tumour, stromal and immune components of the original tumour microenvironment have been successfully generated [23]. Tsai et al. co-cultured primary PDAC cells with cancer-associated fibroblasts from the same tissue and lymphocytes from peripheral blood, which infiltrated the 3D in vitro models [23]. Besides collagen type I and IV, Matrigel is the most commonly used matrix for PDAC organoid growth [11]. While collagen type IV is a major component of the basement membrane of the normal pancreatic epithelium, collagen type I is excessively produced by the PDAC microenvironment forming a dense desmoplastic stroma. Matrigel is a commercially available basement membrane extract that is purified from murine Engelbreth-Holm-Swarm (EHS) sarcomas [11, 24] and contains a complex composition of structural proteins (e.g. collagen and laminin) and various growth factors such as epidermal growth factor (EGF), basic fibroblast growth factor (bFGF) and transforming growth factor beta (TGF-β) [24]. This highly physiologic composition of Matrigel allows patient-derived PDAC cells to form organoids that resemble primary human PDAC much stronger than monolayer cultures [11].

Organoids enable the propagation of large amounts of tumour tissue, providing sufficient material for in-depth genetic and molecular characterisation, as well as drug screening [11]. The efficiency to generate organoids from resected primary PDAC specimen (around 75%) is mostly higher than for cell lines or xenografts [21, 25]. In addition, organoids can be generated from relatively few, or even single, tumour cells [11], which enables the utilization of cancer cells that are obtained by fine needle biopsies and thus allows the generation of personalized tumour models also from PDAC patients that are not eligible for surgical resection [26]. Furthermore, organoids derived from human PDAC can show several distinct morphologies within the same culture [27] and might allow comprehensive modelling of the full spectrum of the disease [3]. Multiple distinct organoid cultures could be generated from distinct geographical regions of the same tumour sample to model intratumoural heterogeneity observed in human PDAC [28].

Patient-derived organoids have already been established as drug testing pipelines for therapeutic profiling in PDAC within a clinically meaningful time frame of less than 6 weeks [25], and the results of a small retrospective analysis confirmed that drug sensitivities observed in patient-derived organoids resemble clinical responses and may thus be used to inform treatment selection [25].

Tumour Slice Cultures

Tumour slice cultures appear to be so far the most physiological approach to model and study individual human PDAC. In contrast to xenografts or cell lines, they exclude species differences and cellular alterations due to adaption to in vitro growth conditions. For the generation of tumour slice cultures, fresh patient-derived tumour samples are cut directly after surgical resection into very thin tissue slices and cultured in the presence of nutrient and growth factor containing media. Membrane filter inserts coated with collagen can be used in order to improve nutrient exchange between slice cultures and culture media and support oxygenation of the tumour slices [29]. The emergence of microtomes with vibrating blades (vibratomes) has enabled the cutting of fresh primary PDAC tissue without the usage of embedding media or fixatives. An ideal slice thickness of 200–400 μm allows for sufficient nutrient diffusion while preserving the original morphology, cellular composition and extracellular matrix components of the primary tumour microenvironment. Therefore, tumour slice cultures also contain various tumour cell subclones that account for tumour heterogeneity observed in human PDAC. A major advantage of tumour slice cultures is that once established, they can be used without any restrictions on any available tumour sample in contrast to xenografts or 2D/3D cell lines, which depend on engraftment success and adaption to growth under culture conditions. However, tumour slice cultures can only be developed when sufficient material is available, and this largely excludes any patient who is not eligible for surgical resection. Tumour slice cultures maintain their baseline morphology and show stable amounts of total cell numbers and a high degree of tissue viability for up to 7 days in culture [29, 30]. In addition, tumour intrinsic immune cell populations such as T cells, macrophages and myeloid-derived suppressor cells were present throughout the culture period [29, 30]. A time frame of 5–6 days is short when compared to other personalized models of PDAC, however sufficient to allow drug testing that might help to identify the optimal treatment for individual patients. As tumour material is limited, tissue slice cultures are not suitable for large-scale drug screens. Noteworthy, also tumour slice cultures are generally produced from only one single region of a human PDAC specimen. In order to address tumour heterogeneity ideally, multiple distinct regions of a single PDAC specimen should be used for the establishment of drug response platforms in precision medicine practices. Further improvements in slice techniques might allow developing tumour slice cultures even from biopsies. Data obtained from these cultures could be used to inform neoadjuvant or palliative treatment choices.

Circulating Tumour Cells

Recently the isolation and culture of circulating tumour cells (CTCs) from peripheral blood of cancer patients has become feasible. The great advantage of this approach in comparison to other personalized models of PDAC lies clearly within its minimal invasiveness [31]. CTCs can be analysed immediately after isolation or stored by "vitrification" – a method of rapid and "ice-free" cryopreservation [32]. The major drawback of CTCs is their paucity, with concentrations as low as 1 CTC in 10^9 blood cells [32]. CTCs have been successfully purified using label-free microfluidic or filter technologies that allow size-based isolation of viable CTCs with depletion rates of white blood cells of up to 99.99% in whole blood [33–35]. These techniques allow fast processing of large patient blood volumes in a cost-effective manner [35]. In addition, antibody-based enrichment methods are applicable such as positive immunoselection for CTC surface markers (e.g. for epithelial cell adhesion molecule; EpCAM) or negative selections depleting leucocytes, usually via anti-CD45 antibodies [36]. The low numbers that are obtained from patient blood make CTCs difficult to culture and expand in vitro. Several studies have recently established culture conditions that enable functional analyses of CTCs in several malignant diseases [31]. While CTCs have been widely used as biomarkers and for molecular characterization of human individual PDAC, only a few studies exist, which have successfully cultured and expanded human CTCs from PDAC ex vivo [37, 38]. Although CTCs cannot be detected in the peripheral blood of all PDAC patients, CTCs have been captured from blood samples of patients with early, advanced or metastatic disease with high efficiency [34, 39]. Once established, the ex vivo culture and expansion of CTCs might be an easy and noninvasive option for testing the sensitivity to drugs in PDAC patients at all disease stages and during the course of therapy over time.

Future Personalized Models of Human PDAC

Since human PDAC shows high genetic heterogeneity and multifaceted interactions with a complex and immunosuppressive tumour microenvironment, future personalized models of human PDAC should preserve most of its original features while supporting survival or even expansion of the tumour tissue ex vivo. New culture methods such as organoids and latest organ-on-a-chip technologies appear to be promising candidates to comprehensively model human PDAC in vitro, but have until now only been partly successful. Even organ-on-a-chip systems, which try to recapitulate the 3D structure of organs and integrate dynamic properties of live tissue, still remain artificial and fail to recapitulate the whole in vivo composition of tissues [40]. Thus, human organ cultures such as patient-derived tumour slice cultures described above might offer a simple and accurate approach to model individual PDACs with practicability on every patient from whom sufficient tissue can be obtained. However, organ cultures are still limited as they only model local disease processes. No technique is currently capable of comprehensively imitating antitumour immune responses in vitro. Also, multi-organ interactions, off-target or systemic side effects of new drugs cannot be infallibly predicted by any model system.

Worldwide, extensive research focuses on the establishment of personalized models of PDAC as a crucial part of precision medicine approaches. However, besides technical challenges that still need to be overcome, there are also numerous practical and organizational problems to be solved in the future. Most importantly, data obtained from personalized models of PDAC would need to be collected and shared between institutions and countries worldwide in order to surmount small cohort sizes for rare genetic alterations. Ideally, data would be centralized in specialized national and international centres with unified definitions for patient and data collection [1].

References

1. Kleeff J, Korc M, Apte M, La Vecchia C, Johnson CD, Biankin AV, et al. Pancreatic cancer. Nat Rev Dis Primers. 2016;2:16022.
2. Strobel O, Neoptolemos J, Jager D, Buchler MW. Optimizing the outcomes of pancreatic cancer surgery. Nat Rev Clin Oncol. 2019;16(1):11–26.
3. Bailey P, Chang DK, Nones K, Johns AL, Patch AM, Gingras MC, et al. Genomic analyses identify molecular subtypes of pancreatic cancer. Nature. 2016;531(7592):47–52.
4. Biankin AV, Waddell N, Kassahn KS, Gingras MC, Muthuswamy LB, Johns AL, et al. Pancreatic cancer genomes reveal aberrations in axon guidance pathway genes. Nature. 2012;491(7424):399–405.
5. Collisson EA, Sadanandam A, Olson P, Gibb WJ, Truitt M, Gu S, et al. Subtypes of pancreatic ductal adenocarcinoma and their differing responses to therapy. Nat Med. 2011;17(4):500–3.
6. Jones S, Zhang X, Parsons DW, Lin JC, Leary RJ, Angenendt P, et al. Core signaling pathways in human pancreatic cancers revealed by global genomic analyses. Science. 2008;321(5897):1801–6.
7. Moffitt RA, Marayati R, Flate EL, Volmar KE, Loeza SG, Hoadley KA, et al. Virtual microdissection identifies distinct tumor- and stroma-specific subtypes of pancreatic ductal adenocarcinoma. Nat Genet. 2015;47(10):1168–78.
8. Waddell N, Pajic M, Patch AM, Chang DK, Kassahn KS, Bailey P, et al. Whole genomes redefine the mutational landscape of pancreatic cancer. Nature. 2015;518(7540):495–501.
9. Friedman AA, Letai A, Fisher DE, Flaherty KT. Precision medicine for cancer with next-generation functional diagnostics. Nat Rev Cancer. 2015;15(12):747–56.
10. Witkiewicz AK, Balaji U, Eslinger C, McMillan E, Conway W, Posner B, et al. Integrated patient-derived models delineate individualized therapeutic vulnerabilities of pancreatic cancer. Cell Rep. 2016;16(7):2017–31.
11. Baker LA, Tiriac H, Clevers H, Tuveson DA. Modeling pancreatic cancer with organoids. Trends Cancer. 2016;2(4):176–90.
12. Delitto D, Pham K, Vlada AC, Sarosi GA, Thomas RM, Behrns KE, et al. Patient-derived xenograft models for pancreatic adenocarcinoma demonstrate retention of tumor morphology through incorporation of murine stromal elements. Am J Pathol. 2015;185(5): 1297–303.
13. Hidalgo M, Amant F, Biankin AV, Budinska E, Byrne AT, Caldas C, et al. Patient-derived xenograft models: an emerging platform for translational cancer research. Cancer Discov. 2014;4(9):998–1013.
14. Mattie M, Christensen A, Chang MS, Yeh W, Said S, Shostak Y, et al. Molecular characterization of patient-derived human pancreatic tumor xenograft models for preclinical and translational development of cancer therapeutics. Neoplasia. 2013;15(10):1138–50.
15. Wege AK. Humanized mouse models for the preclinical assessment of cancer immunotherapy. BioDrugs. 2018;32(3):245–66.

16. Wiekmeijer AS, Pike-Overzet K, Brugman MH, Salvatori DC, Egeler RM, Bredius RG, et al. Sustained engraftment of cryopreserved human bone marrow CD34(+) cells in young adult NSG mice. Biores Open Access. 2014;3(3):110–6.
17. Garrido-Laguna I, Uson M, Rajeshkumar NV, Tan AC, de Oliveira E, Karikari C, et al. Tumor engraftment in nude mice and enrichment in stroma- related gene pathways predict poor survival and resistance to gemcitabine in patients with pancreatic cancer. Clin Cancer Res. 2011;17(17):5793–800.
18. Reyes G, Villanueva A, Garcia C, Sancho FJ, Piulats J, Lluis F, et al. Orthotopic xenografts of human pancreatic carcinomas acquire genetic aberrations during dissemination in nude mice. Cancer Res. 1996;56(24):5713–9.
19. Pergolini I, Morales-Oyarvide V, Mino-Kenudson M, Honselmann KC, Rosenbaum MW, Nahar S, et al. Tumor engraftment in patient-derived xenografts of pancreatic ductal adenocarcinoma is associated with adverse clinicopathological features and poor survival. PLoS One. 2017;12(8):e0182855.
20. Aparicio S, Hidalgo M, Kung AL. Examining the utility of patient-derived xenograft mouse models. Nat Rev Cancer. 2015;15(5):311–6.
21. Boj SF, Hwang CI, Baker LA, Chio II, Engle DD, Corbo V, et al. Organoid models of human and mouse ductal pancreatic cancer. Cell. 2015;160(1–2):324–38.
22. Knudsen ES, Balaji U, Mannakee B, Vail P, Eslinger C, Moxom C, et al. Pancreatic cancer cell lines as patient-derived avatars: genetic characterisation and functional utility. Gut. 2018;67(3):508–20.
23. Tsai S, McOlash L, Palen K, Johnson B, Duris C, Yang Q, et al. Development of primary human pancreatic cancer organoids, matched stromal and immune cells and 3D tumor microenvironment models. BMC Cancer. 2018;18(1):335.
24. Kleinman HK, Martin GR. Matrigel: basement membrane matrix with biological activity. Semin Cancer Biol. 2005;15(5):378–86.
25. Tiriac H, Belleau P, Engle DD, Plenker D, Deschenes A, Somerville TDD, et al. Organoid profiling identifies common responders to chemotherapy in pancreatic cancer. Cancer Discov. 2018;8(9):1112–29.
26. Tiriac H, Bucobo JC, Tzimas D, Grewel S, Lacomb JF, Rowehl LM, et al. Successful creation of pancreatic cancer organoids by means of EUS-guided fine-needle biopsy sampling for personalized cancer treatment. Gastrointest Endosc. 2018;87(6):1474–80.
27. Huang L, Holtzinger A, Jagan I, BeGora M, Lohse I, Ngai N, et al. Ductal pancreatic cancer modeling and drug screening using human pluripotent stem cell- and patient-derived tumor organoids. Nat Med. 2015;21(11):1364–71.
28. Yachida S, Jones S, Bozic I, Antal T, Leary R, Fu B, et al. Distant metastasis occurs late during the genetic evolution of pancreatic cancer. Nature. 2010;467(7319):1114–7.
29. Lim CY, Chang JH, Lee WS, Lee KM, Yoon YC, Kim J, et al. Organotypic slice cultures of pancreatic ductal adenocarcinoma preserve the tumor microenvironment and provide a platform for drug response. Pancreatology. 2018;18(8):913–27.
30. Jiang X, Seo YD, Chang JH, Coveler A, Nigjeh EN, Pan S, et al. Long-lived pancreatic ductal adenocarcinoma slice cultures enable precise study of the immune microenvironment. Oncoimmunology. 2017;6(7):e1333210.
31. Pantel K, Alix-Panabieres C. Functional studies on viable circulating tumor cells. Clin Chem. 2016;62(2):328–34.
32. Sandlin RD, Wong KHK, Tessier SN, Swei A, Bookstaver LD, Ahearn BE, et al. Ultra-fast vitrification of patient-derived circulating tumor cell lines. PLoS One. 2018;13(2):e0192734.
33. Karabacak NM, Spuhler PS, Fachin F, Lim EJ, Pai V, Ozkumur E, et al. Microfluidic, marker-free isolation of circulating tumor cells from blood samples. Nat Protoc. 2014;9(3):694–710.
34. Kulemann B, Pitman MB, Liss AS, Valsangkar N, Fernandez-Del Castillo C, Lillemoe KD, et al. Circulating tumor cells found in patients with localized and advanced pancreatic cancer. Pancreas. 2015;44(4):547–50.

35. Warkiani ME, Khoo BL, Wu L, Tay AK, Bhagat AA, Han J, et al. Ultra-fast, label-free isolation of circulating tumor cells from blood using spiral microfluidics. Nat Protoc. 2016;11(1):134–48.
36. Riva F, Dronov OI, Khomenko DI, Huguet F, Louvet C, Mariani P, et al. Clinical applications of circulating tumor DNA and circulating tumor cells in pancreatic cancer. Mol Oncol. 2016;10(3):481–93.
37. DiPardo BJ, Winograd P, Court CM, Tomlinson JS. Pancreatic cancer circulating tumor cells: applications for personalized oncology. Expert Rev Mol Diagn. 2018;18(9):809–20.
38. Sheng W, Ogunwobi OO, Chen T, Zhang J, George TJ, Liu C, et al. Capture, release and culture of circulating tumor cells from pancreatic cancer patients using an enhanced mixing chip. Lab Chip. 2014;14(1):89–98.
39. Kulemann B, Liss AS, Warshaw AL, Seifert S, Bronsert P, Glatz T, et al. KRAS mutations in pancreatic circulating tumor cells: a pilot study. Tumour Biol. 2016;37(6):7547–54.
40. Al-Lamki RS, Bradley JR, Pober JS. Human organ culture: updating the approach to bridge the gap from in vitro to in vivo in inflammation, cancer, and stem cell biology. Front Med (Lausanne). 2017;4:148.

Chapter 11
Therapeutic Targeting of Stromal Components

Albrecht Neesse

The tumor bulk in pancreatic ductal adenocarcinoma (PDAC) is composed of large amounts of tumor stroma [1] (Fig. 11.1). The tumor stroma or the tumor microenvironment (TME) is a term that describes a complex and highly heterogeneous composition of various nonneoplastic cells and acellular matrix components that surround and embed neoplastic cells, thus shaping a biophysically hard and stiff, yet biochemically highly dynamic matrix scaffold [2–4]. Cancer-associated fibroblasts (CAFs) that originate from various subgroups of myofibroblastic cell types such as pancreatic stellate cells (PSCs) [5–7], resident fibroblasts, mesenchymal stem cells (MSCs), and endothelial cells constitute an important cellular part of the TME [8–10]. CAFs are not a homogeneous cell population itself, and recent reports are only starting to unravel the complexities of several subgroups of CAFs [11], i.e., tumor-promoting CAFs (inflammatory CAFs, iCAFs), tumor-restraining CAFs (myofibroblastic CAFs, myCAFs) [12], or antigen-presenting CAFs (apCAFs) that express MHC class II and CD74 [13] (Fig. 11.2). Besides CAFs, immune cells such as cytotoxic T cells, mature dendritic cells (DCs), macrophages (M1 + M2 subtype), natural killer cells (NKs), myeloid-derived suppressor cells (MDSCs), and T-regulatory cells (Tregs) abundantly accumulate within the stroma and often create an immunosuppressive environment that impedes clearance of neoplastic cells [8]. However, detailed compositions of immune cells and the various emerging immune therapies will be discussed elsewhere in this book. Besides immune cells and CAFs, endothelial cells and neurons can also be found in the TME [14, 15]. Cells from the TME closely interact with epithelial tumor cells either through direct cell-cell interactions and subsequent activation of signalling pathways or via abundantly released growth factors, hormones, and cytokines that generate a highly complicated

A. Neesse (✉)
Department of Gastroenterology and Gastrointestinal Oncology, University Medical Center Göttingen, Center Göttingen, Georg-August-University, Göttingen, Germany
e-mail: albrecht.neesse@med.uni-goettingen.de

© Springer Nature Switzerland AG 2020
C. W. Michalski et al. (eds.), *Translational Pancreatic Cancer Research*,
Molecular and Translational Medicine,
https://doi.org/10.1007/978-3-030-49476-6_11

Fig. 11.1 H&E staining of
a human pancreatic ductal
adenocarcinoma (PDAC)
with a pronounced tumor
stroma (black arrow) and
small nests of neoplastic
cells (white arrow)

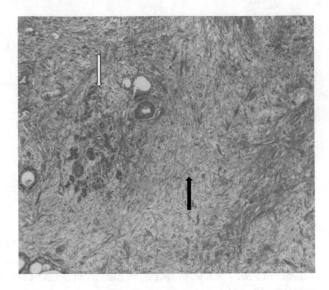

communication network [16, 17]. Apart from the cellular components, the acellular
matrix components make up a large part of the bulk tumor volume. Among others,
collagen, hyaluronic acid (HA), fibronectin, and matricellular proteins such as
secreted protein acidic and rich in cysteine (SPARC), periostin, and tenascin C can
be found in the TME [18, 19].

Historically, the tumor stroma was considered a fibrotic scar that surrounds and
confines neoplastic cells, thus rather preventing than promoting tumor progression
and spread of neoplastic cells to distant organs [1]. Several decades ago, however,
it became increasingly clear that the TME coevolves with transformed epithelial
cells in several carcinomas including PDAC. Since then, numerous studies have
provided evidence that the TME is a highly dynamic, heterogeneous, and complex
arrangement of cells, growth factors, and matrix components that promote tumor
progression, spread, and therapeutic resistance through a complex biochemical and
biophysical cross talk with neoplastic cells [3, 20]. From a clinical point of view,
therapeutic resistance toward chemotherapies remains a major challenge in the
oncological care of PDAC patients, and despite the emergence of novel, intensified
chemotherapies such as nab-paclitaxel + gemcitabine [21] or FOLFIRINOX
(folinic acid, 5-fluorouracil, irinotecan, and oxaliplatin) [22], most patients with
advanced or metastasized disease die during the first 12 months after diagnosis
[16]. Therefore, the idea that the extensive desmoplastic reaction in PDAC could
be causally involved in therapeutic resistance and hence serve as a therapeutic
target seems highly appealing for scientists and clinicians likewise. However, more
than two decades between "hope and hype" for anti-stromal therapies have passed
without the emergence of a single, clinically approved anti-stromal compound [8].
Despite this apparent lack of bench-to-bedside translation, anti-stromal approaches

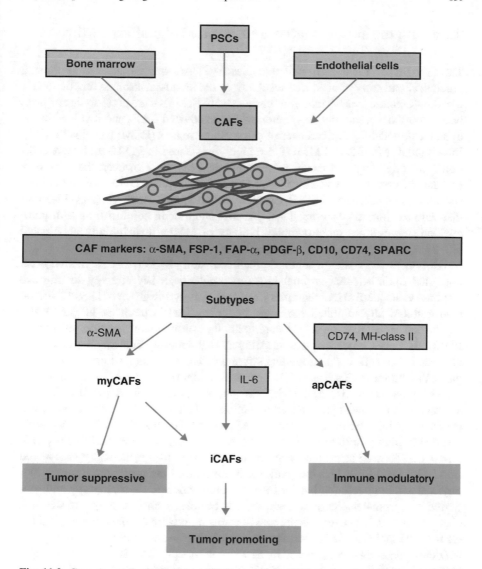

Fig. 11.2 Cancer-associated fibroblast (CAF) evolution, CAF markers, and subtypes in PDAC according to current knowledge. PSC, pancreatic stellate cells; α-SMA, α-smooth muscle actin; FSP-1, fibroblast-specific protein-1; FAP-α, fibroblast activation protein-α; PDGFR-β, platelet-derived growth factor receptor-β, SPARC, secreted protein acidic and rich in cysteine; myCAF, myofibroblastic CAFs; iCAF, inflammatory CAFs; apCAFs, antigen-presenting CAFs

may still constitute powerful and clinically relevant therapeutic options for at least a subset of PDAC patients, and this article will discuss reasons and obstacles that may have led to such apparent failure of preclinical to clinical translation in the past.

Targeting the Tumor Matrix and Stromal Signalling Pathways

The first "hype" for anti-stromal therapies in PDAC was initiated by promising preclinical and early clinical trial results from the broad-spectrum synthetic matrix metalloproteinase (MMP) inhibitor marimastat [23]. MMPs are proteolytic enzymes within the TME predominantly expressed from activated CAFs and involved in the dynamic remodelling and turnover of extracellular matrix (ECM) proteins [24, 25]. In particular, MMP-2 and MMP-9 are highly expressed in PDAC and exert additional pro-migratory and pro-invasive functions [26, 27]. However, the hope of a first anti-stromal therapy was soon squashed by several phase III trials with marimastat as well as selective MMP-2, MMP-3, MMP-9, and MMP-13 (Bay-12-9566) that did not show efficacy in PDAC patients alone or in combination with gemcitabine suggesting a more complex biology of MMPs than initially anticipated [28, 29].

Almost 10 years later, a seminal preclinical study by Olive et al. fuelled great hope and optimism that stromal targeting might be a key strategy to improve response to standard chemotherapies [30]. In this study, the group of David Tuveson pharmacologically inhibited the sonic hedgehog (SHH) pathway in genetically engineered mice that closely recapitulate the stromal composition of human PDAC. SHH is a crucial signalling pathway that centrally controls the cross talk between tumor cells and surrounding stromal cells and promotes tumorigenesis. In particular, tumor cells release SHH ligands that in turn act in a paracrine mode on mesenchymal cells [31, 32]. Using the pharmacological inhibitor IPI-926, the Tuveson group showed pronounced depletion of the tumor stroma that was accompanied by an increase in vessel density and patency. Combination with gemcitabine resulted in higher intra-tumoral levels of gemcitabine, increased rate of apoptotic tumor, cells as well as prolonged survival in tumor-bearing genetically engineered mice (GEMMs) [30]. This hallmark study introduced the tumor stroma as a biophysical and hypovascular barrier for the accumulation of chemotherapy and suggested that stromal depletion strategies would be able to sensitize PDAC to standard chemotherapies. However, despite these promising preclinical data, the clinical trials for SHH inhibitors failed at early stages or had to be suspended prematurely due to decreased survival rates caused by SHH inhibitors [33, 34]. Subsequent in-depth studies of the SHH pathway in various GEMMs revealed that a prolonged inactivation of the pathway resulted in ablation of CAFs, but undifferentiated and more invasive and aggressively growing pancreatic tumors [35, 36]. Very recent data show that *Smo* deletion in fibroblasts leads to increased tumor cell proliferation and proteasomal degradation of the tumor suppressor PTEN with subsequent activation of oncogenic protein kinase B (AKT) in fibroblasts [37]. Interestingly, low stromal PTEN correlated with reduced overall survival in PDAC patients [37]. These studies received great attention in the pancreatic cancer community as they suggested for the first time that stromal cells, in particular CAFs, mediate tumor-restraining rather than tumor-promoting properties. Subsequently, the therapeutic strategy was reconsidered and "stromal reprogramming" rather than "stromal depletion" appeared to be more appropriate. To this end, a number of exciting preclinical studies were recently published that provide insights into stromal biology and the potential to alter biophysical or biochemical properties of the matrix in order to regulate tumor cell tension and contractility and improve therapeutic response [38, 39]. For instance, actomyosin contractility was downregulated in PSCs by all-trans retinoic acid (ATRA), the active metabolite of vitamin A via the retinoic acid receptor [40]. Alternative stromal targets include Rho-kinase (ROCK) [41], the TGF-β pathway [42], and lysyl oxidase (LOX) [43], which have all been tested in preclinical experiments mostly involving various GEMMs. However, translation from preclinical to clinical findings and back is often difficult and exemplified by the stromal depletion hypothesis that was incorrectly suggested for nab-paclitaxel. Nab-paclitaxel is an albumin-coated, nano-formulated drug that was shown to significantly prolong survival in combination with gemcitabine in stage IV PDAC patients in a large, multinational phase III trial [21]. SPARC is an albumin-binding protein that is overexpressed by peritumoral fibroblasts in PDAC [44]. Early clinical trial data and preclinical data indicated that stromal expression of SPARC may predict efficacy of nab-paclitaxel possibly by specifically increasing intratumoral drug accumulation through binding of SPARC and nab-paclitaxel [45]. Furthermore, the interaction between SPARC and nab-paclitaxel was suggested to deplete tumor stroma, thus breaking down the stromal barrier and increasing the accumulation of other drugs such as gemcitabine [46]. However, neither the stromal ablation theory nor the value of SPARC as biomarker for nab-paclitaxel treatment could be confirmed in controlled clinical trials, appropriate GEMMs using SPARC-knockout alleles, and patient-derived xenografts [47–49]. Therefore, the remarkable efficacy of nab-paclitaxel and gemcitabine in PDAC is likely due to improved tolerability of higher doses due to the albumin formulation and possibly also by decreasing the levels of the gemcitabine inactivating enzyme cytidine deaminase in tumor cells [50].

Although stromal depletion approaches have so far failed to achieve meaningful clinical efficacy and caused scepticism to whether it is the most promising therapeutic strategy, the heterogeneity of the stromal composition in human PDAC might be one reason for the conflicting results in murine models and human PDAC. Even though GEMMs recapitulate the tumor stroma quite closely, they are still distinctly different from human PDAC and most likely not as heterogeneous as previously anticipated. Therefore, PDAC patients might benefit from stromal subtyping approaches that could identify certain stromal targets for pharmacological modifications. To this end, pharmacological depletion of hyaluronic acid (HA) by enzymatic degradation using PEGPH20 in combination with gemcitabine was shown to be successful in GEMMs [51, 52]. Interestingly, the corresponding phase I/II study (NCT01839487) showed robust response rates for those patients that highly express HA in the tumor stroma indicating a potential first step toward personalized anti-stromal therapy [53]. Results from a large, randomized phase III trial (NCT02715804) using PEGPH20 in combination with nab-paclitaxel and gemcitabine in stage IV PDAC patients with high levels of HA have not been published yet but are expected to be negative.

Therapeautic Targeting of CAFs

Besides immune cells, CAFs are the predominant cell type within the activated, highly dynamic TME in PDAC [11]. CAFs have been implicated in therapeutic resistance by releasing abundant growth factors and cytokines that act upon surrounding stromal and tumor cells. CAFs are also directly involved in drug metabolism of gemcitabine. To this end, PSCs and CAFs were shown to metabolize and accumulate gemcitabine metabolites intracellularly, thus scavenging large quantities of active metabolites that are not available for tumor cells anymore [54]. Therefore, CAFs are an extremely promising therapeutic target; however, great attention should be paid to the selection of CAF targets as recent preclinical data indicate that broad depletion of CAFs may cause opposite effects with decreased tumor cell differentiation, increased invasiveness, and aggressiveness [35, 36]. Therefore, emerging knowledge about subtyping of CAFs will assist therapeutic target discovery to selectively inhibit tumor-promoting CAFs (e.g., iCAFs) and spare tumor-restraining CAFs (e.g., myCAFs) (Fig. 11.2). The abundance of poorly defined CAF markers such as α-smooth muscle actin (α-SMA), fibroblast-specific protein-1 (FSP-1), fibroblast activating protein-α (FAP-α), platelet-derived growth factor receptor-β (PDGFR-β), CD10, CD74, or SPARC and the potential of CAF plasticity with dynamic states of subtypes pose additional challenges (Fig. 11.2). However, first data are emerging that describe therapeutic targeting of CAF signalling pathways or receptors in experimental models of PDAC. For instance, the vit D receptor (VDR) on PSCs can be activated through VDR ligand calcipotriol and leads to subsequent reduction of PSC activation and fibrosis, thus reprogramming the TME [55]. Similar data regarding the induction of a more quiescent and less motile PSC phenotype were published in vitro and in vivo using ATRA [56]. Ongoing clinical trials in the USA and the UK are currently investigating the safety and efficacy of ATRA and paricalcitol in combination with chemotherapy in PDAC (NCT03307148, NCT03520790). Apart from the vit D receptor, somatostatin receptors (sst1-sst5) are G protein-coupled receptors that are selectively expressed on CAFs and might serve as therapeutic targets in PDAC. To this end, sst1 is overexpressed on CAFs in PDAC and can be pharmacologically targeted by SOM230 (Pasireotide® Novartis) that activates sst1 and subsequently blocks the mTOR/4E-BP1 pathway in CAFs [57, 58]. Targeting of the mTOR/4E-BP1 pathway subsequently led to sensitization to gemcitabine and inhibition of cancer metastasis via Il-6 and other CAF secreted factors [58]. A phase I study (NCT01385956) evaluated Pasireotide in locally advanced and metastatic PDAC ($n = 20$ patients) and found the compound to be well tolerated [59].

CAF-derived exosomes have recently been discovered to mediate chemoresistance in tumor cells via *Snail*, and therapeutic inhibition of exosome release by GW4869 showed beneficial therapeutic effects in co-culture experiments [60]. Further in vivo investigations and possibly clinical trials in combination with chemotherapy are required to comprehensively evaluate inhibition of exosomes as CAF-targeted therapies.

Nanoparticle formulations have also been attempted to selectively kill CAFs. For instance, carboxymethylcellulose-docetaxel nanoparticle (Cellax™-DTX) improved therapeutic response and selectively accumulated in α-SMA-positive CAFs in xenograft models [61]. However, regarding the various molecular subtypes of CAFs that are currently emerging and the use of xenograft models that poorly recapitulate the TME, doubts remain whether this strategy may be sophisticated enough to exclusively target tumor-promoting CAFs.

Another potentially CAF inactivating drug is Minnelide, a water-soluble prodrug of triptolide, a derivate from the Chinese plant *Tripterygium wilfordii*. Following promising experimental data in GEMMs [62], Minnelide is currently investigated in a clinical trial in PDAC patients (NCT03117920).

CAFs not only govern ECM composition and cross talk with tumor cells but also critically affect the composition and function of immune cells. The interaction between CAFs and immune cells often leads to an immunosuppressive TME, thus offering vantage points for future therapies alone or in combination with modern immune therapeutics such as checkpoint antagonists [63]. To this end, the subpopulation of FAP-α CAFs was discovered as major source of CXCL12 that mediated immunosuppression. Using a CXCL12 receptor chemokine (C-X-C motif) receptor 4 inhibitor (AMD3100), rapid T-cell accumulation and response to T-cell checkpoint inhibitors was reported in GEMMs [64]. Two early clinical dose escalation trials (NCT03277209, NCT02179970) were performed recently with AMD3100 (Plerixafor, Sanofi Oncology) to assess the safety, tolerability, and effects on the immune microenvironment, but results have not been reported so far. Table 11.1 summarizes clinical trials and preclinical evidence discussed above.

Table 11.1 Selection of currently active or recently completed clinical trials targeting various stromal components derived from preclinical evidence

NCT number	Phase	Target	Compound	Co-treatment	Preclinical evidence (Ref.)
NCT03117920	II	CAF inactivation	Minnelide	–	[62]
NCT03307148	Ib	CAF inactivation	ATRA	Gemcitabine + nab-paclitaxel	[40, 56]
NCT03331562	II	Vit D receptor agonist	Paricalcitol	Pembrolizumab	[55]
NCT02715804	III	Enzymatic degradation of hyaluronic acid	PEPGH20	Gemcitabine + nab-paclitaxel	[51, 52]
NCT03277209 NCT02179970	I	Antagonist for CXCR4	Plerixafor	–	[64]
NCT01385956	I	Agonist for somatostatin receptor 1	SOM 230 LAR (Pasireotide)	Gemcitabine	[57, 58]

CAF cancer-associated fibroblasts, *CXCR4* C-X-C motif receptor

Concluding Remarks and Future Directions

This article attempts to summarize important developments and current knowledge in the field of therapeutic targeting of the PDAC tumor stroma with a particular focus on acellular matrix components/signalling pathways and CAFs. Despite numerous successful preclinical trials, anti-stromal therapies have so far failed to play a role in clinical routine due to the lack of approved therapies. There are several reasons for this failure: (i) Tumor stroma constitutes a very heterogeneous mass and greatly differs in function and composition among patients. (ii) A variety of model systems have been used in the past to test therapeutic targets and novel drugs (i.e., xenograft models, patient-derived xenografts, orthotopic tumor transplantation, various GEMMs, and more recently organoids). Each of the model systems recapitulates certain features of the TME, but none is universally valid and predictive, and results are often hard to translate from one model to the other. (iii) Treatment schedules and length of treatment are fundamentally different in mouse trials and can only capture a small proportion of real-life oncological treatment outcome in patients as seen for SHH inhibition. (iv) Preclinical trials have no general regulation of required (double-blinded and randomized) controls and often lack sufficient sample size. (v) The complexity of interaction and interdependency of single stromal targets or cells with multiple signalling pathways has been underestimated.

Molecular subtyping of PDAC aims to address the genetic complexity by using high-throughput sequencing technologies such as whole-genome profiling and transcriptome profiling [65]. This molecular taxonomy might provide fundamental molecular characteristics of tumors that are otherwise microscopically indistinguishable. In analogy of the predominant epithelial subtypes [66, 67], "activated" and "normal" stroma subtypes were recently described and independently prognostic [68, 69]. Further discoveries in this field will aim to establish therapeutic implications and individualized therapeutic strategies according to the predominant molecular subtype. Accordingly, clinical trials will have to tackle these issues by providing powerful translational programs to maximize gain in insight. Furthermore, umbrella and basket trials might be more appropriate to identify effective treatment approaches in small subgroups of PDAC patients rather than the traditional phase I–III algorithm.

References

1. Neesse A, Michl P, Frese KK, Feig C, Cook N, Jacobetz MA, et al. Stromal biology and therapy in pancreatic cancer. Gut. 2011;60(6):861–8.
2. Neesse A, Algul H, Tuveson DA, Gress TM. Stromal biology and therapy in pancreatic cancer: a changing paradigm. Gut. 2015;64(9):1476–84.
3. Vennin C, Murphy KJ, Morton JP, Cox TR, Pajic M, Timpson P. Reshaping the tumor stroma for treatment of pancreatic cancer. Gastroenterology. 2018;154(4):820–38.

4. Neuzillet C, Tijeras-Raballand A, Ragulan C, Cros J, Patil Y, Martinet M, et al. Inter- and intra-tumoural heterogeneity in cancer-associated fibroblasts of human pancreatic ductal adenocarcinoma. J Pathol. 2019;248(1):51–65.
5. Apte MV, Haber PS, Applegate TL, Norton ID, McCaughan GW, Korsten MA, et al. Periacinar stellate shaped cells in rat pancreas: identification, isolation, and culture. Gut. 1998;43(1):128–33.
6. Apte MV, Haber PS, Darby SJ, Rodgers SC, McCaughan GW, Korsten MA, et al. Pancreatic stellate cells are activated by proinflammatory cytokines: implications for pancreatic fibrogenesis. Gut. 1999;44(4):534–41.
7. Bachem MG, Schneider E, Gross H, Weidenbach H, Schmid RM, Menke A, et al. Identification, culture, and characterization of pancreatic stellate cells in rats and humans. Gastroenterology. 1998;115(2):421–32.
8. Neesse A, Bauer CA, Ohlund D, Lauth M, Buchholz M, Michl P, et al. Stromal biology and therapy in pancreatic cancer: ready for clinical translation? Gut. 2019;68(1):159–71.
9. Kalluri R. The biology and function of fibroblasts in cancer. Nat Rev Cancer. 2016;16(9):582–98.
10. Waghray M, Yalamanchili M, Dziubinski M, Zeinali M, Erkkinen M, Yang H, et al. GM-CSF mediates mesenchymal-epithelial cross-talk in pancreatic cancer. Cancer Discov. 2016;6(8):886–99.
11. Ohlund D, Elyada E, Tuveson D. Fibroblast heterogeneity in the cancer wound. J Exp Med. 2014;211(8):1503–23.
12. Ohlund D, Handly-Santana A, Biffi G, Elyada E, Almeida AS, Ponz-Sarvise M, et al. Distinct populations of inflammatory fibroblasts and myofibroblasts in pancreatic cancer. J Exp Med. 2017;214(3):579–96.
13. Elyada E, Bolisetty M, Laise P, Flynn WF, Courtois ET, Burkhart RA, et al. Cross-species single-cell analysis of pancreatic ductal adenocarcinoma reveals antigen-presenting cancer-associated fibroblasts. Cancer Discov. 2019;9(8):1102–23.
14. Demir IE, Friess H, Ceyhan GO. Nerve-cancer interactions in the stromal biology of pancreatic cancer. Front Physiol. 2012;3:97.
15. Demir IE, Kujundzic K, Pfitzinger PL, Saricaoglu OC, Teller S, Kehl T, et al. Early pancreatic cancer lesions suppress pain through CXCL12-mediated chemoattraction of Schwann cells. Proc Natl Acad Sci U S A. 2017;114(1):E85–94.
16. Kleeff J, Korc M, Apte M, La Vecchia C, Johnson CD, Biankin AV, et al. Pancreatic cancer. Nat Rev Dis Primers. 2016;2:16022.
17. Vonlaufen A, Phillips PA, Xu Z, Goldstein D, Pirola RC, Wilson JS, et al. Pancreatic stellate cells and pancreatic cancer cells: an unholy alliance. Cancer Res. 2008;68(19):7707–10.
18. Erkan M, Hausmann S, Michalski CW, Fingerle AA, Dobritz M, Kleeff J, et al. The role of stroma in pancreatic cancer: diagnostic and therapeutic implications. Nat Rev Gastroenterol Hepatol. 2012;9(8):454–67.
19. Erkan M, Reiser-Erkan C, Michalski CW, Kong B, Esposito I, Friess H, et al. The impact of the activated stroma on pancreatic ductal adenocarcinoma biology and therapy resistance. Curr Mol Med. 2012;12(3):288–303.
20. Feig C, Gopinathan A, Neesse A, Chan DS, Cook N, Tuveson DA. The pancreas cancer microenvironment. Clin Cancer Res. 2012;18(16):4266–76.
21. Von Hoff DD, Ervin T, Arena FP, Chiorean EG, Infante J, Moore M, et al. Increased survival in pancreatic cancer with nab-paclitaxel plus gemcitabine. N Engl J Med. 2013;369(18):1691–703.
22. Conroy T, Desseigne F, Ychou M, Bouche O, Guimbaud R, Becouarn Y, et al. FOLFIRINOX versus gemcitabine for metastatic pancreatic cancer. N Engl J Med. 2011;364(19):1817–25.
23. Bramhall SR, Rosemurgy A, Brown PD, Bowry C, Buckels JA, Marimastat Pancreatic Cancer Study Group. Marimastat as first-line therapy for patients with unresectable pancreatic cancer: a randomized trial. J Clin Oncol. 2001;19(15):3447–55.
24. Hidalgo M, Eckhardt SG. Development of matrix metalloproteinase inhibitors in cancer therapy. J Natl Cancer Inst. 2001;93(3):178–93.

25. Jones L, Ghaneh P, Humphreys M, Neoptolemos JP. The matrix metalloproteinases and their inhibitors in the treatment of pancreatic cancer. Ann N Y Acad Sci. 1999;880:288–307.
26. Ellenrieder V, Alber B, Lacher U, Hendler SF, Menke A, Boeck W, et al. Role of MT-MMPs and MMP-2 in pancreatic cancer progression. Int J Cancer. 2000;85(1):14–20.
27. Ellenrieder V, Hendler SF, Ruhland C, Boeck W, Adler G, Gress TM. TGF-beta-induced invasiveness of pancreatic cancer cells is mediated by matrix metalloproteinase-2 and the urokinase plasminogen activator system. Int J Cancer. 2001;93(2):204–11.
28. Bramhall SR, Schulz J, Nemunaitis J, Brown PD, Baillet M, Buckels JA. A double-blind placebo-controlled, randomised study comparing gemcitabine and marimastat with gemcitabine and placebo as first line therapy in patients with advanced pancreatic cancer. Br J Cancer. 2002;87(2):161–7.
29. Moore MJ, Hamm J, Dancey J, Eisenberg PD, Dagenais M, Fields A, et al. Comparison of gemcitabine versus the matrix metalloproteinase inhibitor BAY 12-9566 in patients with advanced or metastatic adenocarcinoma of the pancreas: a phase III trial of the National Cancer Institute of Canada Clinical Trials Group. J Clin Oncol. 2003;21(17):3296–302.
30. Olive KP, Jacobetz MA, Davidson CJ, Gopinathan A, McIntyre D, Honess D, et al. Inhibition of Hedgehog signaling enhances delivery of chemotherapy in a mouse model of pancreatic cancer. Science. 2009;324(5933):1457–61.
31. Tian H, Callahan CA, DuPree KJ, Darbonne WC, Ahn CP, Scales SJ, et al. Hedgehog signaling is restricted to the stromal compartment during pancreatic carcinogenesis. Proc Natl Acad Sci U S A. 2009;106(11):4254–9.
32. Yauch RL, Gould SE, Scales SJ, Tang T, Tian H, Ahn CP, et al. A paracrine requirement for hedgehog signalling in cancer. Nature. 2008;455(7211):406–10.
33. Catenacci DV, Junttila MR, Karrison T, Bahary N, Horiba MN, Nattam SR, et al. Randomized phase Ib/II study of gemcitabine plus placebo or vismodegib, a hedgehog pathway inhibitor, in patients with metastatic pancreatic cancer. J Clin Oncol. 2015;33(36):4284–92.
34. Kim EJ, Sahai V, Abel EV, Griffith KA, Greenson JK, Takebe N, et al. Pilot clinical trial of hedgehog pathway inhibitor GDC-0449 (vismodegib) in combination with gemcitabine in patients with metastatic pancreatic adenocarcinoma. Clin Cancer Res. 2014;20(23): 5937–45.
35. Ozdemir BC, Pentcheva-Hoang T, Carstens JL, Zheng X, Wu CC, Simpson TR, et al. Depletion of carcinoma-associated fibroblasts and fibrosis induces immunosuppression and accelerates pancreas cancer with reduced survival. Cancer Cell. 2014;25(6):719–34.
36. Rhim AD, Oberstein PE, Thomas DH, Mirek ET, Palermo CF, Sastra SA, et al. Stromal elements act to restrain, rather than support, pancreatic ductal adenocarcinoma. Cancer Cell. 2014;25(6):735–47.
37. Pitarresi JR, Liu X, Avendano A, Thies KA, Sizemore GM, Hammer AM, et al. Disruption of stromal hedgehog signaling initiates RNF5-mediated proteasomal degradation of PTEN and accelerates pancreatic tumor growth. Life Sci Alliance. 2018;1(5):e201800190.
38. Kai F, Laklai H, Weaver VM. Force matters: biomechanical regulation of cell invasion and migration in disease. Trends Cell Biol. 2016;26(7):486–97.
39. Laklai H, Miroshnikova YA, Pickup MW, Collisson EA, Kim GE, Barrett AS, et al. Genotype tunes pancreatic ductal adenocarcinoma tissue tension to induce matricellular fibrosis and tumor progression. Nat Med. 2016;22(5):497–505.
40. Chronopoulos A, Robinson B, Sarper M, Cortes E, Auernheimer V, Lachowski D, et al. ATRA mechanically reprograms pancreatic stellate cells to suppress matrix remodelling and inhibit cancer cell invasion. Nat Commun. 2016;7:12630.
41. Rath N, Morton JP, Julian L, Helbig L, Kadir S, McGhee EJ, et al. ROCK signaling promotes collagen remodeling to facilitate invasive pancreatic ductal adenocarcinoma tumor cell growth. EMBO Mol Med. 2017;9(2):198–218.
42. Kano MR, Bae Y, Iwata C, Morishita Y, Yashiro M, Oka M, et al. Improvement of cancer-targeting therapy, using nanocarriers for intractable solid tumors by inhibition of TGF-beta signaling. Proc Natl Acad Sci U S A. 2007;104(9):3460–5.

43. Miller BW, Morton JP, Pinese M, Saturno G, Jamieson NB, McGhee E, et al. Targeting the LOX/ hypoxia axis reverses many of the features that make pancreatic cancer deadly: inhibition of LOX abrogates metastasis and enhances drug efficacy. EMBO Mol Med. 2015;7(8):1063–76.
44. Infante JR, Matsubayashi H, Sato N, Tonascia J, Klein AP, Riall TA, et al. Peritumoral fibro-blast SPARC expression and patient outcome with resectable pancreatic adenocarcinoma. J Clin Oncol. 2007;25(3):319–25.
45. Von Hoff DD, Ramanathan RK, Borad MJ, Laheru DA, Smith LS, Wood TE, et al. Gemcitabine plus nab-paclitaxel is an active regimen in patients with advanced pancreatic cancer: a phase I/ II trial. J Clin Oncol. 2011;29(34):4548–54.
46. Alvarez R, Musteanu M, Garcia-Garcia E, Lopez-Casas PP, Megias D, Guerra C, et al. Stromal disrupting effects of nab-paclitaxel in pancreatic cancer. Br J Cancer. 2013;109(4):926–33.
47. Hidalgo M, Plaza C, Musteanu M, Illei P, Brachmann CB, Heise C, et al. SPARC expression did not predict efficacy of nab-paclitaxel plus gemcitabine or gemcitabine alone for metastatic pancreatic cancer in an exploratory analysis of the phase III MPACT trial. Clin Cancer Res. 2015;21(21):4811–8.
48. Neesse A, Frese KK, Chan DS, Bapiro TE, Howat WJ, Richards FM, et al. SPARC indepen-dent drug delivery and antitumour effects of nab-paclitaxel in genetically engineered mice. Gut. 2014;63(6):974–83.
49. Kim H, Samuel S, Lopez-Casas P, Grizzle W, Hidalgo M, Kovar J, et al. SPARC-independent delivery of nab-paclitaxel without depleting tumor stroma in patient-derived pancreatic cancer xenografts. Mol Cancer Ther. 2016;15(4):680–8.
50. Frese KK, Neesse A, Cook N, Bapiro TE, Lolkema MP, Jodrell DI, et al. nab-Paclitaxel poten-tiates gemcitabine activity by reducing cytidine deaminase levels in a mouse model of pancre-atic cancer. Cancer Discov. 2012;2(3):260–9.
51. Jacobetz MA, Chan DS, Neesse A, Bapiro TE, Cook N, Frese KK, et al. Hyaluronan impairs vascular function and drug delivery in a mouse model of pancreatic cancer. Gut. 2013;62(1):112–20.
52. Provenzano PP, Cuevas C, Chang AE, Goel VK, Von Hoff DD, Hingorani SR. Enzymatic tar-geting of the stroma ablates physical barriers to treatment of pancreatic ductal adenocarci-noma. Cancer Cell. 2012;21(3):418–29.
53. Hingorani SR, Zheng L, Bullock AJ, Seery TE, Harris WP, Sigal DS, et al. HALO 202: ran-domized phase II study of PEGPH20 plus nab-paclitaxel/gemcitabine versus nab-paclitaxel/ gemcitabine in patients with untreated, metastatic pancreatic ductal adenocarcinoma. J Clin Oncol. 2018;36(4):359–66.
54. Hessmann E, Patzak MS, Klein L, Chen N, Kari V, Ramu I, et al. Fibroblast drug scaveng-ing increases intratumoural gemcitabine accumulation in murine pancreas cancer. Gut. 2018;67(3):497–507.
55. Sherman MH, Yu RT, Engle DD, Ding N, Atkins AR, Tiriac H, et al. Vitamin D receptor-mediated stromal reprogramming suppresses pancreatitis and enhances pancreatic cancer therapy. Cell. 2014;159(1):80–93.
56. Froeling FE, Feig C, Chelala C, Dobson R, Mein CE, Tuveson DA, et al. Retinoic acid-induced pancreatic stellate cell quiescence reduces paracrine Wnt-beta-catenin signaling to slow tumor progression. Gastroenterology. 2011;141(4):1486–97, 97.e1–14.
57. Duluc C, Moatassim Billah S, Chalabi-Dchar M, Perraud A, Samain R, Breibach F, et al. Pharmacological targeting of the protein synthesis mTOR/4E-BP1 pathway in cancer-associated fibroblasts abrogates pancreatic tumour chemoresistance. EMBO Mol Med. 2015;7(6):735–53.
58. Moatassim-Billah S, Duluc C, Samain R, Jean C, Perraud A, Decaup E, et al. Anti-metastatic potential of somatostatin analog SOM230: indirect pharmacological targeting of pancreatic cancer-associated fibroblasts. Oncotarget. 2016;7(27):41584–98.
59. Suleiman Y, Mahipal A, Shibata D, Siegel EM, Jump H, Fulp WJ, et al. Phase I study of com-bination of pasireotide LAR + gemcitabine in locally advanced or metastatic pancreatic cancer. Cancer Chemother Pharmacol. 2015;76(3):481–7.

60. Richards KE, Zeleniak AE, Fishel ML, Wu J, Littlepage LE, Hill R. Cancer-associated fibro-blast exosomes regulate survival and proliferation of pancreatic cancer cells. Oncogene. 2017;36(13):1770–8.
61. Ernsting MJ, Hoang B, Lohse I, Undzys E, Cao P, Do T, et al. Targeting of metastasis-promoting tumor-associated fibroblasts and modulation of pancreatic tumor-associated stroma with a carboxymethylcellulose-docetaxel nanoparticle. J Control Release. 2015;206:122–30.
62. Dauer P, Zhao X, Gupta VK, Sharma N, Kesh K, Gnamlin P, et al. Inactivation of cancer-associated-fibroblasts disrupts oncogenic signaling in pancreatic cancer cells and promotes its regression. Cancer Res. 2018;78(5):1321–33.
63. Denton AE, Roberts EW, Fearon DT. Stromal cells in the tumor microenvironment. Adv Exp Med Biol. 2018;1060:99–114.
64. Feig C, Jones JO, Kraman M, Wells RJ, Deonarine A, Chan DS, et al. Targeting CXCL12 from FAP-expressing carcinoma-associated fibroblasts synergizes with anti-PD-L1 immunotherapy in pancreatic cancer. Proc Natl Acad Sci U S A. 2013;110(50):20212–7.
65. Collisson EA, Bailey P, Chang DK, Biankin AV. Molecular subtypes of pancreatic cancer. Nat Rev Gastroenterol Hepatol. 2019;16(4):207–20.
66. Bailey P, Chang DK, Nones K, Johns AL, Patch AM, Gingras MC, et al. Genomic analyses identify molecular subtypes of pancreatic cancer. Nature. 2016;531(7592):47–52.
67. Collisson EA, Sadanandam A, Olson P, Gibb WJ, Truitt M, Gu S, et al. Subtypes of pancreatic ductal adenocarcinoma and their differing responses to therapy. Nat Med. 2011;17(4):500–3.
68. Maurer HC, Olive KP. Laser capture microdissection on frozen sections for extraction of high-quality nucleic acids. Methods Mol Biol. 1882;2019:253–9.
69. Moffitt RA, Marayati R, Flate EL, Volmar KE, Loeza SG, Hoadley KA, et al. Virtual microdis-section identifies distinct tumor- and stroma-specific subtypes of pancreatic ductal adenocarci-noma. Nat Genet. 2015;47(10):1168–78.

Chapter 12
Epigenetic Targeting

Svenja Pichlmeier and Ivonne Regel

Historically, pancreatic cancer studies have focused on genetic mutations and classified four frequently mutated genes including *KRAS*, *CDKN2A* (p16), *TP53*, and *SMAD4* as "drivers" for pancreatic carcinogenesis. Numerous other "passenger" mutations with a lower prevalence have been identified with next-generation sequencing (NGS) techniques and affect, among others, epigenetic remodeling enzymes that catalyze histone modifications (*KDM6A*, *SETD2*, *MLL2*, *MLL3*, *ARID1A*, *SMARCA4*) [1, 2]. However, the genetic variants cannot fully explain the different phenotypes of pancreatic cancer, characterized by molecular patterns, therapy resistance, or metastasis formation. Moreover, pancreatic cancer subtypes, defined through gene expression profiles, did not show an association to the identified somatic mutations [1, 3, 4]. In an emerging set of preclinical studies, researchers have investigated epigenetic profiles in pancreatic cancer, which reveal a correlation to pancreatic cancer phenotypes and their characteristics [5, 6]. Consequently, a consideration of the epigenetic status in PDAC tumor tissues could be relevant for prediction and clinical outcome. The reversible nature of epigenetic modifications and a reprogramming of the epigenetic landscape toward a less aggressive tumor phenotype harbor a great potential for pancreatic cancer treatment.

Epigenetics describes structural adaptions in chromatin states that contribute to gene activity without changing the underlying DNA sequence [7]. Particularly, DNA methylation and posttranslational histone modifications, such as methylation or acetylation, determine an open or closed chromatin conformation that is associated with transcriptional active or repressive gene loci (Fig. 12.1). Notably, the epigenetic landscape is highly changed in malignant cells. Probably

S. Pichlmeier · I. Regel (✉)
Department of Medicine II, University Hospital, LMU, Munich, Germany
e-mail: ivonne.regel@med.uni-muenchen.de

© Springer Nature Switzerland AG 2020
C. W. Michalski et al. (eds.), *Translational Pancreatic Cancer Research*,
Molecular and Translational Medicine,
https://doi.org/10.1007/978-3-030-49476-6_12

(a) open chromatin conformation

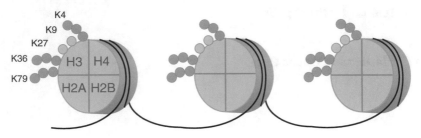

(b) closed chromatin conformation

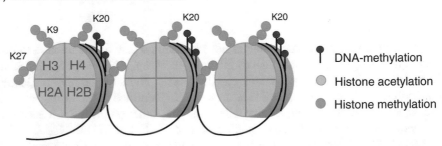

Fig. 12.1 Histone modifications determine open or closed chromatin conformation. (**a**) The acetylation or methylation of specific lysine residues (K4, K9, K27, K36, K79) on histone H3 is associated with transcriptional gene activation and an open chromatin conformation. (**b**) The methylation of the lysine residues K9, K20, and K27 on histone H3 and DNA methylation on CpG islands lead to gene silencing and a closed chromatin conformation

triggered through genetic, environmental, or metabolic factors, the epigenetic alterations can act as an oncogenic stimulus initiating tumor development or accelerating tumor progression [8]. Epigenetic modifications are deposited by "writers," removed by "erasers," and recognized by "readers" (Fig. 12.2). The enzymes are often dysregulated in cancer and are therefore potential targets for an epigenetic-based therapy. The number of epigenetic drugs has highly increased over the last years. The first epigenetic drugs approved by the US Food and Drug Administration (FDA) were the nucleoside analogues 5-azacytidine (5-aza or azacitidine) and 5-aza-2′-deoxycytidine (decitabine), which target DNA methyltransferases (DNMTs) and the histone deacetylase (HDAC) inhibitors vorinostat and romidepsin. In 2014 and 2015, the HDAC inhibitors (HDACi) belinostat and panobinostat were accepted for the indicated diseases, listed in Table 12.1 [9, 10]. Many other epigenetic drugs are currently under investigation in preclinical and clinical trials for various tumor entities (Fig. 12.2). However, the application of these drugs for pancreatic cancer therapies requires a deeper understanding of the epigenetic mechanisms in pancreatic carcinogenesis.

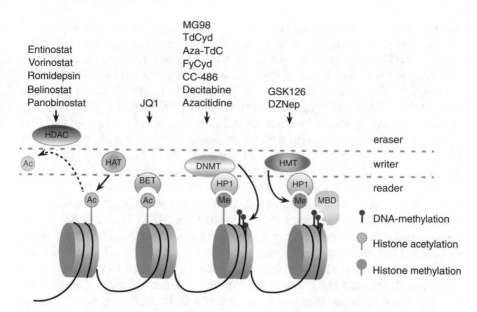

Fig. 12.2 Epigenetic modifiers and their inhibitors. Epigenetic modifications are catalyzed by "writers," such as histone acetyltransferases (HATs), histone methyltransferases (HMTs), and DNA methyltransferases (DNMTs). The marks are removed by "erasers," such as histone deacetylases (HDACs), and recognized by the "readers," bromodomain and extra-terminal (BET) proteins, heterochromatin protein 1 (HP1), and methyl-CpG-binding domain proteins (MBDs). The FDA-approved epigenetic inhibitors are listed in bold; FyCyd, 5-fluoro-2′-deoxycytidine; Aza-TdC, 5-aza-4′-thio-2′-deoxycytidine; TdCyd, 4′-thio-2′-deoxycytidine, DZNep 3-deazaneplanocin

Table 12.1 US Food and Drug Administration (FDA)-approved epigenetic drugs

Epigenetic drug	Classification	Approved year	Proposed indication
Azacitidine	DNMT inhibitor	2004	Myelodysplastic syndromes
Decitabine	DNMT inhibitor	2006	Myelodysplastic syndromes
Vorinostat	HDAC inhibitor	2006	Cutaneous T-cell lymphoma
Romidepsin	HDAC inhibitor	2009	Cutaneous T-cell lymphoma
Belinostat	HDAC inhibitor	2014	Peripheral T-cell lymphoma
Panobinostat	HDAC inhibitor	2015	Multiple myeloma

Modified from Li et al. [10] and updated on the US FDA web page (https://www.fda.gov/Drugs/default.htm)

Preclinical Studies on Epigenetic Alterations

Histone Acetylation

The acetylation and deacetylation of histones is a crucial mechanism for gene regulation and controlled by histone acetyl transferases (HATs) and HDACs, respectively (Fig. 12.2). HATs, such as CREB-binding protein, p300, and KAT2B, catalyze the acetylation of lysine residues on histone tails and promote gene expression, whereas the removal of the acetyl groups, for example, through class I HDAC1, HDAC2, HDAC3, or class III sirtuin (SIRT) enzymes, leads to transcriptional silencing. Particularly, class I HDACs are extensively studied in different tumor entities, including pancreatic cancer. The overexpression of HDACs in pancreatic cancer is associated with poor patient survival, high proliferation activity, increased tumor grade, and epithelial-to-mesenchymal transition (EMT) demonstrating their oncogenic potential [11]. Recent studies have investigated the acetylation of histone H3 on lysine 27 (H3K27ac), a target of class I HDACs, in more detail. Histone acetylation at gene enhancer regions separated low and high-grade PDACs and correlated well with a grade-specific gene expression programs. Thus, high levels of H3K27ac were associated with increased activation of epithelial genes in low-grade tumors [5]. Interestingly, another study showed that an H3K27ac-based reprogramming of enhancer elements occurs predominantly in metastatic lesions. It was noted that a gain of H3K27ac at specific gene enhancers promotes PDAC progression and metastatic potential [12]. These data illustrate that the targeted genomic loci of HATs and HDACs are highly dynamic in tumor evolution and phenotypic variants. Notably, histone acetylation can be found either on differentiation genes or on genes driving metastatic mechanisms. These dynamic and contradictory processes highlight the need for further information on epigenetic regulation and targeting, particularly under which conditions the application of epigenetic drugs would result in a clinical benefit.

In preclinical settings, HDACi show a variety of antitumor effects. HDACi promote cell cycle arrest by regulating the expression of cyclins, cyclin-dependent kinases (CDKs), and CDK inhibitors such as p21. HDACi also induce cell death through the activation of intrinsic and extrinsic apoptotic pathways and inhibit angiogenesis by regulating *HIF1A* and *VEGF* gene expression. Furthermore, some HDACi are able to stimulate the expression of E-cadherin, a potent suppressor of EMT and metastases formation [13]. Besides HDACi, recent experimental data demonstrated that targeting histone acetylation "readers," namely, BET (bromodomain and extra-terminal) proteins, suppresses PDAC development in a pancreatic cancer mouse model (Fig. 12.2). Bromodomain-containing (BRD) proteins, such as BRD2, BRD3, and BRD4, are highly expressed in PDAC and stimulate the expression of the proto-oncogene MYC. Treatment of pancreatic cancer mice with the BET inhibitor JQ1 in combination with the HDACi vorinostat resulted in significant longer overall survival and decreased tumor volume compared to JQ1 monotherapy, revealing promising results for clinical translation [14].

Histone Methylation

While histone acetylation is associated with gene expression, mono-, di-, or trimethylation of lysine residues on histone tails can have different effects. Methylation of H3 lysine 4 (H3K4me), lysine 36 (H3K36me), and lysine 79 (H3K79me) marks active gene loci, whereas methylation of H3 lysine 9 (H3K9me), lysine 27 (H3K27me), and H4 lysine 20 (H4K20me) correlates with gene silencing (Fig. 12.1) [15]. So far, over 50 lysine methyltransferases (KMTs) have been identified, subdivided in DOT1-like proteins and the SET domain-containing protein group [16]. The polycomb repressive complex (PRC) 2 subunit, enhancer of zeste (EZH2), which belongs to the SET domain-containing KMTs, catalyzes the repressive histone modification H3K27me (Fig. 12.2). In experimental approaches, several EZH2 inhibitors (EZH2i) demonstrate therapeutic potential for cancer treatment. The EZH2i 3-deazaneplanocin (DZNep) attenuates EMT and sensitizes pancreatic cancer cells for standard chemotherapy [17, 18]. A more potent EZH2i, GSK126, was tested in a large panel of cancer cell lines, including pancreatic cancer cells [19]. However, it should be noted that in a subset of cells, a loss of H3K27me after GSK126 treatment entailed an increase of transcriptionally active H3K27ac levels targeting preferentially oncogenes, which trigger tumor progression. The oncogenic effect was abandoned after additional BET inhibition [19]. Changing the global epigenetic landscape in a non-stratified manner may cause unintended effects and therapeutic controversies. These data highlight the need for a greater understanding of the molecular mechanisms after epigenetic drug treatment and a possible application of combination therapies for treatment success.

DNA Methylation

Cytosine residues in CG dinucleotide clusters, so-called CpG islands, are targets for DNA methylation. Sixty percent of the human gene promoters are associated with CpG islands and are mostly unmethylated, whereas CpG regions in repetitive elements and heterochromatin are heavily methylated [15]. The DNA methyltransferases 3A and 3B (DNMT3A and DNMT3B) regulate de novo methylation during embryogenesis, whereas DNMT1 catalyzes the methylation of the newly synthesized DNA strand after replication [16]. Methyl-CpG-binding domain proteins (MBDs) are epigenetic "readers" and recruit epigenetic repressor complexes, which mediate further chromatin compaction (Fig. 12.2). Genome-wide alterations of DNA methylation are a common event in tumorigenesis. Malignant cells exhibit an epigenetic silencing of tumor suppressor genes, such as *CDKN2A* (p16), through promoter hypermethylation, whereas the global genome is hypomethylated fostering chromosomal instability and oncogenicity [8]. Early in PDAC development, precursor lesions, such as pancreatic intraepithelial neoplasia (PanINs), show a hypermethylation of *CDKN2A* and other tumor suppressor genes [20]. Further methylated genes, regulating key signaling pathways in cell differentiation, were identified in PDAC patient samples [21] showing the significance of aberrant DNA methylation for pancreatic carcinogenesis.

The nucleoside analog 5-aza was the first synthesized epigenetic drug. It intercalates into the DNA and inhibits DNMT through permanent binding after DNA replication [22]. The treatment of pancreatic cancer cell lines with 5-aza significantly impaired cell proliferation and induced apoptosis in a time- and concentration-dependent manner. Moreover, 5-aza treatment decreased the expression of key molecules of the Wnt signaling pathway, such as β-catenin and MYC, which play an important role in tumor cell migration and metastasis [23]. Further studies have noted that 5-aza has the capability to sensitize cancer cells for chemo- or radiotherapy increasing the effectiveness of antitumor therapy [22, 24].

Although preclinical studies have made significant progress in understanding epigenetic changes in pancreatic cancer, there is still a lack of knowledge of the highly dynamic epigenetic mechanisms and their regulation in pancreatic tumor development and progression. Pharmacologic inhibition of histone-modifying enzymes or DNA methyltransferases has shown promising effects in experimental approaches. However, elucidating the conditions for epigenetic drug treatment and identifying patients who will profit from a certain epigenetic therapy will be the challenge for translating the experimental data into the clinical practice.

Clinical Trials Targeting Epigenetic Alterations

For many years, gemcitabine-based therapies have been the standard of care for patients suffering from PDAC. However, median overall survival stayed below 3 years (35.0 months) after adjuvant chemotherapy with gemcitabine. Admission of the modified FOLFIRINOX combination therapy (folinic acid + 5-fluorouracil + irinotecan + oxaliplatin) was able to raise the overall survival to 54.4 months at the price of increased toxicity [25]. Hence, there is a great need for new therapeutic strategies. Several phase I and II clinical trials address the tolerability and potency of epigenetic drugs as mono- or combination therapy in the setting of advanced disease refractory to standard therapy.

Vorinostat, also known as suberanilohydroxamic acid (SAHA), is an inhibitor of class I and II HDACs and was approved for the treatment of cutaneous T-cell lymphoma in 2006 (Table 12.1). Due to its broad effects on cell cycle arrest, apoptosis, angiogenesis, and tumor microenvironment, vorinostat is currently under investigation in several clinical studies for the treatment of solid tumors (Table 12.2). Although monotherapies of HDACi show a high efficiency in hematologic malignancies, the antitumor effects for solid cancers are mostly unsatisfactory. Thus, combination therapies of epigenetic inhibitors with classical chemotherapeutic agents or small-molecule inhibitors are enrolled for clinical trials [26]. The combination of vorinostat with marizomib, a proteasome inhibitor, was tested in a phase I clinical trial (NCT00667082) in 22 patients with solid cancers, including pancreatic cancer. The data showed stable disease in 61% of evaluable patients [27]. Similarly, the combinatory treatment of vorinostat with the proteasome inhibitor bortezomib in patients with advanced solid tumors (NCT00227513) revealed a stable disease in patients with sarcoma, colorectal cancer, and gastrointestinal stroma tumor (GIST), whereas pancreatic cancer patients were unaffected. The most common adverse events were hematologic and gastrointestinal-related toxicities [28]. Another phase

Table 12.2 Overview of HDAC inhibitors in clinical trials for pancreatic cancer

HDACi	Combination therapy	Phase	Patients	Dosage schedule (HDACi)	Outcome	Serious adverse events	NCT number
Vorinostat	Marizomib	I	22	300 mg/day	SD: 11/18 (61%)	Thrombocytopenia, nausea/vomiting	00667082
	Bortezomib	I	66	Dose escalation (100–300 mg/twice daily)	MTD: 1.3 mg/m^2 iv SD: 5/22 (23%)	Thrombocytopenia, fatigue, increased ALT, diarrhea, nausea	00227513
	Sirolimus	I	249	Dose escalation (100–400 mg/day)	PR: 2/61 (3%) SD: 2/61 (3%) PFS: 9 weeks	Thrombocytopenia, anemia, fatigue, mucositis	01087554
	5-FU, radiation	I/II	10	Varying doses/day, 6 weeks	OS: 6/9 (66.7%) RR: 6/9 (66.7%) PFS: 9.375 months	Hematologic and gastrointestinal, fatigue	00948688
	Capecitabine, radiation	I	21	Dose escalation (100–400 mg/day during radiation and Mon–Fri 2 weeks after radiation)	MTD: 400 mg/day SD: 19/21 (90%)	Lymphopenia, thrombocytopenia, nausea, vomiting, diarrhea	00983268
Belinostat	Carboplatin, paclitaxel	I	23	Dose escalation (600–1000 mg/m^2 Mon–Fri)	PR: 2/23 (9%) SD: 7/23 (30%)	Hematologic	00873119
Panobinostat	Gemcitabine	I	17	Dose escalation	PR: 1/17 (6%) SD: 8/17 (47%)	Hematologic, gastrointestinal, fatigue, rash	00550199
	Bortezomib	II	7	20 mg/3 times a week, 2 weeks	PFS: 2.1 months PD: 5/7 (71%)	Thromboembolic events (2/7), gastrointestinal, fever, dehydration	01056601
Entinostat	Nivolumab	II	54	5 mg 2 lead-in doses 5 mg/week	*Recruiting*		03250273

MTD maximum tolerated dose, *OS* overall survival, *PD* progressive disease, *PFS* progression-free survival, *PR* partial response, *RR* response rate, *SD* stable disease

I dose-escalating study (NCT01087554) evaluated the synergistic effects of the mTOR inhibitor sirolimus and vorinostat in 70 patients, including two patients with pancreatic cancer. They observed two partial responses in patients with refractory Hodgkin lymphoma and perivascular epithelioid cancer. Two patients with hepatocellular carcinoma and fibromyxoid sarcoma had stable disease for at least 12 months. The most common dose-limiting toxicities included grade 4 thrombocytopenia and grade 3 mucositis [29]. A phase I/II clinical trial (NCT00948688) investigated the effects of the antimetabolite 5-fluorouracil (5-FU) in combination with vorinostat and radiation therapy. Ten patients with pancreatic cancer received varying doses of vorinostat for 6 weeks to uncover the highest dosage for safe administration. One year after the study enrollment, 66.7% of the patients were still alive, and the overall response rate was 66.7%. Progression-free survival after 2 years was 9.4 months. Here, the most common serious adverse events were hematologic and gastrointestinal side effects, but no dose-limiting toxicities were observed (unpublished data from https://clinicaltrials.gov/). Furthermore, a phase I dose-escalating trial (NCT00983268) from 2009 to 2012 tested the efficacy of vorinostat and capecitabine as radiosensitizers in 21 patients with pancreatic cancer. Capecitabine was administered at a dosage of 1000 mg on the days of radiation, whereas vorinostat was given orally on the days of radiation and continued for 2 weeks on Monday through Friday after completing the radiation therapy. The maximum tolerated dose of vorinostat was 400 mg/day. They reported thrombocytopenia, nausea and vomiting, diarrhea, and dehydration as dose-limiting toxicities. The most common study-related adverse events with a grade ≥ 3 were lymphopenia (67%) and nausea (14%). Notably, 90% of the patients had stable disease and 33% of patients initially classified as borderline-resectable underwent R0 or R1 resections. The median overall survival in the study was 1.1 years [30]. Even though only a small number of patients were investigated, the study results were encouraging, since advanced PDAC patients rarely show a radiosensitive response.

Belinostat is a pan-HDACi and was approved for the treatment of relapsed or refractory peripheral T-cell lymphoma in 2014 (Table 12.1). Preclinical studies have shown that belinostat inhibits cell growth and initiates apoptosis and cell cycle arrest in a dose-dependent manner. Furthermore, belinostat inactivates downstream signaling of the PI3K-mTOR pathway and blocks hypoxia-induced pro-tumorigenic mechanisms [31, 32]. Along with several experimental approaches to further determine pharmacokinetics and safety of belinostat, first phase I clinical trials are conducted in patients with solid tumors (Table 12.2). In a phase I dose-escalating trial (NCT00873119), 23 patients with solid tumors, including three cases with pancreatic cancer, received 600–1000 mg/m^2 belinostat per day on day one to five of each cycle in combination with carboplatin and/or paclitaxel. No dose-limiting toxicities were observed. Grade 3 adverse events included neutropenia (30%), leukopenia (22%), and thrombocytopenia (13%). Two patients with metastatic pancreatic and metastatic rectal cancer showed a partial response of 7 and 9 months, respectively. Seven patients showed stable disease for ≥ 6 months (range 6–29 months) [33].

Another pan-HDACi, approved for hematologic malignancy (multiple myeloma) (Table 12.1), which is currently under clinical testing for the treatment of solid tumors, is *panobinostat* (Table 12.2). In contrast to other HDACi, panobinostat has a longer elimination time and shows an increased potency against hyperacetylating histone proteins [34]. Therefore, intermittent dosing schedules are needed to reduce common dose-limiting toxicities of HDACi. In a phase I clinical study (NCT00550199), 17 patients with solid tumors received oral panobinostat over five different dose levels (continuous or intermittent dosing) in combination with intravenous gemcitabine treatment. Nevertheless, grade four hematologic side effects, notably thrombocytopenia and neutropenia, occurred at all dose levels and required multiple changes in the study protocol. Other adverse events included anorexia, constipation, diarrhea, fatigue, nausea, vomiting, and rash. Besides one unconfirmed partial response in a patient with ovarian cancer, eight patients including one patient with pancreatic cancer had stable disease (median duration six cycles) [35]. However, another clinical study (NCT01056601) utilizing a combination of panobinostat and bortezomib showed progressive disease in >70% of the participants. More preclinical studies are urgently needed to identify panobinostat treatment strategies and combinatory agents improving patient outcome.

Several other new HDACi are currently under investigation in various combinatory trials. For example, an ongoing clinical study (NCT03250273) is testing the safety and efficiency of *entinostat*, a class I HDACi, in combination with nivolumab, an IgG4 monoclonal antibody, on patients with pancreatic cancer or with tumors of the biliary tract (Table 12.2). The first results are eagerly awaited.

Azacitidine (5-azacytidine) and decitabine (*5-aza-2'-deoxycytidine*) are DNMT inhibitors (DNMTi) and approved for the treatment of myelodysplastic syndrome (MDS), acute myeloid leukemia (AML), and chronic myelomonocytic leukemia (CMML), respectively (Table 12.1). The nucleoside analogues share structural similarities with cytidine and are incorporated into the DNA during the replication of cancer cells, which causes direct cytotoxicity [22]. In several clinical trials, DNMTi are investigated as mono- or combinatory therapy (Table 12.3). The combination of 5-aza and gemcitabine was tested in a phase I dose escalation study on nine patients with advanced pancreatic cancer (NCT01167816). Furthermore, two phase II studies with 5-aza and pembrolizumab, an immune checkpoint inhibitor, are ongoing (NCT03264404, NCT01845805). Due to the rapid deamination of (deoxy-) cytidine to (deoxy-) uridine, cytidine deaminase inhibitors like tetrahydrouridine (THU) are co-administered with cytidine analogues [36]. In a phase I clinical trial (NCT00359606), 58 patients with refractory solid tumors received the cytidine analogue *5-fluoro-2'-deoxycytidine* (FyCyd). The DNMTi was administered intravenously on days 1–5 every 3 weeks or on days 1–5 and 8–12 every 4 weeks together with a fixed dose of 350 mg/m²/day THU. In the 3-week schedule, no dose-limiting toxicities were observed. In the 4-week schedule, one dose-limiting grade 3 colitis was reported during the first cycle. The MTD was defined as 134 mg/m²/day. Fifty percent of the patients (20/40) included in this study reached stable disease as best outcome (1.4–13.3 months). One partial response was reported in a heavily pretreated breast cancer patient (>90% decrease in tumor size) and maintained for 15.2 months. Unfortunately, no patients with pancreatic cancer were included in this study [37]. A second phase I trial (NCT01534598) investigates the effects of a

Table 12.3 Overview of DNMT inhibitors in clinical trials for solid tumors

DNMTi	Combination therapy	Phase	Patients	Dosage schedule (DNMTi)	Outcome	NCT number
5-Azacytidine (azacitidine)	Gemcitabine	I	9	Dose escalation, 5 consecutive days each 4-week cycle	*Terminated*	01167816
	Pembrolizumab	II	31	50 mg/m^2 subcutaneous daily, 5 days each 4-week cycle	*Recruiting*	03264404
		II	80	300 mg daily on days 1–21 of each 4-week cycle	*Recruiting*	01845805
5-Fluoro-2′-deoxycytidine (FyCyd)	Tetrahydrouridine (THU)	I	58	Dose escalation, days 1–5 of each 3-week cycle or days 1–5 and 8–12 of each 4-week cycle	MTD: 134 mg/m^2 SD: 20/40 (50%) PR: 1/40 (3%)	00359606
	Tetrahydrouridine (THU)	I	68	Dose escalation, days 1 to 3 and 8 to 10 of a 3-week cycle, oral administration	*Recruiting*	01534598
CC-486	Carboplatin, Nab-paclitaxel	I	169	Dose escalation	PR: 5/57 (9%) RR: 6/57 (11%)	01478685
5-Aza-2′-deoxycytidine (decitabine)	Gemcitabine	I	42	Dose escalation starting at 0.1 mg/kg subcutaneously, two times a week for 3 weeks of a 4-week cycle	*Recruiting*	02959164
	Tetrahydrouridine (THU)	I	13	Starting dose by weight (10–20 mg daily) two times a week on consecutive days	*Active*	02847000
MG98		I	20	Dose escalation (40–360 mg/m^2), 21 consecutive days of 4-week cycle	No changes in DNMT1 levels	
		I	33	Dose escalation, 7 consecutive days of a 2-week cycle	PR: 1/33 (3%)	

MTD maximum tolerated dose, *PR* partial response, *RR* response rate, *SD* stable disease different dosage schedule of FyCyd and THU in 68 patients with advanced solid tumors. Moreover, pharmacokinetics and efficacy of an oral formulation of 5-azacytidine (*CC-486*) were explored in patients with relapsed or refractory solid tumors in a phase I clinical trial (NCT01478685). The first part of the trial included a dose escalation study of CC-486 alone or in combination with carboplatin or nab-paclitaxel in 57 patients. In the second part of the study, 112 patients were assigned to treatment arms according to the tumor type and received CC-486 at the recommended dose alone or in combination with carboplatin or nab-paclitaxel. Thus, patients with pancreatic cancer received 200 mg CC-486 orally for 2 weeks and 100 mg/m^2 nab-paclitaxel intravenously on days 1 and 14. The objective response rate in the first part of the study was 10.5% (6/57), and five partial responses were reported in the study arms with CC-486 monotherapy and CC-486 in combination with nab-paclitaxel. In the second part, partial responses were detected in patients with bladder cancer, ovarian cancer, non-small cell lung carcinoma (NSCLC), nasopharyngeal carcinoma (NPC), and other virus-associated tumors (OVAT). Disease control rates reached 45.8% in pancreatic cancer. The most common adverse event with grade $\geq$ 3 in all study arms was neutropenia. The study showed promising effects and partial response rates for several tumor entities; however, the CC-486 combination therapy with carboplatin or nab-paclitaxel did not improve the overall response in comparison to the CC-486 monotherapy [38].

New treatment strategies for solid tumors also implement the use of the DNMTi *decitabine* (Table 12.3). Two ongoing phase I clinical trials aim at determining the maximum tolerated dose, as well as outcome and dose-limiting toxicities in combination with the classic chemotherapeutic agent gemcitabine (NCT02959164) or with the cytidine deaminase inhibitor THU (NCT02847000). Most clinical studies for DNMTi are phase I trials testing drug safety in patients with advanced solid tumors. Thus, different dosage regimens of new agents, such as *5-aza-4'-thio-2'-deoxycytidine* (Aza-TdC) (NCT03366116) and *4'-thio-2'-Deoxycytidine* (TdCyd) (NCT02423057), are elucidated for safe drug administration. A second-generation DNMT1 inhibitor, which was tested in clinical trials, is *MG98*. This is a phosphorothioate antisense oligonucleotide, which inhibits DNMT1 translation with a high specificity [39]. Fourteen patients with solid cancers received MG98 in a dose-escalating phase I study. MG98 was administered intravenously for 21 consecutive days, followed by 1-week rest period. A significant number of patients experienced dose-limiting transaminase elevations. Other dose-limiting toxicities included fatigue, anorexia, and thrombocytopenia. Although the mean plasma drug concentrations of MG98 were ten times higher than the IC$_{50}$ values determined in vitro (50–70 nM), no significant changes in DNMT1 levels were observed [40]. Later on, another phase I dose escalation clinical trial investigated the effects of MG98 on DNMT1 expression in 33 patients with advanced solid tumors, including four patients with tumors of the pancreas or biliary system. Here, MG98 was administered by continuous intravenous infusion over 7 days in a 2-week cycle. The most common observed drug-related toxicities were grade 3 transaminitis and grade 3 thrombocytopenia. Other side effects included fatigue, headaches, myalgia, and nausea. One patient with esophageal cancer achieved a partial response, and another patient with GIST showed prolonged disease stabilization for more than 3 years [39].

Although DNMTi are tested in a variety of clinical studies with different co-medications, only one study protocol using a combination of FyCyd and THU [35] showed promising results in solid tumors. However, this study did not include patients with pancreatic cancer. Hence, there is a great need to include more patients with advanced pancreatic cancer in clinical trials investigating safety and efficacy of DNMTi.

Conclusion

Hematologic malignancies have been successfully treated with epigenetic drugs, such as vorinostat or azacitidine, for several years. Although more and more clinical studies exhibited promising effects of epigenetic drugs in solid tumor therapy regimens, there are many aspects not uncovered yet transferring experimental data into a successful clinical approach. Notably, broad antitumorigenic effects of HDACi and DNMTi were detected in experimental settings, but most clinical trials testing epigenetic treatment strategies in pancreatic cancer patients demonstrated rather disappointing results on overall survival and response rates. One aspect might be a required stratification of pancreatic cancer patients according to their epigenetic landscape to identify those patients who would benefit from an epigenetic treatment. Furthermore, the molecular mechanisms affected by epigenetic drugs are barely understood. The influence of unknown regulators, activated in response to epigenetic treatment, might limit the efficiency of epigenetic therapies. Moreover, the dynamic nature of epigenetic modifications targeting either tumor suppressor genes or oncogenes makes the application of epigenetic drugs sometimes unpredictable. An additional complication of epigenetic remodeler inhibition is the complete blockage of their enzymatic activity without the possibility to rescue the physiological function. Consequently, more preclinical and clinical studies are needed to investigate the molecular mechanisms controlled by epigenetic modifiers. Revealing the functional consequences of epigenetic drug treatment, under the consideration of various pancreatic cancer subtypes, will be a future challenge. Nevertheless, several phase I clinical trials were able to determine the maximum tolerated dose for HDACi, DNMTi, and other epigenetic inhibitors, building a foundation for further epigenetic treatment strategies.

References

1. Bailey P, Chang DK, Nones K, Johns AL, Patch AM, Gingras MC, et al. Genomic analyses identify molecular subtypes of pancreatic cancer. Nature. 2016;531(7592):47–52.

2. Waddell N, Pajic M, Patch AM, Chang DK, Kassahn KS, Bailey P, et al. Whole genomes redefine the mutational landscape of pancreatic cancer. Nature. 2015;518(7540):495–501.
3. Moffitt RA, Marayati R, Flate EL, Volmar KE, Loeza SG, Hoadley KA, et al. Virtual microdissection identifies distinct tumor- and stroma-specific subtypes of pancreatic ductal adenocarcinoma. Nat Genet. 2015;47(10):1168–78.
4. Collisson EA, Sadanandam A, Olson P, Gibb WJ, Truitt M, Gu S, et al. Subtypes of pancreatic ductal adenocarcinoma and their differing responses to therapy. Nat Med. 2011;17(4):500–3.
5. Diaferia GR, Balestrieri C, Prosperini E, Nicoli P, Spaggiari P, Zerbi A, et al. Dissection of transcriptional and cis-regulatory control of differentiation in human pancreatic cancer. EMBO J. 2016;35(6):595–617.
6. Lomberk G, Blum Y, Nicolle R, Nair A, Gaonkar KS, Marisa L, et al. Distinct epigenetic landscapes underlie the pathobiology of pancreatic cancer subtypes. Nat Commun. 2018;9(1):1978.
7. Bird A. Perceptions of epigenetics. Nature. 2007;447(7143):396–8.
8. Flavahan WA, Gaskell E, Bernstein BE. Epigenetic plasticity and the hallmarks of cancer. Science. 2017;357(6348):eaal2380.
9. Berdasco M, Esteller M. Clinical epigenetics: seizing opportunities for translation. Nat Rev Genet. 2019;20(2):109–27.
10. Li J, Hao D, Wang L, Wang H, Wang Y, Zhao Z, et al. Epigenetic targeting drugs potentiate chemotherapeutic effects in solid tumor therapy. Sci Rep. 2017;7(1):4035.
11. Schneider G, Kramer OH, Schmid RM, Saur D. Acetylation as a transcriptional control mechanism-HDACs and HATs in pancreatic ductal adenocarcinoma. J Gastrointest Cancer. 2011;42(2):85–92.
12. Roe JS, Hwang CI, Somerville TDD, Milazzo JP, Lee EJ, Da Silva B, et al. Enhancer reprogramming promotes pancreatic cancer metastasis. Cell. 2017;170(5):875–88.e20.
13. Feng W, Zhang B, Cai D, Zou X. Therapeutic potential of histone deacetylase inhibitors in pancreatic cancer. Cancer Lett. 2014;347(2):183–90.
14. Mazur PK, Herner A, Mello SS, Wirth M, Hausmann S, Sanchez-Rivera FJ, et al. Combined inhibition of BET family proteins and histone deacetylases as a potential epigenetics-based therapy for pancreatic ductal adenocarcinoma. Nat Med. 2015;21(10):1163–71.
15. Bernstein BE, Meissner A, Lander ES. The mammalian epigenome. Cell. 2007;128(4):669–81.
16. Lomberk GA, Iovanna J, Urrutia R. The promise of epigenomic therapeutics in pancreatic cancer. Epigenomics. 2016;8(6):831–42.
17. Hung SW, Mody H, Marrache S, Bhutia YD, Davis F, Cho JH, et al. Pharmacological reversal of histone methylation presensitizes pancreatic cancer cells to nucleoside drugs: in vitro optimization and novel nanoparticle delivery studies. PLoS One. 2013;8(8):e71196.
18. Mody HR, Hung SW, Pathak RK, Griffin J, Cruz-Monserrate Z, Govindarajan R. miR-202 diminishes TGFbeta receptors and attenuates TGFbeta1-induced EMT in pancreatic cancer. Mol Cancer Res. 2017;15(8):1029–39.
19. Huang X, Yan J, Zhang M, Wang Y, Chen Y, Fu X, et al. Targeting epigenetic crosstalk as a therapeutic strategy for EZH2-aberrant solid tumors. Cell. 2018;175(1):186–99.e19.
20. Sato N, Fukushima N, Hruban RH, Goggins M. CpG island methylation profile of pancreatic intraepithelial neoplasia. Mod Pathol. 2008;21(3):238–44.
21. Nones K, Waddell N, Song S, Patch AM, Miller D, Johns A, et al. Genome-wide DNA methylation patterns in pancreatic ductal adenocarcinoma reveal epigenetic deregulation of SLIT-ROBO, ITGA2 and MET signaling. Int J Cancer. 2014;135(5):1110–8.
22. Paradise BD, Barham W, Fernandez-Zapico ME. Targeting epigenetic aberrations in pancreatic cancer, a new path to improve patient outcomes? Cancers. 2018;10(5):128.
23. Zhang H, Zhou WC, Li X, Meng WB, Zhang L, Zhu XL, et al. 5-Azacytidine suppresses the proliferation of pancreatic cancer cells by inhibiting the Wnt/beta-catenin signaling pathway. Genet Mol Res. 2014;13(3):5064–72.
24. Gailhouste L, Liew LC, Hatada I, Nakagama H, Ochiya T. Epigenetic reprogramming using 5-azacytidine promotes an anti-cancer response in pancreatic adenocarcinoma cells. Cell Death Dis. 2018;9(5):468.

25. Conroy T, Hammel P, Hebbar M, Ben Abdelghani M, Wei AC, Raoul JL, et al. FOLFIRINOX or gemcitabine as adjuvant therapy for pancreatic cancer. N Engl J Med. 2018;379(25):2395–406.
26. Hessmann E, Johnsen SA, Siveke JT, Ellenrieder V. Epigenetic treatment of pancreatic cancer: is there a therapeutic perspective on the horizon? Gut. 2017;66(1):168–79.
27. Millward M, Price T, Townsend A, Sweeney C, Spencer A, Sukumaran S, et al. Phase 1 clinical trial of the novel proteasome inhibitor marizomib with the histone deacetylase inhibitor vorinostat in patients with melanoma, pancreatic and lung cancer based on in vitro assessments of the combination. Investig New Drugs. 2012;30(6):2303–17.
28. Deming DA, Ninan J, Bailey HH, Kolesar JM, Eickhoff J, Reid JM, et al. A phase I study of intermittently dosed vorinostat in combination with bortezomib in patients with advanced solid tumors. Investig New Drugs. 2014;32(2):323–9.
29. Park II, Garrido-Laguna I, Naing A, Fu S, Falchook GS, Piha-Paul SA, et al. Phase I dose-escalation study of the mTOR inhibitor sirolimus and the HDAC inhibitor vorinostat in patients with advanced malignancy. Oncotarget. 2016;7(41):67521–31.
30. Chan E, Arlinghaus LR, Cardin DB, Goff L, Berlin JD, Parikh A, et al. Phase I trial of vorinostat added to chemoradiation with capecitabine in pancreatic cancer. Radiother Oncol. 2016;119(2):312–8.
31. Chien W, Lee DH, Zheng Y, Wuensche P, Alvarez R, Wen DL, et al. Growth inhibition of pancreatic cancer cells by histone deacetylase inhibitor belinostat through suppression of multiple pathways including HIF, NFkB, and mTOR signaling in vitro and in vivo. Mol Carcinog. 2014;53(9):722–35.
32. Dovzhanskiy DI, Arnold SM, Hackert T, Oehme I, Witt O, Felix K, et al. Experimental in vivo and in vitro treatment with a new histone deacetylase inhibitor belinostat inhibits the growth of pancreatic cancer. BMC Cancer. 2012;12:226.
33. Lassen U, Molife LR, Sorensen M, Engelholm SA, Vidal L, Sinha R, et al. A phase I study of the safety and pharmacokinetics of the histone deacetylase inhibitor belinostat administered in combination with carboplatin and/or paclitaxel in patients with solid tumours. Br J Cancer. 2010;103(1):12–7.
34. Singh A, Patel VK, Jain DK, Patel P, Rajak H. Panobinostat as pan-deacetylase inhibitor for the treatment of pancreatic cancer: recent progress and future prospects. Oncol Ther. 2016;4(1):73–89.
35. Jones SF, Bendell JC, Infante JR, Spigel DR, Thompson DS, Yardley DA, et al. A phase I study of panobinostat in combination with gemcitabine in the treatment of solid tumors. Clin Adv Hematol Oncol. 2011;9(3):225–30.
36. Beumer JH, Parise RA, Newman EM, Doroshow JH, Synold TW, Lenz HJ, et al. Concentrations of the DNA methyltransferase inhibitor 5-fluoro-2′-deoxycytidine (FdCyd) and its cytotoxic metabolites in plasma of patients treated with FdCyd and tetrahydrouridine (THU). Cancer Chemother Pharmacol. 2008;62(2):363–8.
37. Newman EM, Morgan RJ, Kummar S, Beumer JH, Blanchard MS, Ruel C, et al. A phase I, pharmacokinetic, and pharmacodynamic evaluation of the DNA methyltransferase inhibitor 5-fluoro-2′-deoxycytidine, administered with tetrahydrouridine. Cancer Chemother Pharmacol. 2015;75(3):537–46.
38. Von Hoff DD, Rasco DW, Heath EI, Munster PN, Schellens JHM, Isambert N, et al. Phase I study of CC-486 alone and in combination with carboplatin or nab-paclitaxel in patients with relapsed or refractory solid tumors. Clin Cancer Res. 2018;24(17):4072–80.
39. Plummer R, Vidal L, Griffin M, Lesley M, de Bono J, Coulthard S, et al. Phase I study of MG98, an oligonucleotide antisense inhibitor of human DNA methyltransferase 1, given as a 7-day infusion in patients with advanced solid tumors. Clin Cancer Res. 2009;15(9):3177–83.
40. Davis AJ, Gelmon KA, Siu LL, Moore MJ, Britten CD, Mistry N, et al. Phase I and pharmacologic study of the human DNA methyltransferase antisense oligodeoxynucleotide MG98 given as a 21-day continuous infusion every 4 weeks. Investig New Drugs. 2003;21(1):85–97.

Chapter 13
Targeting Metabolism

Yoshiaki Sunami

Understanding Metabolic Reprogramming to Improve Therapeutic Strategies in Pancreatic Cancer

Pancreatic ductal adenocarcinoma (PDAC) is a devastating disease with an unfavorable outcome and is projected to become the second deadliest cancer by 2030, and currently the overall 5-year survival rate is less than 7% [1, 2]. PDAC arises through multistage genetic and histological progression from precursors such as pancreatic intraepithelial neoplasia (PanIN). Activating mutations in the *KRAS* oncogene are observed in over 90% of PDAC patients, and using genetically engineered mouse models, it has been demonstrated that *KRAS* mutations influence tumor initiation, progression, and maintenance [3, 4]. Tumorigenesis is dependent on the reprogramming of cellular metabolism which can be a consequence of oncogenic mutations. In line with this, a profound rewiring of metabolic pathways involved in, e.g., glucose, glutamine, and lipid metabolisms, is activated downstream of oncogenic *KRAS* [5]. In general, metabolic reprogramming has now been recognized as a hallmark of cancer [6]. Cancer cells manipulate metabolisms to keep generating their own cellular components such as DNA, proteins, and lipids for maintaining rapid cell growth. Understanding and identification of metabolic reprogramming strategies of individual cancers could uncover novel potential personalized targets. This chapter provides a background of cancer metabolism focusing on glucose, glutamine, acetate, and lipid metabolism and targeting strategies for modulating enzymes/factors involved in key metabolic pathways.

Y. Sunami (✉)
Department of Visceral, Vascular and Endocrine Surgery, Martin-Luther-University
Halle-Wittenberg, University Medical Center Halle, Halle (Saale), Germany
e-mail: yoshiaki.sunami@uk-halle.de

© Springer Nature Switzerland AG 2020
C. W. Michalski et al. (eds.), *Translational Pancreatic Cancer Research*,
Molecular and Translational Medicine,
https://doi.org/10.1007/978-3-030-49476-6_13

183

Glucose Metabolism and Pentose Phosphate Pathway in Pancreatic Cancer

Warburg Effect and Reprogramming of Glucose Metabolism: The Role of Gene Mutations

A pioneer of the study of cancer metabolic reprogramming, Otto Heinrich Warburg made a striking discovery known as Warburg effect that many cancer cells preferentially convert glucose into lactate (fermentation) rather than respiration – transporting pyruvate into mitochondria and converted it into acetyl-CoA for subsequent ATP production via the citric acid cycle and electron transport chain – even in the presence of oxygen [7–10]. Glycolysis, a metabolic pathway that converts glucose into pyruvate (and lactate) in the cytoplasm, is a sequence of ten enzyme-catalyzed reactions (Fig. 13.1). The three reactions converting glucose into glucose 6-phosphate by hexokinase (HK), fructose 6-phosphate into fructose 1,6-bisphosphate by phosphofructokinase (PFK), and phosphoenolpyruvate into pyruvate by pyruvate kinase are key steps. Oncogenic KRAS^{G12D} plays a role in upregulating gene expression of the glucose transporter (GLUT) *Slc2a1* (SLC: solute carrier), *Hk1*, *Hk2*, and *Pfk1* as well as *Ldha* coding lactate dehydrogenase (LDH), an enzyme for converting pyruvate to lactate. Concomitantly oncogenic KRAS enhances glucose uptake and lactate production in a pancreatic cancer mouse model [11]. The transcription factor p53 is recognized as a key tumor suppressor and also frequently mutated in human tumors. Missense mutations such as R175H, R248Q, and R273H not only result in loss of the tumor suppressive function of p53 but also in oncogenic functions that promote invasion, metastasis, proliferation, and cell survival [12]. Mutation of p53 also enhances glucose uptake by GLUT1 translocation, glycolytic rate, and lactate production in R172H mutant-expressing p53 in murine cancer cells or fibroblasts (R172H is equivalent to human R175H) [13]. Deficiency of another tumor suppressor gene, *SMAD4*, increases GLUT1 levels and lactate production in cancer cells [14]. *KRAS*, *TP53*, *CDKN2A,* and *SMAD4* are the most prevalent genetic mutations in pancreatic cancer [1]; yet these genes are currently not druggable. However, targeting glucose metabolic reprogramming may provide a selective mechanism for eliminating cancer cells.

Targeting Enzymes and Factors Involved in Glucose Metabolism

Inhibition of GLUT, especially GLUT1 expression, can be an option to halt the proliferation of cancers. A small-molecule GLUT1 inhibitor WZB117 has been shown to block glucose uptake and tumor growth in a tumor xenograft model [15, 16]. Furthermore, WZB117 administration inhibits tumor initiation after implantation of cancer stemlike cells derived from pancreatic cancer cells without causing adverse events in host mice [17]. Overexpression of GLUT1 correlates with poor

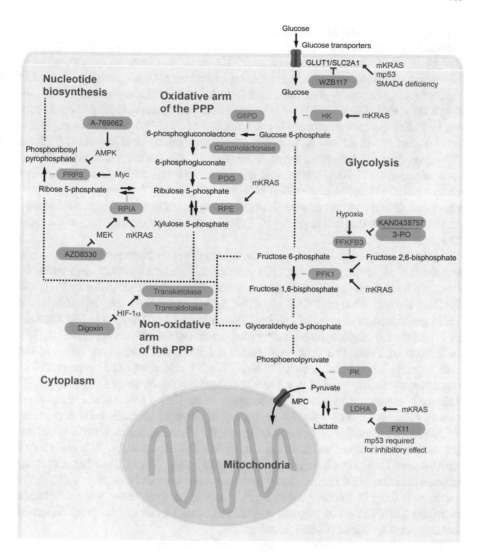

Fig. 13.1 Regulation of glycolysis, pentose phosphate pathway, and nucleotide biosynthesis. AMPK AMP-activated protein kinase, G6PD glucose 6-phosphate dehydrogenase, HIF hypoxia-inducible factor, HK hexokinase, LDH lactate dehydrogenase, mKRAS mutant KRAS, mp53 mutant p53, MPC mitochondria pyruvate carrier, PFK phosphofructokinase, PGD 6-phosphogluconate dehydrogenase PK pyruvate kinase, PPP pentose phosphate pathway, PRPS phosphoribosylpyrophosphate synthetase, RPE ribose 5-phosphate-3-epimerase, RPIA ribose 5-phosphate isomerase A, SLC solute carrier

overall survival of several solid tumors [18], and high GLUT1 expression is also suggested to predict shorter overall survival in patients with pancreatic cancer [19].

In the mammalian glycolytic pathway, PFK1 is rate-limiting and the most important control element. When PFK1 is inactive, the concentration of fructose

6-phosphate rises, and in equilibrium, the level of glucose 6-phosphate also rises. Hexokinase, another key enzyme in the glycolytic pathway, is allosterically inhibited by glucose 6-phosphate; therefore, PFK1 inhibition leads to the inhibition of hexokinase. Activity of PFK1 is stimulated by fructose 2,6-bisphosphate, which is derived from fructose 6-phosphate catalyzed by PFK2. There are four PFK2 isoforms (PFKFB1–4), and PFKFB3 is highly expressed in many types of human cancer including pancreatic cancer [20]. Expression of PFKFB3 can also be regulated by hypoxia [21]. PFKFB3 also regulates angiogenesis and vessel branching [22] and can be an emerging anticancer target. In this line, KAN0438757 has been considered as a selective PFKFB3 inhibitor, and treatment with this inhibitor radioscnsitizcs cancer cells [23]. Another PFKFB3 blocker 3-(3-pyridinyl)-1-(4-pyridinyl)-2-propen-1-one (3PO) reduces orthotopically implanted pancreatic cancer cell development [24], suggesting that targeting PFKFB3 can be an option for pancreatic cancer treatment.

In the late step in glycolysis, pyruvate kinase plays an important role as catalyzing the last physiological irreversible reaction to produce pyruvate. In mammals, there are four pyruvate kinase isoforms encoded by two genes: isoforms PKL and PKR are derived from the PKLR gene, and PKM1 and PKM2 are derived from the PKM gene through alternative splicing. The amino acid differences in PKM2 result in a fructose 1,6-bisphosphate-binding pocket for positive allosteric regulation [25]. Activation of PFK1 (for producing fructose 1,6-bisphosphate) can therefore not only regulate hexokinase activity but also PKM2 activity. PKM2 is expressed during embryogenesis, regeneration processes, and in cancer, suggesting that PKM2 activity is important in actively proliferating cells [25]. Orthotopically implanted cancer cells expressing PKM2 support tumorigenesis, whereas cells expressing PKM1 reduce tumorigenicity, suggesting that the PKM2 splice isoform is important for cancer metabolism and tumor growth [26]. On the contrary, in some studies activation of PKM2 can inhibit cancer cell proliferation [27, 28]. Furthermore, conditional deletion of PKM2 in a pancreatic cancer mouse model (oncogenic KRAS^{G12D} expression and p53 deletion) does not affect mouse survival, tumor weight, or tumor histology [29]. Therefore, targeting PKM2 might not be suitable for pancreatic cancer treatment and needs further investigation.

Pyruvate is a key metabolite in the network of metabolic pathways. Pyruvate in the cytoplasm can be converted into alanine by alanine aminotransferase (ALT) or transported into the mitochondria via mitochondria pyruvate carrier (MPC) and converted there into oxaloacetate by pyruvate carboxylase for gluconeogenesis or converted into acetyl-CoA by the pyruvate dehydrogenase (PDH) complex for the citric acid cycle. Pyruvate decarboxylase catalyzes a reaction converting pyruvate into acetaldehyde in the cytoplasm and mitochondria. Cancer cells however preferentially convert pyruvate into lactate, which is catalyzed by LDH. LDH is a tetramer of two subunits LDHA and LDHB, which assemble into five different combinations [30]. LDHA has a higher affinity for pyruvate than LDHB, and elevated levels of LDHA are a hallmark of many cancer types; hence targeting LDHA can be a promising strategy for cancer therapeutics. Consistently, FX11 (3-dihydroxy-6-methyl-7-(phenylmethyl)-4-propylnaphthalene-1-carboxylic   acid),   a   small-molecule inhibitor of LDHA, inhibits the progression of pancreatic cancer xenografts [31]. Interestingly, the inhibitory effect of FX11 requires mutant p53, and FX11 treatment does not inhibit tumor progression of patient-derived PDAC xenografts without p53 mutation [32], suggesting that targeting LDHA in pancreatic cancer can be an attractive stratification option since drug responsiveness in PDAC patients may depend on the genetic status.

Pentose Phosphate Pathway: Helper of Cancer's Anabolic Demands

The pentose phosphate pathway (PPP) is another pathway in the cytoplasm for glucose catabolism starting from glucose 6-phosphate. The major function of the PPP is not energy production, but generating extramitochondrial nicotinamide adenine dinucleotide phosphate (NADPH), which is required for fatty acid synthesis and for scavenging reactive oxygen species (ROS). The PPP also supports the synthesis of ribonucleotides. The PPP is divided into two parts, namely, the oxidative arm and non-oxidative arm. The oxidative arm is initiated by conversion of glucose 6-phosphate to 6-phosphogluconolactone by glucose 6-phosphate dehydrogenase (G6PD), which is converted into 6-phosphogluconate by gluconolactonase and further converted into ribulose 5-phosphate by 6-phosphogluconate dehydrogenase (PGD). In the non-oxidative phase of the PPP, ribulose 5-phosphate is either reversibly catalyzed by ribose 5-phosphate isomerase A (RPIA) for producing ribose 5-phosphate or reversibly catalyzed by ribose 5-phosphate-3-epimerase (RPE) for producing xylulose 5-phosphate [33]. Ribose 5-phosphate is converted by phosphoribosylpyrophosphate synthetase (PRPS) to phosphoribosyl pyrophosphate, which serves as the backbone for nucleotide synthesis. Oncogenic KRAS^{G12D} upregulates *RPIA* and *RPE* gene expression in murine primary cells of a pancreatic cancer model with oncogenic KRAS^{G12D} and p53 deficiency. Knockdown of *Rpia* or *Rpe* genes in primary cells reduces the flux of glucose into DNA/RNA synthesis and xenograft pancreatic tumor growth [11], and knockdown of *Rpia* gene inhibits human PDAC cell growth [34]. Ribose 5-phosphate and xylulose 5-phosphate in the non-oxidative branch of the PPP can also be reversibly catalyzed by transketolase and aldolase to fructose 6-phosphate or glyceraldehyde 3-phosphate, which can be utilized in the glycolysis [33]. Vice versa, fructose 6-phosphate and glyceraldehyde 3-phosphate in the glycolytic pathway can be incorporated into the PPP pathway, and many cancer cells generate ribose 5-phosphate through the non-oxidative branch of the PPP for de novo nucleotide biosynthesis [35]. Fructose induces transketolase flux and proliferation of pancreatic cancer cells [36]. High fructose intake has been suggested to be associated with increased pancreatic cancer risk [37]. A key regulator of the non-oxidative branch of the PPP is hypoxia-inducible factor (HIF)-1α which increases the carbon flux into the PPP [35], and HIF-1α directly regulates transketolase gene expression [38]. Taken together, the PPP especially the non-oxidative arm plays an important role in de novo nucleotide biosynthesis, and directly or indirectly targeting enzymes and factors involved in the PPP is a promising therapeutic strategy against pancreatic cancer.

Targeting Enzymes and Factors Involved in the Pentose Phosphate Pathway and Nucleotide Synthesis

Oncogenic KRAS[G12D] reprograms metabolism of the PPP in PDAC through MAPK and Myc pathways [11, 34]. Myc has been further shown to control PRPS2, but not PRPS1, and functional loss of PRPS2 delays Myc-dependent tumor initiation [39]. Since KRAS and Myc are currently not druggable, targeting RPIA, RPE of the non-oxidative branch of the PPP, as well as targeting PRPS2 in the nucleotide biosynthesis pathway can be considered as therapeutic options. Inhibitors of RPIA, RPE, or PRPS remain largely undiscovered. Especially selective PRPS2 inhibitors are challenging to identify, since PRPS2 shares more than 97% amino acid identity with the PRPS1 [40]. So far, pharmacological inhibitors of effector pathways on cancer metabolism have been used. For example, treatment with the MEK inhibitor AZD8330 decreases *Rpia* gene expression in murine primary cells of a pancreatic cancer model with oncogenic KRAS[G12D] and p53 deficiency [11]. AMP-activated protein kinase (AMPK) phosphorylation leads to conversion of PRPS hexamer to monomer resulting in inhibition of nucleotide synthesis in cancer cells (AMPK activator: A-769662) [41]. Digoxin is an HIF-1α synthesis inhibitor [42], and targeting HIF-1α leads to reduction of transketolase gene expression and improved gemcitabine sensitivity in pancreatic cancer cells [38]. MEK/MAPK, AMPK, and HIF-1α regulate not only the PPP and/or nucleotide biosynthesis. However, reprogramming the reprogrammed metabolism of the PPP and nucleotide biosynthesis in cancer by modulating effectors is also a promising targeting strategy.

Lipid Metabolism in Pancreatic Cancer

Fatty Acid Synthesis as an Entrance of Lipid Metabolism and Critical for Cancer Cell Proliferation

The most prominent metabolic alteration is known as the Warburg effect. However, cancer cells manipulate many other metabolic pathways for building up their own cellular components. Especially, activating lipid synthesis is highly important for cancer cells, because lipids such as phospholipid bilayers are fundamental structural components enabling cellular proliferation. It has been shown that extracellular lipids can sufficiently stimulate pancreatic cancer cell proliferation [43]. However, in a wide variety of tumors, de novo synthesis of fatty acids (FAs) is activated irrespective of the levels of circulating lipids. In contrast to normal cells, cancer cells may gain more than 93% of triacylglycerol FAs via de novo synthesis [44]. In the first step of FA synthesis, cytoplasmic acetyl-CoA is generated from citrate by ATP-citrate lyase (ACLY) and then converted into malonyl-CoA by acetyl-CoA carboxylase (ACC). Malonyl-CoA and acetyl-CoA are coupled to the acyl-carrier protein (ACP) domain of the multienzyme protein fatty acid synthase (FASN) (Fig. 13.2). Via repeated condensations of acetyl groups by the FASN in an

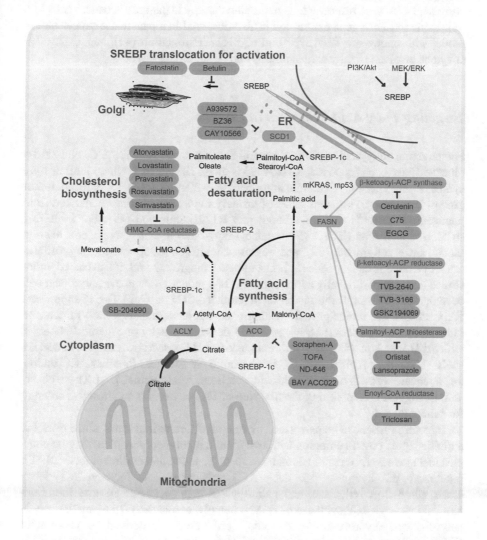

Fig. 13.2 Regulation of fatty acid synthesis, cholesterol synthesis, fatty acid desaturation, and SREBP translocation. ACC acetyl-CoA carboxylase, ACLY ATP-citrate lyase, ER endoplasmic reticulum, FASN fatty acid synthase, HMG-CoA 3-hydroxy-3-methylglutaryl-CoA or β-hydroxy-β-methylglutaryl-CoA, SCD Δ^9-stearoyl-CoA desaturase, SREBP sterol regulatory element-binding protein

NADPH-dependent manner, a basic 16-carbon saturated FA called palmitic acid is generated [45]. In cancer cells, expression of ACLY and ACC is also markedly increased [44]. Furthermore, serum FASN levels are higher in patients with PDAC, in patients with intraductal papillary mucinous neoplasm (IPMN), and in patients with chronic pancreatitis in comparison to healthy controls [46]. Pancreatic cancer patients with high FASN expression in the pancreas show a shorter overall survival than patients with low FASN expression [47]. Furthermore, FASN expression is correlated with poor response to gemcitabine therapy in pancreatic cancer cells [47, 48]. Increased *Fasn* gene expression is also observed in a pancreatic cancer mouse model with oncogenic KRAS^{G12D} and p53 R172H mutation [47], suggesting that enzymes involved in fatty acid synthesis can be important targets.

Targeting Fatty Acid Synthesis in Cancer

For targeting fatty acid synthesis, several inhibitors for ACLY, ACC, and FASN blockade have been proposed. SB-204990 is an ACLY inhibitor which inhibits lipid synthesis. Intraperitoneal administration of SB-204990 leads to reduced tumor growth in mice carrying xenografts of primary mouse PDAC lines generated from oncogenic KRAS^{G12D} with or without p53 R172H mutation [49]. For inhibiting ACC, soraphen A and TOFA (5-(tetradecyloxy)-2-furoic acid) have been shown to block cancer cell growth [50], and treatment with TOFA suppresses the proliferation of pancreatic cancer cells [51]. In a mouse xenograft model, it has been demonstrated that intraperitoneally administered TOFA reduces human ovarian cancer cell development [52]. Oral administration of another ACC inhibitor ND-646 suppresses FA synthesis and tumor growth in lung cancer mouse models where tumors are induced by oncogenic KRAS^{G12D} with p53 deficiency or by oncogenic KRAS^{G12D} with *Stk11* knockout [53]. Serine/threonine kinase 11, also known as liver kinase B1 (LKB1), activates AMPK for ACC inhibition. BAY ACC022 (another ACC inhibitor) attenuates growth of pancreatic cancer cell xenograft in mice [54]. These observations suggest that inhibiting the first step of FA synthesis is an attractive strategy for cancer therapy.

Targeting FASN can be performed by several different inhibitors, since FASN is a multienzyme protein complex with two identical polypeptides. The enzyme complex includes several catalytic domains with ACP, malonyl/acetyltransferase (MAT), β-ketoacyl-ACP synthase, β-ketoacyl-ACP reductase, 3-hydroxyacyl-ACP dehydrase, enoyl-CoA reductase, and palmitoyl-ACP thioesterase. Several inhibitors block β-ketoacyl-ACP synthase of FASN, namely, cerulenin, C75 (4-methylene-2-octyl-5-oxotetrahydrofuran-3-carboxylic acid, cerulenin-derived semisynthetic FASN inhibitor with improved stability), and epigallocatechin-3 gallate (EGCG) [44]. Cerulenin and C75 have been tested in several cancer xenograft models like for ovary, prostate, mesothelioma, breast, and colon cancer. Intraperitoneally administered cerulenin also suppresses liver metastasis of colon cancer cells in mice [55]. Blockage of FASN with EGCG has been considered for a broad range of cancer types such as prostate, lung, breast, and colorectal cancer [56, 57]. EGCG inhibits pancreatic cancer cell proliferation, and antiproliferative effects are also observed with catechin gallate (CG) and epicatechin gallate (ECG) [58]. EGCG inhibits growth of pancreatic tumor cells orthotopically implanted in mice [59]. For inhibiting β-ketoacyl-ACP reductase, several compounds like TVB-2640, TVB-3166, and GSK2194069 have been proposed. TVB-2640 has entered clinical trials, e.g., for colon cancer, breast cancer, and astrocytoma. Treatment with TVB-3166 leads to inhibition of proliferation and reduction in tumor growth of multiple cancer cell lines and pancreatic cancer xenografts [57, 60]. The β-lactone orlistat blocks palmitoyl-ACP thioesterase, and enoyl-CoA reductase can be blocked by triclosan [44, 61]. Orlistat is a US food and Drug Administration (FDA)-approved anti-obesity drug, and it has been shown that orlistat reduces human pancreatic cancer cell growth [47, 62]. Inhibition of FASN with orlistat suppresses growth of EGFR tyrosine kinase inhibitor-resistant cancer cells and also tumors in EGFR mutant transgenic mice [63]. One main limitation of orlistat is its low oral bioavailability, and improved formulation of orlistat-like inhibitors may be required in the future. Alternatively, other inhibitors of palmitoyl-ACP thioesterase can be identified via in silico screening of FDA-approved drugs. Lansoprazole, rabeprazole, omeprazole, and pantoprazole are proton pump inhibitors, but also function as inhibitors of thioesterase activity, which can induce pancreatic cancer cell death [64]. In conclusion, a number of inhibitors of ACLY, ACC, and FASN have been proposed and show significant effects in cancer therapy.

Fatty Acid Desaturases: Not Just a Modifier

The main product of FA synthesis in the cytoplasm is 16-carbon saturated palmitic acid. Longer FAs are formed by reactions catalyzed by several enzymes on the cytosolic side of the endoplasmic reticulum (ER). The desaturation of fatty acids occurs also in ER membranes. These modifications support the production of a wide variety of FAs and lipids. In mammalian cells, three types of fatty acid desaturases introduce carbon double bonds at Δ^5 (Δ^5-eicosatrienoyl-CoA desaturase), Δ^6 (Δ^6-oleoyl(linolenoyl)-CoA desaturase), or Δ^9 (Δ^9-stearoyl-CoA desaturase) (SCD). SCD is the rate-limiting enzyme catalyzing the synthesis of monounsaturated 16- or 18-carbon-like palmitoleate and oleate from palmitoyl-CoA and stearoyl-CoA [65]. Enhanced FA synthesis in cancer cells also increases the requirement of enzymes for modifying FAs and lipids. SCD1 (the main isoform) has been associated with insulin resistance and diabetes. Expression of SCD1 is associated with tumor promotion, shorter survival of lung cancer patients [66], and with sorafenib resistance in liver cancer patients [67]. SCD1 expression is upregulated in human colorectal cancer tissues, and patients with high SCD1 expression levels have a shorter overall survival [68]. It has also been suggested that increased SCD1 expression is associated with shorter survival of pancreatic cancer patients [69]. SCD1 contributes to the maintenance of cancer cell stemness, and knockdown of SCD1 reduces the expression of stemness markers like *SOX2* and *NANOG* [70]. Cancer stemness may be responsible not only for tumor initiation but also for metastasis [71]. Taken together, targeting SCD1 could be a promising option.

Targeting Fatty Acid Desaturases

However, the role of SCD1 remains controversial and requires further investigation. In a murine intestinal cancer model with a mutant allele Min (multiple intestinal neoplasia) of the Apc (adenomatous polyposis coli) locus (called Apc$^{Min/+}$ mice), conditional deletion of *Scd1* in the intestinal epithelium promotes inflammation and tumorigenesis [72]. On the other hand, the inhibitor A939572 has been applied for renal cell carcinoma treatment. Oral administration of A939572 inhibits the development of tumor xenografts in mice [73]. Intraperitoneal injection with another SCD1 inhibitor (BZ36) reduces prostate cancer xenografts in mice [74]. Furthermore, pretreatment with the SCD1 inhibitor CAY10566 suppresses ovarian tumor growth after inoculation of cancer stem cells, where inhibition of SCD1 impairs cancer cell stemness [70]. The effects these inhibitors have on pancreatic cancer cells are currently not known.

Sterol Regulatory Element-Binding Proteins: Master Regulators of Lipid Biogenesis and Cholesterol Metabolism

Expression of genes involved in FA synthesis and modification such as *ACLY*, *ACACA/B* (coding ACCs), *FASN*, and *SCD* is regulated by the transcription factor sterol regulatory element-binding protein 1c (SREBP-1c) that is itself regulated transcriptionally and/or posttranslationally by several signaling pathways and factors such as PI3K/Akt and MEK/ERK [75]. EGFR signaling is required for oncogenic KRAS^{G12D}-induced pancreatic tumorigenesis [76, 77], and EGFR activation also induces upregulation of FASN in pancreatic cancer cells in an ERK-dependent manner [78]. Along this line, PDAC patients with high SREBP1 expression have a shorter overall survival than patients with low SREBP1 expression, and knockdown of *SREBF1* (for SREBP1 expression) decreases pancreatic cancer cell viability and proliferation [79]. Taken together, oncogenic signaling pathways activate expression of lipogenic enzymes leading to aberrant activation of FA synthesis, which supports cancer cell development.

There are three SREBP isoforms, SREBP-1a, SREBP-1c, and SREBP-2. Both SREBP-1a and SREBP-1c are derived from a single gene but through alternative transcription start sites. Whereas SREBP-1c preferentially regulates genes of FA metabolism, SREBP-1a is a potent activator of all SREBP-responsive genes, and SREBP-2 regulates cholesterol biosynthesis [80]. Cholesterol is an essential structural component of cell membranes together with various phospholipids, sphingomyelin, and glycolipids. Cholesterol is de novo synthesized from cytoplasmic acetyl-CoA through the mevalonate pathway. The rate-limiting step of the pathway is the conversion of 3-hydroxy-3-methylglutaryl-CoA (HMG-CoA, also known as β-hydroxy-β-methylglutaryl-CoA) to mevalonate by HMG-CoA reductase [81]. In addition to the mevalonate pathway, cells can increase their cholesterol contents thought receptor-mediated endocytosis of low-density lipoproteins (LDLs) [82]. The LDL receptor (LDLR) and HMG-CoA reductase are both transcriptional targets of SREBP-2 [80]. Expression of HMG-CoA reductase and LDLR is elevated in an oncogenic KRAS^{G12D} pancreatic cancer mouse model [83]. It has been suggested that cholesterol intake is associated with increased risk of pancreatic cancer [84]. Increased expression of *Ldlr* has no significant effect on overall survival of pancreatic cancer patients, but high *Ldlr* expression is associated with an increased risk of tumor recurrence. Since LDLR silencing reduces ERK signaling as well as proliferation of PDAC cells, silencing also enhances response to gemcitabine chemotherapy [83].

Targeting Cholesterol Synthesis and SREBP

The development of LDLR-inactivating agents is currently an ongoing issue. Alternatively, SREBP-1c and SREBP-2 can be potential targets for cancer therapy, since these are key regulators of FASN expression and other enzymes in fatty acid synthesis like ACLY and ACC, and it also regulates expression of SCD, LDLR, and HMG-CoA reductase. SREBPs interact with the SREBP cleavage-activating protein (SCAP), and the complex stays with the ER membrane proteins INSIG1 and INSIG2. Under physiological conditions, reduction of cellular lipid levels results in conformational change of SCAP that abrogates its interaction with INSIGs. Dissociation of the SREBP/SCAP complex from INSIGs leads to transport of the complex from the ER to the Golgi where SREBP is cleaved and activated [85]. Glucose can enhance SCAP stability and reduce its association with INSIGs allowing transport of the SREBP/SCAP complex to the Golgi [86]. Betulin and fatostatin have been proposed as SREBP inhibitors through inhibition of ER-Golgi translocation. Betulin has initially been shown to improve hyperlipidemia and insulin resistance and to reduce atherosclerotic plaques [87]. Intraperitoneal injection of betulinic acid combined with mithramycin A (DNA and RNA polymerase inhibitor) blocks the development of pancreatic cancer xenografts in mice [88]. Fatostatin injection reduces expression of FASN, ACC, SCD1, ACLY, and also Hmgcr (HMG-CoA reductase) and *Ldlr* transcription to a lesser extent in obese mice [85]. The inhibitor has been tested in glioblastoma and prostate cancer cell xenografts. There, intraperitoneal treatment with fatostatin reduced xenograft growth in mice [89, 90]. Inhibiting de novo cholesterol synthesis by blockage of the rate-limiting enzyme HMG-CoA reductase has also been considered for cancer therapy. Several statin derivatives such as atorvastatin, lovastatin, pravastatin, rosuvastatin, and simvastatin have entered clinical trials. Among the derivatives, atorvastatin and simvastatin have been considered for pancreatic cancer treatment [57]. Taken together, there are several therapeutic options targeting SREBP and the mevalonate pathway, and a number of cancer studies are currently ongoing.

Glutamine and Acetate Metabolism in Pancreatic Cancer

Glutamine Metabolism: It Works Also Without Mitochondria

By modulating the activity of several metabolic pathways including glutamine metabolism, cancer cells aim for continuous generation of FAs necessary for cell growth. Glutamine is the most abundant and nonessential amino acid that can be synthesized from glucose. In the canonical route of mitochondrial glutamine catabolism (glutaminolysis), glutaminase (GLS) catalyzes glutamine to glutamate (Fig. 13.3). Glutamate is further converted by glutamate dehydrogenase (GLUD1)

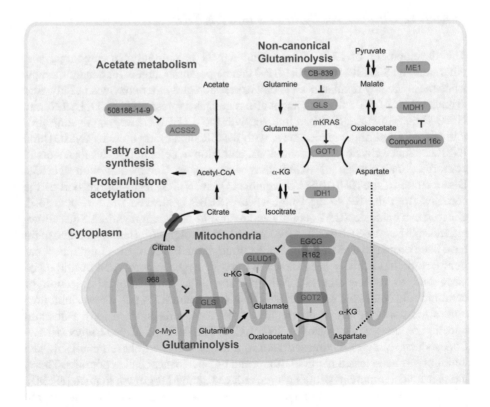

Fig. 13.3 Regulation of glutaminolysis and acetate metabolism. ACSS short-chain acyl-CoA synthetase, GLS glutaminase, GLUD glutamate dehydrogenase, GOT aspartate transaminase, IDH isocitrate dehydrogenase, MDH malate dehydrogenase, ME malate enzyme

to α-ketoglutarate (α-KG), and α-KG can then be integrated into the tricarboxylic acid cycle (TCA cycle). Glutamine is an essential nutrient for the proliferation of human cancer cells [91], and several oncogenes which activate glutaminolysis have been identified. Oncogenic c-Myc enhances expression of mitochondrial GLS supporting canonical glutaminolysis [92]. Pancreatic cancer cells rely on a cytoplasmic noncanonical glutaminolysis pathway producing pyruvate via aspartate transaminase (GOT1, catalyzes aspartate/oxaloacetate), malate dehydrogenase (MDH1, catalyzes malate/oxaloacetate), and malate enzyme (ME1, catalyzes malate/pyruvate). Oncogenic KRAS induces a shift from canonical to noncanonical glutaminolysis by inhibiting mitochondrial GLUD1 and activating cytoplasmic GOT1 [93]. By reprogramming of glutamine metabolism from the mitochondrial to the cytoplasmic system, pancreatic cancer can keep synthesis of FAs intact, because cytoplasmic isocitrate dehydrogenase (IDH1) can catalyze α-KG/isocitrate under hypoxic conditions or even with defective mitochondria [94–96].

Targeting Glutamine Metabolism

Several drugs such as 968, BPTES, and CB-839 have been developed to inhibit GLS glutamate synthesis. Treatment with 968 or with BPTES reduces pancreatic cancer cell viability [93]. Intravenous injection of BPTES nanoparticles reduces pancreatic cancer xenograft growth in mice, and combination with intraperitoneal injection of metformin enhances therapeutic effects [97]. CB-839 has already been tested in several clinical studies including a broad range of cancer types, such as clear cell renal carcinoma, breast cancer, and colorectal cancer. However, oral gavage of CB-839 has no antitumor activity in mice with oncogenic KRAS^{G12D} combined with Trp53 deficiency. In addition, mice treated with CB-839 show marginally shorter survival than the group without CB-839 treatment [98]. Further investigations are therefore required to judge whether GLS inhibition is a potential therapeutic option for pancreatic cancer patients. EGCG and R162 have been considered to inhibit GLUD1 [99]. EGCG has been described as a FASN β-ketoacyl-ACP synthase inhibitor and shown to inhibit pancreatic cancer cell proliferation (see Targeting Fatty Acid Synthesis in Cancer), and it is also recognized as a GLUD1 inhibitor. Treatment with R162 inhibits proliferation of several cancer cells including primary leukemia cells. Furthermore, intraperitoneal injection of R162 inhibits the development of lung cancer xenografts in mice [100]. Oncogenic KRAS^{G12D} has been suggested to inhibit GLUD1 and preferentially activate the noncanonical glutaminolysis pathway (see Glutamine Metabolism: It Works Also Without Mitochondria); thus, GLUD1 inhibition might be ineffective in pancreatic cancer. Methyl 3-(3-(4-(2,4,4-trimethylpentan-2-yl)phenoxy)-propanamido)benzoate (named compound 16c) has been synthesized to inhibit the noncanonical glutaminolysis pathway as a MDH inhibitor. This inhibitor blocks both cytoplasmic MDH1 and mitochondrial MDH2 enzymes. It has been shown that intraperitoneal administration of this inhibitor attenuates the development of colon cancer xenografts [101]. Since inhibition of

MDH1 activity leads to suppression of glutamine metabolism and reduction of pancreatic cancer cell growth [102], inhibitors for the noncanonical glutaminolysis pathway could be potential candidates for pancreatic cancer therapy.

Acetate Metabolism: Cancer Cells Are Experts in Bridging the Gap

Acetyl CoA represents a central metabolite not only for lipid synthesis but also for regulating gene expression as a key determinant of protein/histone acetylation [103, 104]. Cancer cells preferentially convert pyruvate into lactate rather than to transport it into the mitochondria for PDH reaction and the TCA cycle. Although the IDH1-mediated non-canonical glutaminolysis pathway (see Glutamine Metabolism: It Works Also Without Mitochondria) may compensate to provide acetyl-CoA in the cytoplasm, alternative sources of acetyl-CoA could still be necessary for sufficient supporting lipid synthesis and cancer cell growth. Cells with ACLY deficiency remain viable and proliferate, where acetate supports acetyl-CoA generation and de novo lipid synthesis is supported by the enzyme called ACSS2 [105]. There have been 26 acyl-CoA synthetases (ACS) identified in the human genome. Among those, three enzymes, the short-chain ACS (ACSS) family (acetyl-CoA synthetase), are capable of catalyzing synthesis of acetyl-CoA from acetate in an ATP-dependent manner [106]. ACSS1 and ACSS3 are mitochondrial enzymes, and ACSS2 localizes to both the cytoplasmic and nuclear compartments. Silencing of ACSS2 in cancer cells reduces incorporation of acetyl units from acetate into either lipids or histones. ACSS2 is highly expressed in several human tumors, and loss of ACSS2 suppresses tumor development in certian mouse liver cancer models including c-Myc combined with PTEN knockout [107]. Under metabolic stress such as hypoxia and/or low-nutrition conditions, expression of ACSS2 is elevated, and it promotes acetate uptake for lipid synthesis and membrane phospholipids in several cancers including pancreatic cancer cells [108, 109].

Inhibitors specifically targeting ACSS2 remain largely unexplored. So far a compound 1-(2,3-di(thiophen-2-yl)quinoxalin-6-yl)-3-(2-methoxyethyl)urea (PubChem CID: 2300455; here referred to as 508186-14-9) has been proposed as a ACSS2-specific inhibitor [107]. The inhibitor has been tested and showed decreased lipid contents in bladder cancer cells, but not in non-cancer cells [110]. Targeting ACSS2 and acetate metabolism would be a highly interesting concept for treating pancreatic cancer.

Conclusion

Extensive research on cancer metabolism has revealed that a number of enzymes and metabolites are involved in reprogramming strategies of many cancer types including pancreatic cancer. Furthermore, it is evident that overexpression of specific enzymes is not only related with metabolic reprogramming but also with cellular stemness. Several studies with inhibitors targeting specific catalyzing steps in selected metabolic pathways have shown convincing effects in inhibiting cancer development and progression. Cancers may however still find other ways to generate necessary metabolic intermediates and cellular components. Therefore, it is important to further understand not only the cross talk between oncogenic signaling pathways and metabolism but also between metabolic pathways for offering stratified and more effective therapies in the future.

References

1. Kleeff J, Korc M, Apte M, La Vecchia C, Johnson CD, Biankin AV, et al. Pancreatic cancer. Nat Rev Dis Primers. 2016;2:16022.
2. Rahib L, Smith BD, Aizenberg R, Rosenzweig AB, Fleshman JM, Matrisian LM. Projecting cancer incidence and deaths to 2030: the unexpected burden of thyroid, liver, and pancreas cancers in the United States. Cancer Res. 2014;74:2913–21.
3. Hingorani SR, Petricoin EF, Maitra A, Rajapakse V, King C, Jacobetz MA, et al. Preinvasive and invasive ductal pancreatic cancer and its early detection in the mouse. Cancer Cell. 2003;4(6):437–50.
4. Perera RM, Bardeesy N. Pancreatic cancer metabolism: breaking it down to build it Back up. Cancer Discov. 2015;5(12):1247–61.
5. White E. Exploiting the bad eating habits of Ras-driven cancers. Genes Dev. 2013;27(19):2065–71.
6. Hanahan D, Weinberg RA. Hallmark of cancer: the next generation. Cell. 2011;144:646–74.
7. Warburg O, Minami S. Versuche an Überlebendem Carcinomgewebe. Klin Wochenschr. 1923;2(17):776–7.
8. Warburg O, Posener K, Negelein E. Über den Stoffwechsel der Carcinomzelle. Biochem Z. 1924;152:309–44.
9. Warburg O, Wind F, Negelein E. The metabolism of tumors in the body. J Gen Physiol. 1927;8(6):519–30.
10. Warburg O. On respiratory impairment in cancer cells. Science. 1956;124(3215):269–70.
11. Ying H, Kimmelman AC, Lyssiotis CA, Hua S, Chu GC, Fletcher-Sananikone E, et al. Oncogenic Kras maintains pancreatic tumors through regulation of anabolic glucose metabolism. Cell. 2012;149(3):656–70.
12. Muller PA, Vousden KH. p53 mutations in cancer. Nat Cell Biol. 2013;15(1):2–8.
13. Zhang C, Liu J, Liang Y, Wu R, Zhao Y, Hong X, et al. Tumour-associated mutant p53 drives the Warburg effect. Nat Commun. 2013;4:2935.
14. Papageorgis P, Cheng K, Ozturk S, Gong Y, Lambert AW, Abdolmaleky HM, et al. Smad4 inactivation promotes malignancy and drug resistance of colon cancer. Cancer Res. 2011;71(3):998–1008.
15. Zhang W, Liu Y, Chen X, Bergmeier SC. Novel inhibitors of basal glucose transport as potential anticancer agents. Bioorg Med Chem Lett. 2010;20(7):2191–4.
16. Liu Y, Cao Y, Zhang W, Bergmeier S, Qian Y, Akbar H, et al. A small-molecule inhibitor of glucose transporter 1 downregulates glycolysis, induces cell-cycle arrest, and inhibits cancer cell growth in vitro and in vivo. Mol Cancer Ther. 2012;11(8):1672–82.
17. Shibuya K, Okada M, Suzuki S, Seino M, Seino S, Takeda H, et al. Targeting the facilitative glucose transporter GLUT1 inhibits the self-renewal and tumor-initiating capacity of cancer stem cells. Oncotarget. 2015;6(2):651–61.

18. Wang J, Ye C, Chen C, Xiong H, Xie B, Zhou J, et al. Glucose transporter GLUT1 expression and clinical outcome in solid tumors: a systematic review and meta-analysis. Oncotarget. 2017;8(10):16875–86.
19. Sharen G, Peng Y, Cheng H, Liu Y, Shi Y, Zhao J. Prognostic value of GLUT-1 expression in pancreatic cancer: results from 538 patients. Oncotarget. 2017;8(12):19760–7.
20. Atsumi T, Chesney J, Metz C, Leng L, Donnelly S, Makita Z, et al. High expression of inducible 6-phosphofructo-2-kinase/fructose-2,6-bisphosphatase (iPFK-2; PFKFB3) in human cancers. Cancer Res. 2002;62(20):5881–7.
21. Minchenko A, Leshchinsky I, Opentanova I, Sang N, Srinivas V, Armstead V, et al. Hypoxia-inducible factor-1-mediated expression of the 6-phosphofructo-2-kinase/fructose-2,6-bisphosphatase-3 (PFKFB3) gene. Its possible role in the Warburg effect. J Biol Chem. 2002;277(8):6183–7
22. De Bock K, Georgiadou M, Schoors S, Kuchnio A, Wong BW, Cantelmo AR, et al. Role of PFKFB3-driven glycolysis in vessel sprouting. Cell. 2013;154(3):651–63.
23. Gustafsson NMS, Färnegårdh K, Bonagas N, Ninou AH, Groth P, Wiita E, et al. Targeting PFKFB3 radiosensitizes cancer cells and suppresses homologous recombination. Nat Commun. 2018;9(1):3872.
24. Conradi LC, Brajic A, Cantelmo AR, Bouché A, Kalucka J, Pircher A, et al. Tumor vessel disintegration by maximum tolerable PFKFB3 blockade. Angiogenesis. 2017;20(4):599–613.
25. Dayton TL, Jacks T, Vander Heiden MG. PKM2, cancer metabolism, and the road ahead. EMBO Rep. 2016;17(12):1721–30.
26. Christofk HR, Vander Heiden MG, Harris MH, Ramanathan A, Gerszten RE, Wei R, et al. The M2 splice isoform of pyruvate kinase is important for cancer metabolism and tumour growth. Nature. 2008;452(7184):230–3.
27. Anastasiou D, Yu Y, Israelsen WJ, Jiang JK, Boxer MB, Hong BS, et al. Pyruvate kinase M2 activators promote tetramer formation and suppress tumorigenesis. Nat Chem Biol. 2012;8(10):839–47.
28. Luengo A, Gui DY, Vander Heiden MG. Targeting metabolism for cancer therapy. Cell Chem Biol. 2017;24(9):1161–80.
29. Hillis AL, Lau AN, Devoe CX, Dayton TL, Danai LV, Di Vizio D, et al. PKM2 is not required for pancreatic ductal adenocarcinoma. Cancer Metab. 2018;6:17.
30. Doherty JR, Cleveland JL. Targeting lactate metabolism for cancer therapeutics. J Clin Invest. 2013;123(9):3685–92.
31. Le A, Cooper CR, Gouw AM, Dinavahi R, Maitra A, Deck LM, et al. Inhibition of lactate dehydrogenase A induces oxidative stress and inhibits tumor progression. Proc Natl Acad Sci U S A. 2010;107(5):2037–42.
32. Rajeshkumar NV, Dutta P, Yabuuchi S, de Wilde RF, Martinez GV, Le A, et al. Therapeutic targeting of the Warburg effect in pancreatic cancer relies on an absence of p53 function. Cancer Res. 2015;75(16):3355–64.
33. Patra KC, Hay N. The pentose phosphate pathway and cancer. Trends Biochem Sci. 2014;39(8):347–54.
34. Santana-Codina N, Roeth AA, Zhang Y, Yang A, Mashadova O, Asara JM, et al. Oncogenic KRAS supports pancreatic cancer through regulation of nucleotide synthesis. Nat Commun. 2018;9(1):4945.
35. Tong X, Zhao F, Thompson CB. The molecular determinants of de novo nucleotide biosynthesis in cancer cells. Curr Opin Genet Dev. 2009;19(1):32–7.
36. Liu H, Huang D, McArthur DL, Boros LG, Nissen N, Heaney AP. Fructose induces transketolase flux to promote pancreatic cancer growth. Cancer Res. 2010;70(15):6368–76.
37. Aune D, Chan DS, Vieira AR, Navarro Rosenblatt DA, Vieira R, Greenwood DC, et al. Dietary fructose, carbohydrates, glycemic indices and pancreatic cancer risk: a systematic review and meta-analysis of cohort studies. Ann Oncol. 2012;23(10):2536–46.

38. Shukla SK, Purohit V, Mehla K, Gunda V, Chaika NV, Vernucci E, et al. MUC1 and HIF-1alpha signaling crosstalk induces anabolic glucose metabolism to impart gemcitabine resistance to pancreatic cancer. Cancer Cell. 2017;32(1):71–87.e7.
39. Cunningham JT, Moreno MV, Lodi A, Ronen SM, Ruggero D. Protein and nucleotide biosynthesis are coupled by a single rate-limiting enzyme, PRPS2, to drive cancer. Cell. 2014;157(5):1088–103.
40. Becker MA, Heidler SA, Bell GI, Seino S, Le Beau MM, Westbrook CA, et al. Cloning of cDNAs for human phosphoribosylpyrophosphate synthetases 1 and 2 and X chromosome localization of PRPS1 and PRPS2 genes. Genomics. 1990;8(3):555–61.
41. Qian X, Li X, Tan L, Lee JH, Xia Y, Cai Q, et al. Conversion of PRPS hexamer to monomer by AMPK-mediated phosphorylation inhibits nucleotide synthesis in response to energy stress. Cancer Discov. 2018;8(1):94–107.
42. Zhang H, Qian DZ, Tan YS, Lee K, Gao P, Ren YR, et al. Digoxin and other cardiac glycosides inhibit HIF-1alpha synthesis and block tumor growth. Proc Natl Acad Sci U S A. 2008;105(50):19579–86.
43. Clerc P, Bensaadi N, Pradel P, Estival A, Clemente F, Vaysse N. Lipid-dependent proliferation of pancreatic cancer cell lines. Cancer Res. 1991;51:3633–8.
44. Menendez JA, Lupu R. Fatty acid synthase and the lipogenic phenotype in cancer pathogenesis. Nat Rev Cancer. 2007;7:763–77.
45. Baenke F, Peck B, Miess H, Schulze A. Hooked on fat: the role of lipid synthesis in cancer metabolism and tumour development. Dis Model Mech. 2013;6:1353–63.
46. Walter K, Hong SM, Nyhan S, Canto M, Fedarko N, Klein A, et al. Serum fatty acid synthase as a marker of pancreatic neoplasia. Cancer Epidemiol Biomark Prev. 2009;18:2380–5.
47. Tadros S, Shukla SK, King RJ, Gunda V, Vernucci E, Abrego J, et al. De novo lipid synthesis facilitates gemcitabine resistance through endoplasmic reticulum stress in pancreatic cancer. Cancer Res. 2017;77:5503–17.
48. Yang Y, Liu H, Li Z, Zhao Z, Yip-Schneider M, Fan Q, et al. Role of fatty acid synthase in gemcitabine and radiation resistance of pancreatic cancers. Int J Biochem Mol Biol. 2011;2:89–98.
49. Hatzivassiliou G, Zhao F, Bauer DE, Andreadis C, Shaw AN, Dhanak D, et al. ATP citrate lyase inhibition can suppress tumor cell growth. Cancer Cell. 2005;8:311–21.
50. Currie E, Schulze A, Zechner R, Walther TC, Farese RV Jr. Cellular fatty acid metabolism and cancer. Cell Metab. 2013;18:153–61.
51. Nishi K, Suzuki K, Sawamoto J, Tokizawa Y, Iwase Y, Yumita N, et al. Inhibition of fatty acid synthesis induces apoptosis of human pancreatic cancer cells. Anticancer Res. 2016;36(9):4655–60.
52. Li S, Qiu L, Wu B, Shen H, Zhu J, Zhou L, et al. TOFA suppresses ovarian cancer cell growth in vitro and in vivo. Mol Med Rep. 2013;8:373–8.
53. Svensson RU, Parker SJ, Eichner LJ, Kolar MJ, Wallace M, Brun SN, et al. Inhibition of acetyl-CoA carboxylase suppresses fatty acid synthesis and tumor growth of non-small-cell lung cancer in preclinical models. Nat Med. 2016;22:1108–19.
54. Petrova E, Scholz A, Paul J, Sturz A, Haike K, Siegel F, et al. Acetyl-CoA carboxylase inhibitors attenuate WNT and Hedgehog signaling and suppress pancreatic tumor growth. Oncotarget. 2017;8:48660–70.
55. Murata S, Yanagisawa K, Fukunaga K, Oda T, Kobayashi A, Sasaki R, et al. Fatty acid synthase inhibitor cerulenin suppresses liver metastasis of colon cancer in mice. Cancer Sci. 2010;101:1861–5.
56. Niedzwiecki A, Roomi MW, Kalinovsky T, Rath M. Anticancer efficacy of polyphenols and their combinations. Nutrients. 2016;8(9):pii: E552.
57. Sunami Y, Rebelo A, Kleeff J. Lipid metabolism and lipid droplets in pancreatic cancer and stellate cells. Cancers (Basel). 2017;10(1):pii: E3.

58. Kürbitz C, Heise D, Redmer T, Goumas F, Arlt A, Lemke J, et al. Epicatechin gallate and catechin gallate are superior to epigallocatechin gallate in growth suppression and anti-inflammatory activities in pancreatic tumor cells. Cancer Sci. 2011;102(4):728–34.
59. Shankar S, Marsh L, Srivastava RK. EGCG inhibits growth of human pancreatic tumors orthotopically implanted in Balb C nude mice through modulation of FKHRL1/FOXO3a and neuropilin. Mol Cell Biochem. 2013;372:83–94.
60. Röhrig F, Schulze A. The multifaceted roles of fatty acid synthesis in cancer. Nat Rev Cancer. 2016;16(11):732–49.
61. Jones SF, Infante JR. Molecular pathways: fatty acid synthase. Clin Cancer Res. 2015;21:5434–8.
62. Sokolowska E, Presler M, Goyke E, Milczarek R, Swierczynski J, Sledzinski T. Orlistat reduces proliferation and enhances apoptosis in human pancreatic cancer cells (PANC-1). Anticancer Res. 2017;37:6321–7.
63. Ali A, Levantini E, Teo JT, Goggi J, Clohessy JG, Wu CS, et al. Fatty acid synthase mediates EGFR palmitoylation in EGFR mutated non-small cell lung cancer. EMBO Mol Med. 2018;10(3):pii: e8313.
64. Fako VE, Wu X, Pflug B, Liu JY, Zhang JT. Repositioning proton pump inhibitors as anticancer drugs by targeting the thioesterase domain of human fatty acid synthase. J Med Chem. 2015;58:778–84.
65. Peck B, Schulze A. Lipid desaturation – the next step in targeting lipogenesis in cancer? FEBS J. 2016;283(15):2767–78.
66. Huang J, Fan XX, He J, Pan H, Li RZ, Huang L, et al. SCD1 is associated with tumor promotion, late stage and poor survival in lung adenocarcinoma. Oncotarget. 2016;7:39970–9.
67. Ma MKF, Lau EYT, Leung DHW, Lo J, Ho NPY, Cheng LKW, et al. Stearoyl-CoA desaturase regulates sorafenib resistance via modulation of ER stress-induced differentiation. J Hepatol. 2017;67:979–90.
68. Ran H, Zhu Y, Deng R, Zhang Q, Liu X, Feng M, et al. Stearoyl-CoA desaturase-1 promotes colorectal cancer metastasis in response to glucose by suppressing PTEN. J Exp Clin Cancer Res. 2018;37(1):54.
69. Macášek J, Vecka M, Žák A, Urbánek M, Krechler T, Petružželka L, et al. Plasma fatty acid composition in patients with pancreatic cancer: correlations to clinical parameters. Nutr Cancer. 2012;64:946–55.
70. Li J, Condello S, Thomes-Pepin J, Ma X, Xia Y, Hurley TD, et al. Lipid desaturation is a metabolic marker and therapeutic target of ovarian cancer stem cells. Cell Stem Cell. 2017;20:303–314.e5.
71. Marquardt JU, Thorgeirsson SS. Stem cells in hepatocarcinogenesis: evidence from genomic data. Semin Liver Dis. 2010;30(1):26–34.
72. Ducheix S, Peres C, Härdfeldt J, Frau C, Mocciaro G, Piccinin E, et al. Deletion of stearoyl-CoA desaturase-1 from the intestinal epithelium promotes inflammation and tumorigenesis, reversed by dietary oleate. Gastroenterology. 2018;155(5):1524–1538.e9.
73. Von Roemeling CA, Marlow LA, Wei JJ, Cooper SJ, Caulfield TR, Wu K, et al. Stearoyl-CoA desaturase 1 is a novel molecular therapeutic target for clear cell renal cell carcinoma. Clin Cancer Res. 2013;19:2368–80.
74. Fritz V, Benfodda Z, Rodier G, Henriquet C, Iborra F, Avancès C, et al. Abrogation of de novo lipogenesis by stearoyl-CoA desaturase 1 inhibition interferes with oncogenic signaling and blocks prostate cancer progression in mice. Mol Cancer Ther. 2010;9:1740–54.
75. Wang Y, Viscarra J, Kim SJ, Sul HS. Transcriptional regulation of hepatic lipogenesis. Nat Rev Mol Cell Biol. 2015;16(11):678–89.
76. Ardito CM, Grüner BM, Takeuchi KK, Lubeseder-Martellato C, Teichmann N, Mazur PK, et al. EGF receptor is required for KRAS-induced pancreatic tumorigenesis. Cancer Cell. 2012;22:304–17.

77. Navas C, Hernández-Porras I, Schuhmacher AJ, Sibilia M, Guerra C, Barbacid M. EGF receptor signaling is essential for k-Ras oncogene-driven pancreatic ductal adenocarcinoma. Cancer Cell. 2012;22:318–30.
78. Bian Y, Yu Y, Wang S, Li L. Up-regulation of fatty acid synthase induced by EGFR/ERK activation promotes tumor growth in pancreatic cancer. Biochem Biophys Res Commun. 2015;463:612–7.
79. Sun Y, He W, Luo M, Zhou Y, Chang G, Ren W, et al. SREBP1 regulates tumorigenesis and prognosis of pancreatic cancer through targeting lipid metabolism. Tumor Biol. 2015;36:4133–41.
80. Horton JD, Goldstein JL, Brown MS. SREBPs: activators of the complete program of cholesterol and fatty acid synthesis in the liver. J Clin Invest. 2002;109:1125–31.
81. Ikonen E. Cellular cholesterol trafficking and compartmentalization. Nat Rev Mol Cell Biol. 2008;9:125–38.
82. Goldstein JL, Brown MS, Anderson RG, Russell DW, Schneider WJ. Receptor-mediated endocytosis: concepts emerging from the LDL receptor system. Annu Rev Cell Biol. 1985;1:1–39.
83. Guillaumond F, Bidaut G, Ouaissi M, Servais S, Gouirand V, Olivares O, et al. Cholesterol uptake disruption, in association with chemotherapy, is a promising combined metabolic therapy for pancreatic adenocarcinoma. Proc Natl Acad Sci U S A. 2015;112:2473–8.
84. Chen H, Qin S, Wang M, Zhang T, Zhang S. Association between cholesterol intake and pancreatic cancer risk: evidence from a meta-analysis. Sci Rep. 2015;5:8243.
85. Soyal SM, Nofziger C, Dossena S, Paulmichl M, Patsch W. Targeting SREBPs for treatment of the metabolic syndrome. Trends Pharmacol Sci. 2015;36(6):406–16.
86. Cheng C, Ru P, Geng F, Liu J, Yoo JY, Wu X, et al. Glucose-mediated N-glycosylation of SCAP is essential for SREBP-1 activation and tumor growth. Cancer Cell. 2015;28(5):569–81.
87. Tang JJ, Li JG, Qi W, Qiu WW, Li PS, Li BL, et al. Inhibition of SREBP by a small molecule, betulin, improves hyperlipidemia and insulin resistance and reduces atherosclerotic plaques. Cell Metab. 2011;13:44–56.
88. Gao Y, Jia Z, Kong X, Li Q, Chang DZ, Wie D, et al. Combining betulinic acid and mithramycin a effectively suppresses pancreatic cancer by inhibiting proliferation, invasion, and angiogenesis. Cancer Res. 2011;71:5182–93.
89. Williams KJ, Argus JP, Zhu Y, Wilks MQ, Marbois BN, York AG, et al. An essential requirement for the SCAP/SREBP signaling axis to protect cancer cells from lipotoxicity. Cancer Res. 2013;73:2850–62.
90. Li X, Chen YT, Hu P, Huang WC. Fatostatin displays high antitumor activity in prostate cancer by blocking SREBP-regulated metabolic pathways and androgen receptor signaling. Mol Cancer Ther. 2014;13(4):855–66.
91. Eagle H. Nutrition needs of mammalian cells in tissue culture. Science. 1955;122:501–14.
92. Gao P, Tchernyshyov I, Chang TC, Lee YS, Kita K, Ochi T, et al. c-Myc suppression of miR-23a/b enhances mitochondrial glutaminase expression and glutamine metabolism. Nature. 2009;458:762–5.
93. Son J, Lyssiotis CA, Ying H, Wang X, Hua S, Ligorio M, et al. Glutamine supports pancreatic cancer growth through a KRAS-regulated metabolic pathway. Nature. 2013;496:101–5.
94. Metallo CM, Gameiro PA, Bell EL, Mattaini KR, Yang J, Hiller K, et al. Reductive glutamine metabolism by IDH1 mediates lipogenesis under hypoxia. Nature. 2011;481:380–4.
95. Mullen AR, Wheaton WW, Jin ES, Chen PH, Sullivan LB, Cheng T, et al. Reductive carboxylation supports growth in tumour cells with defective mitochondria. Nature. 2011;481:385–8.
96. Anastasiou D, Cantley LC. Breathless cancer cells get fat on glutamine. Cell Res. 2012;22:443–6.
97. Elgogary A, Xu Q, Poore B, Alt J, Zimmermann SC, Zhao L, et al. Combination therapy with BPTES nanoparticles and metformin targets the metabolic heterogeneity of pancreatic cancer. Proc Natl Acad Sci U S A. 2016;113:E5328–36.

98. Biancur DE, Paulo JA, Małachowska B, Quiles Del Rey M, Sousa CM, Wang X, et al. Compensatory metabolic networks in pancreatic cancers upon perturbation of glutamine metabolism. Nat Commun. 2017;8:15965.
99. Altman BJ, Stine ZE, Dang CV. From Krebs to clinic: glutamine metabolism to cancer therapy. Nat Rev Cancer. 2016;16:619–34.
100. Jin L, Li D, Alesi GN, Fan J, Kang HB, Lu Z, et al. Glutamate dehydrogenase 1 signals through antioxidant glutathione peroxidase 1 to regulate redox homeostasis and tumor growth. Cancer Cell. 2015;27:257–70.
101. Naik R, Ban HS, Jang K, Kim I, Xu X, Harmalkar D, et al. Methyl 3-(3-(4-(2,4,4-Trimeth ylpentan-2-yl)phenoxy)-propanamido)benzoate as a novel and dual malate dehydrogenase (MDH) 1/2 inhibitor targeting cancer metabolism. J Med Chem. 2017;60:8631–46.
102. Wang YP, Zhou W, Wang J, Huang X, Zuo Y, Wang TS, et al. Arginine methylation of MDH1 by CARM1 inhibits glutamine metabolism and suppresses pancreatic cancer. Mol Cell. 2016;64:673–87.
103. Choudhary C, Weinert BT, Nishida Y, Verdin E, Mann M. The growing landscape of lysine acetylation links metabolism and cell signaling. Nat Rev Mol Cell Biol. 2014;15:536–50.
104. Pietrocola F, Galluzzi L, Bravo-San Pedro JM, Madeo F, Kroemer G. Acetyl coenzyme A: a central metabolite and second messenger. Cell Metab. 2015;21:805–21.
105. Zhao S, Torres A, Henry RA, Trefely S, Wallace M, Lee JV, et al. ATP-citrate lyase controls a glucose-to-acetate metabolic switch. Cell Rep. 2016;17(4):1037–52.
106. Watkins PA, Maiguel D, Jia Z, Pevsner J. Evidence for 26 distinct acyl-coenzyme A synthetase genes in the human genome. J Lipid Res. 2007;48:2736–50.
107. Comerford SA, Huang Z, Du X, Wang Y, Cai L, Witkiewicz AK, et al. Acetate dependence of tumors. Cell. 2014;159:1591–602.
108. Schug ZT, Peck B, Jones DT, Zhang Q, Grosskurth S, Alam IS, et al. Acetyl-CoA synthetase 2 promotes acetate utilization and maintains cancer cell growth under metabolic stress. Cancer Cell. 2015;27:57–71.
109. Bulusu V, Tumanov S, Michalopoulou E, van den Broek NJ, MacKay G, Nixon C, et al. Acetate recapturing by nuclear acetyl-CoA synthetase 2 prevents loss of histone acetylation during oxygen and serum limitation. Cell Rep. 2017;18:647–58.
110. Lee MY, Yeon A, Shahid M, Cho E, Sairam V, Figlin R, et al. Reprogrammed lipid metabolism in bladder cancer with cisplatin resistance. Oncotarget. 2018;9(17):13231–43.

Chapter 14
Targeting the Immune System in Pancreatic Cancer

D. Kabacaoglu, D. A. Ruess, and Hana Algül

The Immune Response in Pancreatic Cancer and Its Major Players

The immune system can be both harmful and beneficial during carcinogenesis and progression of pancreatic cancer (PC). The ability of both innate and adaptive immune cells to exert either tumor-suppressive or tumor-promoting properties yields a mosaic pattern of immune cell composition in the tumor microenvironment (TME). Therefore, an understanding of the individual components of this mosaic is required to develop efficient therapeutics.

Chronic inflammation is an important characteristic of PC, which is maintained by a complex interplay of immune cells in the TME [1, 2]. The myeloid compartment has many components, undoubtedly the most important one of them being tumor-associated macrophages (TAM). TAMs are found as M1 or M2 macrophages, which are classified according to the cytokine profile and surface markers they express [3]. Both M1 and M2 macrophages derive from monocytes. M1 macrophages, as "good cops," produce pro-inflammatory cytokines like TNF, IL12, IL-1β, and IFN-γ and show tumoricidal activity and induce an antitumor Th1 immune response. On the other hand, M2 macrophages, as the "bad cops," produce anti-inflammatory tumor-promoting cytokines like TGFβ and IL-10 and stimulate a Th2 immune response [3]. Next to TAMs, myeloid-derived suppressor cells (MDSC) are produced from immature myeloid cells and are known to suppress

D. Kabacaoglu · H. Algül (✉)
Department of Internal Medicine II, Klinikum rechts der Isar,
Technische Universitat München, Munich, Germany
e-mail: hana.alguel@mri.tum.de

D. A. Ruess
Department of Surgery, Faculty of Medicine, Medical Center,
University of Freiburg, Freiburg, Germany

© Springer Nature Switzerland AG 2020
C. W. Michalski et al. (eds.), *Translational Pancreatic Cancer Research*,
Molecular and Translational Medicine,
https://doi.org/10.1007/978-3-030-49476-6_14

adaptive immunity with the recruitment of regulatory T cells (T_{reg}) to the TME and by reducing antitumor T cell activation [4, 5]. In line with this, the presence of immunosuppressive cells like M2 macrophages, MDSCs, and T_{reg} cells in the pancreatic TME has been shown to negatively correlate with overall survival [6–11]. Although both pro- and antitumorigenic abilities of neutrophils are reported, the inhibition of neutrophil recruitment to the TME remains a promising option in preclinical studies [12–14].

In the adaptive immune system, antigen-presenting cells (APC) such as dendritic cells (DC) can prime naïve T cells broadly into functional CD4+ helper T cells (Th) or CD8+ cytotoxic T cells (CTL) [15]. Th cells are further mainly characterized as Th_1, Th_2, and T_{reg}, and their coordination is highly deterministic for the type of tumor immune response [15]. Th_1 cells as conductors of an antitumorigenic response promote antigen presentation on APCs and cytolytic activity of CD8+ T cells and boost M1 macrophages [16, 17]. However, Th_2 and T_{reg} cells are pro-tumorigenic since they can oppose the Th_1 immune response and escalate T cell exhaustion. Their presence is correlated with reduced survival in PC patients [18–23]. CD8+ CTLs are the "best cops" in tumors, since they can directly recognize tumor cell-specific antigens and induce cancer cell death [15, 24].

Immunotherapy for PC: Obstacles and Potential Solutions

Boosting the adaptive immune response is one of the most attractive goals in cancer therapeutics: Other than generating a repertoire of T cells recognizing tumor-specific antigens, the ability of the adaptive immune system to form an immunological memory holds promise for long-term disease control [25]. Immunotherapeutic approaches, currently being established as a fourth pillar of cancer therapeutics (next to chemo-/targeted therapy, radiotherapy, and surgery), augment the antitumor adaptive immune response [26]. Immune checkpoint inhibitors are the best studied candidates in immunotherapeutic options so far. While checkpoint inhibitors like anti-CTLA-4 and anti-PD-1 antibodies showed very promising results in clinical studies for many solid tumors and hematologic malignancies, as single agents or in combination, they appear to be ineffective in PC [27–36]. Therefore, precise understanding of the immune cell network in PC is essential to explore ways to exploit immunotherapeutic approaches for treatment of patients with PC.

Immune Checkpoint Inhibition

CTLA-4 and PD-1 were the first immune checkpoint targets discovered and evaluated for cancer immunotherapeutics [37–39]. During APC:MHC molecule engagement with T cell receptor (TCR) on T cells, axes of co-stimulatory and co-inhibitory signals in T cells mediate T cell activity. These co-signaling pathways are essential for physiological homeostasis since an imbalance can cause either autoimmunity or disability to fight invaders. Tumors may evolve the ability to skew this balance by reducing co-stimulation and inducing co-inhibition to impair antitumor T cell activity [40]. CTLA-4 and PD-1 are such co-inhibitory molecules leading to T cell anergy and exhaustion [41–44]. Antibodies targeting CTLA-4 and PD-1 can impair such signaling pathways in T cells and boost an antitumor cytotoxic immune response in tumors.

The question is though, why checkpoint inhibitors are not effective in PC as opposed to other solid tumor entities. PC owes this to its extreme immune-privileged nature [45]. Immune privilege is the ability to retain the production of antigens, without creating an anti-tumor immune response [46]. Normally, during carcinogenesis, tumor cells produce unique antigens (de novo mutations, re-expression of embryonic stage proteins), which may be recognized by the immune system, potentially leading to tumor cell elimination. During the immunosurveillance process (a hypothesis developed by Paul Ehrlich), the immune system continuously inspects the body for any malignant transformation [47–49]. However, some transformed cells have the ability to escape detection in a process called immunoediting. Immunoediting proposed by Schreiber and colleagues comprises three phases (triple E): elimination, equilibrium, and escape [50]. During the elimination phase, most of the transformed somatic cells die due to immunosurveillance, while the remaining survivors in the equilibrium step no more respond to immune reaction. Through a Darwinian-like selection, these clones proliferate and expand within the escape phase. While many tumors undergo the triple E of immunoediting process, PC holds a unique state [51, 52].

PC carcinogenesis is different in terms of the immunoediting process compared to many other solid tumors. With the use of genetically engineered mouse models (GEMMs), PC was shown to have an immunosuppressive microenvironment and a scarcity of antitumor T cells already during the carcinogenesis process [45]. Due to immunosuppression, the adaptive immune system is not educated toward recognition of any tumor-specific antigens, bypassing the elimination phase of triple E. With this rather immune quiescence-like phenotype, PC limits the entry of antitumor immune cells into the microenvironment maintaining its immune privileged status [51].

Overall, an approach to augment T cell entry and activity in the PC microenvironment may have the ability to render PC cells responsive toward immune checkpoint inhibitors. The factors which will determine such responsiveness are (1st) antigenicity of cancer cells and (2nd) immunogenicity of the tumor in general [53].

Antigenicity is the degree to which tumor cells produce and present neoantigens to generate an antitumor adaptive immune response [53]. These antigens can be divided into tumor-specific antigens (TSA) and tumor-associated antigens (TAA). TSAs are produced upon tumor-specific mutations of genes or reactivation of genes for embryonic development, which are not occurring in healthy somatic cells, while TAAs are wild-type proteins but expressed higher in tumor cells compared to somatic ones [54]. Production and MHC-mediated presentation of such antigens determine the level of antigenicity of tumors [53, 54].

Tumors carrying a high mutational burden generally respond better to checkpoint inhibition since they have a diverse tumor-antigen responsive T cell repertoire [55–57]. PC on the other hand doesn't carry such mutational load, compared to other entities [58, 59]. However, a subgroup of PC patients, representing around 1% of a patient cohort, carry mutations leading to mismatch repair (MMR) deficiency and microsatellite instability (MSI) and may profit from checkpoint inhibitors [60, 61]. As a result, anti PD-1 immunotherapy is approved by FDA for solid tumors including PC with MMR deficiency and MSI [62]. Moreover, one study identified long-term survivors in a PC patient cohort based on their ability to express good quality neoantigens, but not quantity [63]. Most importantly, a decrease in neoantigen quality of metastatic tumors compared to their respective primaries implied the importance of immunosurveillance in cancer metastasis and its implication in therapeutics [63]. Other than antigen production, presentation of these antigens via MHC molecules has been shown to be reduced in PC through the activation of oncogenic drivers like RAS [64–66]. Also, reduced MHC expression in disseminated PC cells appears to be an important driver of metastasis [67]. Since a correlation between antigenic load and immune checkpoint inhibition efficacy is absent in PC, as opposed by other solid tumor entities, in addition, factors determining immunogenicity of PC require exploitation.

Tumors with better ability to induce an adaptive immune response are considered immunogenic. This ability can be modulated both at the tumor cell level and at the level of cross talk of tumor cells with cells of the TME [53]. Transcriptomic analyses revealed an immunogenic subtype of PC, showing higher cytolytic T cell activity, antigen presentation, and CTLA-4 and PD-1 signatures [68]. Signatures as those may help to predetermine the prognostic value of checkpoint inhibitor therapy in the context of "personalized medicine" [69].

Tumor cell-specific immunogenicity can be decreased upon co-inhibitory checkpoint ligand expression in tumor cells, such as PD-L1. In various solid tumors, PD-L1 expression by tumor cells is increased due to oncogenic signaling pathways like PI3K, Hippo, Myc, and JAK-STAT [70–74]. In PC, the myeloid compartment was shown to induce EGFR-dependent MAPK signaling, leading to an increase of PD-L1 production in tumor cells [75]. An imbalance of autophagic modulation in mitochondrial iron homeostasis also may induce PD-L1 expression by pancreatic cancer cells [76].

Reprogramming the Tumor Microenvironment

Even if specific cancer cells are sufficiently antigenic and immunogenic, they may still not respond well to checkpoint inhibition due to an overall impaired immunogenicity mediated by the corresponding tumor tissue. The immunosuppressive TME is the main player in this context. An understanding of the responsible TME compartments, and of their cross talk with antitumor adaptive immune cells, is essential to reveal options for boosting immune checkpoint inhibitor response (Fig. 14.1).

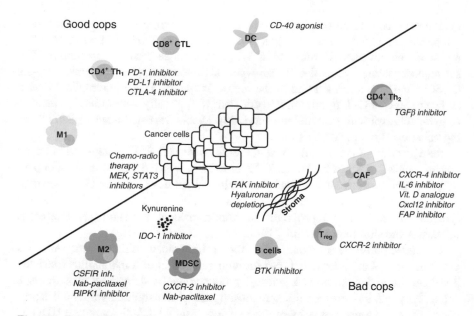

Fig. 14.1 The good and the bad cops of the tumor microenvironment and how to target them to boost a favorable immune response in PC. M1: M1 macrophages, M2: M2 macrophages, MDSC: myeloid-derived suppressor cells, CTL: cytotoxic T lymphocytes, DC: dendritic cells, T$_{reg}$: regulatory T cells, CAF: cancer-associated fibroblasts

Cancer-associated fibroblasts (CAFs) are the leading actors regarding the characteristic desmoplastic stroma formation in PC. Various studies revealed a binary action of stromal cells in the immunogenicity of PC. One study revealed a positive correlation between type-I collagen production and CTL infiltration in tumor specimens of PC patients, whereas another showed the inhibition of CTL activity by αSMA$^+$ CAFs [77]. Other studies demonstrated an inhibitory action of CAFs toward CD8$^+$ T cell infiltration [78]. While most of the research so far implies the prognostic value of "stromal remodeling" in PC, an understanding of CAF action heterogeneity in the TME may provide options to improve the efficacy of immune checkpoint inhibitors. For example, with the use of preclinical mouse models, impairment of CXCR4 or IL-6 signaling in CAFs was shown to be synergistic with anti PD-L1 therapy [79, 80]. Stromal remodeling with FAK inhibitors reduced the immunosuppressive milieu in the TME, increasing chemotherapy-checkpoint inhibitor combination therapy efficacy [81]. Previous studies showed the benefit of hyaluronan depletion and vitamin D receptor activation in stromal remodeling [82–85]. Here, a combination therapy with immune checkpoint inhibitors may have therapeutic impact.

The myeloid compartment is a double-edged sword as also mentioned earlier. Years of research dissected the complex roles of individual components in PC. Studies focusing on CD40 agonist treatment of PC actually revealed the quite unique properties of PC. Treatment of preclinical mouse models with a CD40 agonist (acting on APCs increasing their capability to prime CTL) in combination with gemcitabine created an only mild response by remodeling the stroma and repro-gramming immunosuppressive myeloid cells inside the TME [86]. However, this regimen was not enough to create an adaptive immune response in tumors. The subsequent studies identified a subtype of immunosuppressive macrophages (Ly6C^{low} F4/80$^+$), accumulating in the tumor periphery. These macrophages were shown to prevent CTL migration into the TME [87]. Finally, a combination therapy of nab-paclitaxel with gemcitabine and CD40 agonist revealed a synergism allow-ing penetration of active CTLs [88].

Re-education of neutrophils, MDSCs, and TAMs can also be achieved via vari-ous inhibitors targeting CSF1R, CXCR2, or RIPK1, which demonstrated synergism with immune checkpoint inhibitors in preclinical studies [14, 89, 90]. Other than directly targeting the myeloid compartment, inhibition of B cell-specific Bruton's tyrosine kinase (BTK) reprogrammed tumor resident macrophages indirectly, increasing the antitumor immunity [91].

Immunosuppressive immune cells impair immunosurveillance not only via cytokine-chemokine release but also through generation of a metabolite-restricted TME. Arginine depletion via arginase-1 produced by TAMs and MDSCs limits T cell activity [92, 93]. Further, the immunosuppressive metabolite kynurenine is pro-duced from tryptophan as a by-product of indoleamine 2,3-dioxygenase (IDO-1) enzymatic activity. IDO-1 expression from cancer cells, TAMs, and MDSCs not only limits tryptophan availability for antitumor T cells but also increases inhibition of T cell activity by kynurenine [94]. Adenosine production by T$_{reg}$ cells and prosta-glandin E2 production from TAMs and MDSCs are also responsible for antitumor T cell activity impairment [95, 96].

Immunotherapeutic Properties of "Classical" Treatment Approaches

Other than targeted inhibitors, chemotherapeutic agents and radiotherapy also have the ability to convert nonresponsive, "immunologically cold," tumors to responsive, "immunologically hot," tumors. Chemo- and radiotherapy can boost both, antigenic properties of cancer cells due to their mutagenic effect and also immunogenicity of the tumor due to the induction of immunogenic cell death and subsequently enhanced inflammation [97, 98]. Next to their direct effect on cancer cells, such treatments may also alter the composition of immunosuppressive immune cells in the TME [88, 99]. Strikingly, immune checkpoint inhibition in cancer may not only enhance the response to radiation therapy in primary tumors but also has the potential for an abscopal response in metastatic sites [100, 101]. In conclusion, while chemotherapy and radio-therapy still are the gold standard therapies for cancer treatment, their combination with checkpoint inhibitors may be the next step to both increase the treatment response and T cell memory for long-term disease control, even for PC. Essentially, analysis of respective clinical trials may inform about dosing, sequence of treatment, and specific subgroups profiting most from the expected synergism.

Other Strategies for Boosting the Antitumor Immune Response

Immunotherapeutic approaches are not only limited to immune checkpoint inhibitors.

Oncolytic viruses (OV) can be designed to only target tumor cells, but not healthy somatic ones. This specificity can be achieved at multiple levels [102]. At the physiological level, OVs are not equipped to win a combat against healthy cells. Tumor cells, however, already may have imbalanced interferon signaling and increased cellular metabolism coupled with proliferation making them vulnerable towards viral infection. OVs can also be designed to take advantage of tumor-specific expression of cell entry receptors or transcription factors, limiting their action on healthy cells.

Cancer vaccines aim to boost adaptive immune response in the host against tumors. They can be produced as either whole cell (e.g. GVAX) or antigen-specific vaccines. GVAX is composed of pancreatic cancer cells genetically engineered to secrete GM-CSF with the aim to convert "cold" tumors to "hot" ones, and these cells are irradiated to prevent further proliferation [103]. *Listeria* vaccine is an engineered bacterial strain to secrete TAAs such as human mesothelin, boosting antitumor CTL activity. An approach with total cell followed by antigen-specific vaccine may recapitulate a "prime and boost" scenario [104].

Chimeric antigen receptor T cells (CAR-T) are genetically designed to express a receptor construct comprising an antibody-like ectodomain targeting TSAs and a TCR-like endodomain, bypassing the need for MHC engagement [105]. Upon antigen recognition they exert their cytotoxic properties. CAR-T cell therapy requires adoptive T cell transfer (ATC), in which patient's T cells have to be isolated, expanded, and genetically engineered. Without a genetic manipulation, in vitro induction and expansion of TILs (TIL-ATC) is also a valuable approach to exploit tumor targeting not only by a single antigen but a pool of them [106, 107].

Currently Ongoing Clinical Trials for Immunotherapy of Patients with PC

An overview of clinical trials based on abovementioned preclinical studies is given in Table 14.1. Overall, these studies reveal that PC is actually antigenic enough to create an antitumor adaptive immune response. However, the main barrier to be exceeded is the immunosuppressive microenvironment, which blocks the antitumor T cell priming and infiltration. One important factor is that many of these studies for PC are still in their early stages. Thorough analysis of each of these trials will pave the way to dissect individual rationales for combination therapies.

Table 14.1 Selected clinical trials aiming to induce an antitumor immune response in pancreatic cancer

Combination-arm 1	Combination-arm 2	Status	Patient eligibility criteria	Trial ID
Ipilimumab (αCTLA-4), gemcitabine	–	Phase 1	Stage III–IV or recurrent pancreatic cancer, uneligible to surgery	NCT01473940
Nab-paclitaxel, gemcitabine, nivolumab (αPD-1)	Nab-paclitaxel and nivolumab	Completed/ phase 1	Multiple solid tumors including pancreatic cancer	NCT01473941
Cyclophosphamide, GVAX, pembrolizumab (αPD-1), radiation (SBRT-6.6 Gy)	–	Recruiting/ phase 2	Locally advanced pancreatic ductal adenocarcinoma upon standard chemotherapy	NCT02648282
Durvalumab (αPD-L1), radiation (SBRT-6.6 Gy)	–	Recruiting/ phase 1–2	Borderline resectable and locally advanced pancreatic adenocarcinoma, treated with standard of care (SOC)	NCT03245541
Cyclophosphamide, GVAX, nivolumab (αPD-1), radiation (SBRT-6.6 Gy)	–	Recruiting/ phase 2	Borderline resectable pancreatic cancer	NCT03161379
Durvalumab (αPD-L1), radiation (SBRT-6.6 Gy)	–	Recruiting/ phase 1–2	SOC treated, borderline resectable, and locally advanced pancreatic adenocarcinoma	NCT03245541
Durvalumab (αPD-L1), tremelimumab (αCTLA4), radiation (SBRT-6.6 Gy)	Radiation (SBRT-6.6 Gy) with either durvalumab or tremelimumab	Recruiting/ phase 1	Uunresectable, nonmetastatic, locally advanced adenocarcinoma of pancreas	NCT02868632
Avelumab (αPD-L1), binimetinib (MEK inhibitor), talazoparib (PARP inhibitor)	Avelumab, binimetinib	Recruiting/ phase 2	Locally advanced or metastatic Ras-mutant solid tumors, including pancreatic cancer	NCT03637491
Durvalumab (αPD-L1), AZD9150 (STAT3 antisense)	–	Recruiting/ phase 2	Advanced pancreatic cancer	NCT02983578
Pembrolizumab (αPD-1), paricalcitol (vit D analogue)	Pembrolizumab, placebo	Recruiting/ early phase 2	Stage IV pancreatic cancer	NCT03331562

Table 14.1   (continued)

Combination-arm 1	Combination-arm 2	Status	Patient eligibility criteria	Trial ID
PEGPH20 (hyaluronidase), pembrolizumab (αPD-1)	–	Phase 2	Hyaluronan high (HA-high) metastatic pancreatic ductal adenocarcinoma	NCT03634332
PEGPH20 (hyaluronidase), avelumab (αPD-L1)	–	Recruiting/ early phase 1	Chemotherapy-resistant advanced or locally advanced pancreatic ductal adenocarcinoma	NCT03481920
Galunisertib (TGFβ inhibitor), durvalumab (αPD-L1)	–	Phase 1	Metastatic pancreatic cancer	NCT02734160
Spartalizumab (αPD-1), NIS793 (TGFβ inhibitor)	NIS793 (TGFβ inhibitor)	Recruiting/ phase 1	Advanced malignancies including pancreatic cancer	NCT02947165
Pembrolizumab (αPD-1), defactinib (FAK inhibitor)	–	Recruiting/ phase 1–2	Advanced solid malignancies including pancreatic neoplasms	NCT02758587
Pembrolizumab (αPD-1), defactinib (FAK inhibitor), gemcitabine	–	Recruiting/ phase 1	Advanced solid malignancies including pancreatic cancer	NCT02546531
Pembrolizumab (αPD-1), defactinib (FAK inhibitor)	Pembrolizumab (αPD-1)	Recruiting/ phase 2	SOC treated, neoadjuvant, and adjuvant treatment for resectable pancreatic ductal adenocarcinoma	NCT03727880
Cyclophosphamide, GVAX, pembrolizumab (αPD-1), IMC-CS4 (CSF1R inhibitor)	–	Recruiting/ early phase 1	Borderline resectable pancreatic ductal adenocarcinoma	NCT03153410
Durvalumab (αPD-L1), pexidartinib (CSF1R, FLT3, and KIT inhibitor)	–	Recruiting/ phase 1	Metastatic/ advanced pancreatic or colorectal cancers	NCT02777710
Nivolumab (αPD-1), cabiralizumab (αCSF1R)	Cabiralizumab	Phase 1	Advanced solid tumors including pancreatic cancer	NCT02526017

(continued)

Table 14.1 (continued)

Combination-arm 1	Combination-arm 2	Status	Patient eligibility criteria	Trial ID
Pembrolizumab (αPD-1), AMG820 (CSF1R inhibitor)	–	Phase 1–2	Advanced solid tumors including pancreatic cancer	NCT02713529
Pembrolizumab (αPD-1), BL-8040 (CXCR4 inhibitor)	BL-8040	Phase 2	Metastatic pancreatic adenocarcinoma	NCT02826486
Olaptesed pegol (CXCL12 inhibitor) + Pembrolizumab	Olaptesed pegol	Phase 1–2	Metastatic colorectal and pancreatic cancer	NCT03168139
APX005M (CD40 agonist), gemcitabine, nab-paclitaxel, nivolumab (αPD-1)	APX005M, gemcitabine, nab-paclitaxel	Recruiting/ phase 1–2	Previously untreated metastatic pancreatic adenocarcinoma	NCT03214250
CDX-1140 (CD40 agonist), CDX-301 (CD135 agonist)	CDX-1140	Recruiting/ phase 1	Advanced malignancies including pancreatic adenocarcinoma	NCT03329950
Pembrolizumab (αPD-1), acalabrutinib (BTK inhibitor)	Acalabrutinib	Phase 2	Metastatic pancreatic cancer	NCT02362048
Durvalumab (αPD-L1), ibritunib (BTK inhibitor)	–	Completed/ phase 1–2	Relapsed or refractory solid tumors including pancreatic cancer	NCT02403271
Epacadostat (IDO-1 inhibitor), pembrolizumab (αPD-1)	–	Phase 2/ withdrawn	Advanced pancreatic cancer with chromosomal instability/ homologous recombination repair deficiency (HRRD)	NCT03432676

Table 14.1 (continued)

Combination-arm 1	Combination-arm 2	Status	Patient eligibility criteria	Trial ID
Atezolizumab (αPD-L1), chemotherapy, selicrelumab (CD40 agonist)	Nab-paclitaxel, gemcitabine (chemotherapy)	Recruiting/ phase 1–2	Cohort 1 treatment to be performed on patients with no prior systemic therapy for metastatic pancreatic ductal adenocarcinoma	NCT03193190
Atezolizumab (αPD-L1), chemotherapy, selicrelumab (CD40 agonist), bevacizumab (αVEGF)				
Atezolizumab (αPD-L1) + chemotherapy + bevacizumab (αVEGF)				
Atezolizumab (αPD-L1) + chemotherapy + emactuzumab (αCSF1R)				
Atezolizumab (αPD-L1) + cobimetinib (MEK inhibitor)	Nab-paclitaxel and gemcitabine or mFOLFOX6 (chemotherapy)		Cohort 2 treatment to be performed on patients with disease progression upon control chemotherapy of cohort 1	
Atezolizumab (αPD-L1) + PEGPH20 (hyaluronidase)				
Atezolizumab + BL-8040 (CXCR4 inhibitor)				
Atezolizumab (αPD-L1) + RO6874281 (FAP-IL2 fusion protein)				
Atezolizumab (αPD-L1) + emactuzumab (αCSF1R)				

References

1. Guerra C, Schuhmacher AJ, Cañamero M, Grippo PJ, Verdaguer L, Pérez-Gallego L, Dubus P, Sandgren EP, Barbacid M. Chronic pancreatitis is essential for induction of pancreatic ductal adenocarcinoma by K-Ras oncogenes in adult mice. Cancer Cell. 2007;11:291–302.
2. McKay CJ, Glen P, McMillan DC. Chronic inflammation and pancreatic cancer. Best Pract Res Clin Gastroenterol. 2008;22:65–73.
3. Ruffell B, Affara NI, Coussens LM. Differential macrophage programming in the tumor microenvironment. Trends Immunol. 2012;33:119–26.
4. Ostrand-Rosenberg S, Sinha P. Myeloid-derived suppressor cells: linking inflammation and cancer. J Immunol. 2009;182:4499–506.
5. Gabrilovich DI. Myeloid-derived suppressor cells. Cancer Immunol Res. 2017;5:3–8.
6. Hiraoka N, Onozato K, Kosuge T, Hirohashi S. Prevalence of FOXP3+ regulatory T cells increases during the progression of pancreatic ductal adenocarcinoma and its premalignant lesions. Clin Cancer Res. 2006;12:5423–34.
7. Tjomsland V, Niklasson L, Sandström P, Borch K, Druid H, Bratthäll C, Messmer D, Larsson M, Spångeus A. The desmoplastic stroma plays an essential role in the accumulation and modulation of infiltrated immune cells in pancreatic adenocarcinoma. Clin Dev Immunol. 2011;2011:212810.

8. Kurahara H, Shinchi H, Mataki Y, Maemura K, Noma H, Kubo F, Sakoda M, Ueno S, Natsugoe S, Takao S. Significance of M2-polarized tumor-associated macrophage in pancreatic cancer. J Surg Res. 2011;167:e211–9.
9. Greten TF, Manns MP, Korangy F. Myeloid derived suppressor cells in human diseases. Int Immunopharmacol. 2011;11:802–7.
10. Ino Y, Yamazaki-Itoh R, Shimada K, Iwasaki M, Kosuge T, Kanai Y, Hiraoka N. Immune cell infiltration as an indicator of the immune microenvironment of pancreatic cancer. Br J Cancer. 2013;108:914–23.
11. Goedegebuure P, Mitchem JB, Porembka MR, Tan MCB, Belt BA, Wang-Gillam A, Gillanders WE, Hawkins WG, Linehan DC. Myeloid-derived suppressor cells: general characteristics and relevance to clinical management of pancreatic cancer. Curr Cancer Drug Targets. 2011;11:734–51.
12. Leliefeld PHC, Koenderman L, Pillay J. How neutrophils shape adaptive immune responses. Front Immunol. 2015;6:471.
13. Fridlender ZG, Sun J, Kim S, Kapoor V, Cheng G, Ling L, Worthen GS, Albelda SM. Polarization of tumor-associated neutrophil phenotype by TGF-beta: "N1" versus "N2" TAN. Cancer Cell. 2009;16:183–94.
14. Steele CW, Karim SA, Leach JDG, et al. CXCR2 inhibition profoundly suppresses metastases and augments immunotherapy in pancreatic ductal adenocarcinoma. Cancer Cell. 2016;29:832–45.
15. Gao GF, Rao Z, Bell JI. Molecular coordination of alphabeta T-cell receptors and coreceptors CD8 and CD4 in their recognition of peptide-MHC ligands. Trends Immunol. 2002;23:408–13.
16. Steimle V, Siegrist CA, Mottet A, Lisowska-Grospierre B, Mach B. Regulation of MHC class II expression by interferon-gamma mediated by the transactivator gene CIITA. Science. 1994;265:106–9.
17. Stout RD, Bottomly K. Antigen-specific activation of effector macrophages by IFN-gamma producing (TH1) T cell clones. Failure of IL-4-producing (TH2) T cell clones to activate effector function in macrophages. J Immunol. 1989;142:760–5.
18. Tanaka A, Sakaguchi S. Regulatory T cells in cancer immunotherapy. Cell Res. 2017;27:109–18.
19. Dobrzanski MJ. Expanding roles for CD4 T cells and their subpopulations in tumor immunity and therapy. Front Oncol. 2013;3:63.
20. Tassi E, Gavazzi F, Albarello L, Senyukov V, Longhi R, Dellabona P, Doglioni C, Braga M, Di Carlo V, Protti MP. Carcinoembryonic antigen-specific but not antiviral CD4+ T cell immunity is impaired in pancreatic carcinoma patients. J Immunol. 2008;181:6595–603.
21. De Monte L, Reni M, Tassi E, Clavenna D, Papa I, Recalde H, Braga M, Di Carlo V, Doglioni C, Protti MP. Intratumor T helper type 2 cell infiltrate correlates with cancer-associated fibroblast thymic stromal lymphopoietin production and reduced survival in pancreatic cancer. J Exp Med. 2011;208:469–78.
22. Gabitass RF, Annels NE, Stocken DD, Pandha HA, Middleton GW. Elevated myeloid-derived suppressor cells in pancreatic, esophageal and gastric cancer are an independent prognostic factor and are associated with significant elevation of the Th2 cytokine interleukin-13. Cancer Immunol Immunother. 2011;60:1419–30.
23. Formentini A, Prokopchuk O, Sträter J, Kleeff J, Grochola LF, Leder G, Henne-Bruns D, Korc M, Kornmann M. Interleukin-13 exerts autocrine growth-promoting effects on human pancreatic cancer, and its expression correlates with a propensity for lymph node metastases. Int J Color Dis. 2009;24:57–67.
24. Nathan CF, Murray HW, Wiebe ME, Rubin BY. Identification of interferon-gamma as the lymphokine that activates human macrophage oxidative metabolism and antimicrobial activity. J Exp Med. 1983;158:670–89.
25. Pardoll DM. The blockade of immune checkpoints in cancer immunotherapy. Nat Rev Cancer. 2012;12:252–64.

26. Iwai Y, Hamanishi J, Chamoto K, Honjo T. Cancer immunotherapies targeting the PD-1 signaling pathway. J Biomed Sci. 2017;24:26.
27. Royal RE, Levy C, Turner K, et al. Phase 2 trial of single agent Ipilimumab (anti-CTLA-4) for locally advanced or metastatic pancreatic adenocarcinoma. J Immunother. 2010;33:828–33.
28. Brahmer JR, Tykodi SS, Chow LQM, et al. Safety and activity of anti-PD-L1 antibody in patients with advanced cancer. N Engl J Med. 2012;366:2455–65.
29. Hodi FS, O'Day SJ, McDermott DF, et al. Improved survival with ipilimumab in patients with metastatic melanoma. N Engl J Med. 2010;363:711–23.
30. Weber JS, D'Angelo SP, Minor D, et al. Nivolumab versus chemotherapy in patients with advanced melanoma who progressed after anti-CTLA-4 treatment (CheckMate 037): a randomised, controlled, open-label, phase 3 trial. Lancet Oncol. 2015;16:375–84.
31. Ribas A, Puzanov I, Dummer R, et al. Pembrolizumab versus investigator-choice chemotherapy for ipilimumab-refractory melanoma (KEYNOTE-002): a randomised, controlled, phase 2 trial. Lancet Oncol. 2015;16:908–18.
32. Rizvi NA, Mazières J, Planchard D, et al. Activity and safety of nivolumab, an anti-PD-1 immune checkpoint inhibitor, for patients with advanced, refractory squamous non-small-cell lung cancer (CheckMate 063): a phase 2, single-arm trial. Lancet Oncol. 2015;16:257–65.
33. Motzer RJ, Rini BI, McDermott DF, et al. Nivolumab for metastatic renal cell carcinoma: results of a randomized phase II trial. J Clin Oncol. 2015;33:1430–7.
34. Powles T, O'Donnell PH, Massard C, et al. Efficacy and safety of durvalumab in locally advanced or metastatic urothelial carcinoma: updated results from a phase 1/2 open-label study. JAMA Oncol. 2017;3:e172411.
35. Powles T, Eder JP, Fine GD, et al. MPDL3280A (anti-PD-L1) treatment leads to clinical activity in metastatic bladder cancer. Nature. 2014;515:558–62.
36. Ansell SM, Lesokhin AM, Borrello I, et al. PD-1 blockade with nivolumab in relapsed or refractory Hodgkin's lymphoma. N Engl J Med. 2015;372:311–9.
37. Dong H, Strome SE, Salomao DR, et al. Tumor-associated B7-H1 promotes T-cell apoptosis: a potential mechanism of immune evasion. Nat Med. 2002;8:793–800.
38. Ishida Y, Agata Y, Shibahara K, Honjo T. Induced expression of PD-1, a novel member of the immunoglobulin gene superfamily, upon programmed cell death. EMBO J. 1992;11:3887–95.
39. Leach DR, Krummel MF, Allison JP. Enhancement of antitumor immunity by CTLA-4 blockade. Science. 1996;271:1734–6.
40. Topalian SL, Drake CG, Pardoll DM. Immune checkpoint blockade: a common denominator approach to cancer therapy. Cancer Cell. 2015;27:450–61.
41. Crespo J, Sun H, Welling TH, Tian Z, Zou W. T cell anergy, exhaustion, senescence, and stemness in the tumor microenvironment. Curr Opin Immunol. 2013;25:214–21.
42. Walunas TL, Lenschow DJ, Bakker CY, Linsley PS, Freeman GJ, Green JM, Thompson CB, Bluestone JA. CTLA-4 can function as a negative regulator of T cell activation. Immunity. 1994;1:405–13.
43. Krummel MF, Allison JP. CD28 and CTLA-4 have opposing effects on the response of T cells to stimulation. J Exp Med. 1995;182:459–65.
44. Freeman GJ, Long AJ, Iwai Y, et al. Engagement of the PD-1 immunoinhibitory receptor by a novel B7 family member leads to negative regulation of lymphocyte activation. J Exp Med. 2000;192:1027–34.
45. Clark CE, Hingorani SR, Mick R, Combs C, Tuveson DA, Vonderheide RH. Dynamics of the immune reaction to pancreatic cancer from inception to invasion. Cancer Res. 2007;67:9518–27.
46. Hong S, Van Kaer L. Immune privilege: keeping an eye on natural killer T cells. J Exp Med. 1999;190:1197–200.
47. Ehrlich P, Himmelweit F, Marquadt M, Dale HH. The collected papers of Paul Ehrlich of Paul Ehrlich: immunology and cancer research. London: Pergamon Press; 1957.
48. Burnet FM. The concept of immunological surveillance. Prog Exp Tumor Res. 1970;13:1–27.
49. Thomas L. On immunosurveillance in human cancer. Yale J Biol Med. 1982;55:329–33.

50. Dunn GP, Old LJ, Schreiber RD. The three Es of cancer immunoediting. Annu Rev Immunol. 2004;22:329–60.
51. Evans RA, Diamond MS, Rech AJ, et al. Lack of immunoediting in murine pancreatic cancer reversed with neoantigen. JCI Insight. 2016. https://doi.org/10.1172/jci.insight.88328.
52. Kabacaoglu D, Ciecielski KJ, Ruess DA, Algül H. Immune checkpoint inhibition for pancreatic ductal adenocarcinoma: current limitations and future options. Front Immunol. 2018;9:1878.
53. Beatty GL, Gladney WL. Immune escape mechanisms as a guide for cancer immunotherapy. Clin Cancer Res. 2015;21:687–92.
54. Yarchoan M, Hopkins A, Jaffee EM. Tumor mutational burden and response rate to PD-1 inhibition. N Engl J Med. 2017;377:2500–1.
55. Goodman AM, Kato S, Bazhenova L, Patel SP, Frampton GM, Miller V, Stephens PJ, Daniels GA, Kurzrock R. Tumor mutational burden as an independent predictor of response to immunotherapy in diverse cancers. Mol Cancer Ther. 2017;16:2598–608.
56. Rizvi NA, Hellmann MD, Snyder A, et al. Cancer immunology. Mutational landscape determines sensitivity to PD-1 blockade in non-small cell lung cancer. Science. 2015;348:124–8.
57. Yarchoan M, Johnson BA, Lutz ER, Laheru DA, Jaffee EM. Targeting neoantigens to augment antitumour immunity. Nat Rev Cancer. 2017;17:569.
58. Campbell BB, Light N, Fabrizio D, et al. Comprehensive analysis of hypermutation in human cancer. Cell. 2017;171:1042–1056.e10.
59. Vogelstein B, Papadopoulos N, Velculescu VE, Zhou S, Diaz LA, Kinzler KW. Cancer genome landscapes. Science. 2013;339:1546–58.
60. Germano G, Lamba S, Rospo G, et al. Inactivation of DNA repair triggers neoantigen generation and impairs tumour growth. Nature. 2017;552:116–20.
61. Humphris JL, Patch A-M, Nones K, et al. Hypermutation in pancreatic cancer. Gastroenterology. 2017;152:68–74.e2.
62. Le DT, Durham JN, Smith KN, et al. Mismatch repair deficiency predicts response of solid tumors to PD-1 blockade. Science. 2017;357:409–13.
63. Balachandran VP, Łuksza M, Zhao JN, et al. Identification of unique neoantigen qualities in long-term survivors of pancreatic cancer. Nature. 2017;551:512–6.
64. Delp K, Momburg F, Hilmes C, Huber C, Seliger B. Functional deficiencies of components of the MHC class I antigen pathway in human tumors of epithelial origin. Bone Marrow Transplant. 2000;25(Suppl 2):S88–95.
65. Lohmann S, Wollscheid U, Huber C, Seliger B. Multiple levels of MHC class I downregulation by ras oncogenes. Scand J Immunol. 1996;43:537–44.
66. Seliger B, Harders C, Wollscheid U, Staege MS, Reske-Kunz AB, Huber C. Suppression of MHC class I antigens in oncogenic transformants: association with decreased recognition by cytotoxic T lymphocytes. Exp Hematol. 1996;24:1275–9.
67. Pommier A, Anaparthy N, Memos N, et al. Unresolved endoplasmic reticulum stress engenders immune-resistant, latent pancreatic cancer metastases. Science. 2018. https://doi.org/10.1126/science.aao4908.
68. Bailey P, Chang DK, Nones K, et al. Genomic analyses identify molecular subtypes of pancreatic cancer. Nature. 2016;531:47–52.
69. Zhang J, Wolfgang CL, Zheng L. Precision immuno-oncology: prospects of individualized immunotherapy for pancreatic cancer. Cancers (Basel). 2018. https://doi.org/10.3390/cancers10020039.
70. Feng J, Yang H, Zhang Y, Wei H, Zhu Z, Zhu B, Yang M, Cao W, Wang L, Wu Z. Tumor cell-derived lactate induces TAZ-dependent upregulation of PD-L1 through GPR81 in human lung cancer cells. Oncogene. 2017;36:5829–39.
71. Casey SC, Tong L, Li Y, et al. MYC regulates the antitumor immune response through CD47 and PD-L1. Science. 2016;352:227–31.
72. Parsa AT, Waldron JS, Panner A, et al. Loss of tumor suppressor PTEN function increases B7-H1 expression and immunoresistance in glioma. Nat Med. 2007;13:84–8.

73. Lastwika KJ, Wilson W, Li QK, et al. Control of PD-L1 expression by oncogenic activation of the AKT-mTOR pathway in non-small cell lung cancer. Cancer Res. 2016;76:227–38.
74. Song TL, Nairismägi M-L, Laurensia Y, et al. Oncogenic activation of the STAT3 pathway drives PD-L1 expression in natural killer/T-cell lymphoma. Blood. 2018;132:1146–58.
75. Zhang Y, Velez-Delgado A, Mathew E, Li D, Mendez FM, Flannagan K, Rhim AD, Simeone DM, Beatty GL, Pasca di Magliano M. Myeloid cells are required for PD-1/PD-L1 checkpoint activation and the establishment of an immunosuppressive environment in pancreatic cancer. Gut. 2017;66:124–36.
76. Li C, Zhang Y, Cheng X, et al. PINK1 and PARK2 suppress pancreatic tumorigenesis through control of mitochondrial iron-mediated immunometabolism. Dev Cell. 2018;46:441–455.e8.
77. Carstens JL, Correa de Sampaio P, Yang D, Barua S, Wang H, Rao A, Allison JP, LeBleu VS, Kalluri R. Spatial computation of intratumoral T cells correlates with survival of patients with pancreatic cancer. Nat Commun. 2017;8:15095.
78. Ene-Obong A, Clear AJ, Watt J, et al. Activated pancreatic stellate cells sequester CD8+ T cells to reduce their infiltration of the juxtatumoral compartment of pancreatic ductal adenocarcinoma. Gastroenterology. 2013;145:1121–32.
79. Feig C, Jones JO, Kraman M, et al. Targeting CXCL12 from FAP-expressing carcinoma-associated fibroblasts synergizes with anti-PD-L1 immunotherapy in pancreatic cancer. Proc Natl Acad Sci U S A. 2013;110:20212–7.
80. Mace TA, Shakya R, Pitarresi JR, et al. IL-6 and PD-L1 antibody blockade combination therapy reduces tumour progression in murine models of pancreatic cancer. Gut. 2018;67:320–32.
81. Jiang H, Hegde S, Knolhoff BL, et al. Targeting focal adhesion kinase renders pancreatic cancers responsive to checkpoint immunotherapy. Nat Med. 2016;22:851–60.
82. Jacobetz MA, Chan DS, Neesse A, et al. Hyaluronan impairs vascular function and drug delivery in a mouse model of pancreatic cancer. Gut. 2013;62:112–20.
83. Provenzano PP, Cuevas C, Chang AE, Goel VK, Von Hoff DD, Hingorani SR. Enzymatic targeting of the stroma ablates physical barriers to treatment of pancreatic ductal adenocarcinoma. Cancer Cell. 2012;21:418–29.
84. Thompson CB, Shepard HM, O'Connor PM, et al. Enzymatic depletion of tumor hyaluronan induces antitumor responses in preclinical animal models. Mol Cancer Ther. 2010;9:3052–64.
85. Sherman MH, Yu RT, Engle DD, et al. Vitamin D receptor-mediated stromal reprogramming suppresses pancreatitis and enhances pancreatic cancer therapy. Cell. 2014;159:80–93.
86. Beatty GL, Chiorean EG, Fishman MP, et al. CD40 agonists alter tumor stroma and show efficacy against pancreatic carcinoma in mice and humans. Science. 2011;331:1612–6.
87. Beatty GL, Winograd R, Evans RA, et al. Exclusion of T cells from pancreatic carcinomas in mice is regulated by Ly6C(low) F4/80(+) extratumoral macrophages. Gastroenterology. 2015;149:201–10.
88. Byrne KT, Vonderheide RH. CD40 stimulation obviates innate sensors and drives T cell immunity in cancer. Cell Rep. 2016;15:2719–32.
89. Zhu Y, Knolhoff BL, Meyer MA, Nywening TM, West BL, Luo J, Wang-Gillam A, Goedegebuure SP, Linehan DC, DeNardo DG. CSF1/CSF1R blockade reprograms tumor-infiltrating macrophages and improves response to T-cell checkpoint immunotherapy in pancreatic cancer models. Cancer Res. 2014;74:5057–69.
90. Wang W, Marinis JM, Beal AM, et al. RIP1 kinase drives macrophage-mediated adaptive immune tolerance in pancreatic cancer. Cancer Cell. 2018;34:757–774.e7.
91. Gunderson AJ, Kaneda MM, Tsujikawa T, et al. Bruton tyrosine kinase-dependent immune cell cross-talk drives pancreas cancer. Cancer Discov. 2016;6:270–85.
92. Rodriguez PC, Hernandez CP, Quiceno D, Dubinett SM, Zabaleta J, Ochoa JB, Gilbert J, Ochoa AC. Arginase I in myeloid suppressor cells is induced by COX-2 in lung carcinoma. J Exp Med. 2005;202:931–9.
93. Rodriguez PC, Ernstoff MS, Hernandez C, Atkins M, Zabaleta J, Sierra R, Ochoa AC. Arginase I-producing myeloid-derived suppressor cells in renal cell carcinoma are a subpopulation of activated granulocytes. Cancer Res. 2009;69:1553–60.

94. Platten M, Wick W, Van den Eynde BJ. Tryptophan catabolism in cancer: beyond IDO and tryptophan depletion. Cancer Res. 2012;72:5435–40.
95. Ohta A. A metabolic immune checkpoint: adenosine in tumor microenvironment. Front Immunol. 2016;7:109.
96. Sreeramkumar V, Fresno M, Cuesta N. Prostaglandin E2 and T cells: friends or foes? Immunol Cell Biol. 2012;90:579–86.
97. Brown JS, Sundar R, Lopez J. Combining DNA damaging therapeutics with immunotherapy: more haste, less speed. Br J Cancer. 2018;118:312–24.
98. Azad A, Yin Lim S, D'Costa Z, et al. PD-L1 blockade enhances response of pancreatic ductal adenocarcinoma to radiotherapy. EMBO Mol Med. 2017;9:167–80.
99. Zheng Y, Dou Y, Duan L, Cong C, Gao A, Lai Q, Sun Y. Using chemo-drugs or irradiation to break immune tolerance and facilitate immunotherapy in solid cancer. Cell Immunol. 2015;294:54–9.
100. Golden EB, Demaria S, Schiff PB, Chachoua A, Formenti SC. An abscopal response to radiation and ipilimumab in a patient with metastatic non-small cell lung cancer. Cancer Immunol Res. 2013;1:365–72.
101. Formenti SC, Demaria S. Combining radiotherapy and cancer immunotherapy: a paradigm shift. J Natl Cancer Inst. 2013;105:256–65.
102. Naik S, Russell SJ. Engineering oncolytic viruses to exploit tumor specific defects in innate immune signaling pathways. Expert Opin Biol Ther. 2009;9:1163–76.
103. Lutz ER, Wu AA, Bigelow E, et al. Immunotherapy converts nonimmunogenic pancreatic tumors into immunogenic foci of immune regulation. Cancer Immunol Res. 2014;2:616–31.
104. Le DT, Wang-Gillam A, Picozzi V, et al. Safety and survival with GVAX pancreas prime and Listeria Monocytogenes-expressing mesothelin (CRS-207) boost vaccines for metastatic pancreatic cancer. J Clin Oncol. 2015;33:1325–33.
105. Akce M, Zaidi MY, Waller EK, El-Rayes BF, Lesinski GB. The potential of CAR T cell therapy in pancreatic cancer. Front Immunol. 2018;9:2166.
106. Poschke I, Faryna M, Bergmann F, et al. Identification of a tumor-reactive T-cell repertoire in the immune infiltrate of patients with resectable pancreatic ductal adenocarcinoma. Onco Targets Ther. 2016;5:e1240859.
107. Hall M, Liu H, Malafa M, Centeno B, Hodul PJ, Pimiento J, Pilon-Thomas S, Sarnaik AA. Expansion of tumor-infiltrating lymphocytes (TIL) from human pancreatic tumors. J Immunother Cancer. 2016;4:61.

Chapter 15
Phase I Trials in Pancreatic Cancer

Thomas Seufferlein, Angelika Kestler, Alica Beutel, Lukas Perkhofer, and Thomas Ettrich

For a long time pancreatic ductal adenocarcinoma (PDAC) has been a largely neglected entity in clinical research. Only recently there has been a substantial increase in the number, but also the spectrum of clinical trials for the treatment of pancreatic cancer in different clinical settings. This is partly due to a better understanding of the molecular setup of pancreatic cancer and consequently the definition of subgroups that allow a more specific targeting.

In this chapter we will highlight recent trends in the very early phase of clinical trials in pancreatic cancer. There are substantial activities in targeting specific signaling pathways overexpressed or active in PDAC, the cell cycle, and DNA damage repair, but also the tumor microenvironment including the stromal compartment and the immune system. Given the still poor prognosis of pancreatic cancer, even rather novel approaches such as CarT cells are tried in pancreatic cancer.

Interfering with Signaling Pathways

Targeting Receptor Tyrosine Kinases

"Classical" approaches targeting receptor tyrosine kinases are still examined in phase I trials for PDAC. The PDGFRa inhibitor olaratumab is examined in combination with gemcitabine plus nab-paclitaxel in metastatic PDAC (mPDAC) (NCT03086369).

T. Seufferlein (✉) · A. Kestler · A. Beutel · L. Perkhofer · T. Ettrich
Department of Internal Medicine I, Gastroenterology-Endocrinology-Nephrology-Nutrition and Metabolic Diseases, Ulm University Hospital, Ulm, Germany
e-mail: Thomas.seufferlein@uniklinik-ulm.de

© Springer Nature Switzerland AG 2020
C. W. Michalski et al. (eds.), *Translational Pancreatic Cancer Research*,
Molecular and Translational Medicine,
https://doi.org/10.1007/978-3-030-49476-6_15

HER2 3+ overexpression and/or gene amplification is observed in about 10% of patients with pancreatic cancer [1]. A previous study using trastuzumab in patients with pancreatic cancer exhibiting overexpression of the human epidermal growth factor receptor 2 (HER2) did not demonstrate a benefit for adding trastuzumab to chemotherapy. A phase I/II trial examines a novel approach. A166 is an antibody drug conjugate composed of a monoclonal antibody (mAb) targeting HER2 and conjugated to a cytotoxic agent that has not been disclosed so far. A166 is examined in locally advanced/metastatic solid tumors including PDAC with HER2 expression or amplification (NCT03602079).

The HGF/c-MET signaling module plays a major role in the interaction between pancreatic stellate cells and the tumor cells in pancreatic cancer. Ficlatuzumab, a mAb that binds soluble HGF and thereby interrupts this interaction [2], is currently examined in combination with nab-paclitaxel and gemcitabine in patients with previously untreated PDAC (NCT03316599).

Overexpression of B-type ephrins correlates with progression of PDAC and is involved in angiogenesis and tumor growth. Currently, a recombinant EphB4-HSA fusion protein (sEphB4-HSA) is under investigation in a multi-arm study in combination with various chemotherapy regimens in patients with advanced solid tumors including PDAC. sEphB4-HAS is a recombinant fusion protein composed of the extracellular domain of human receptor tyrosine kinase ephrin type-B receptor 4 (sEphB4) and fused to full-length human serum albumin (HSA) [3]. sEphB4-HSA acts a decoy receptor for the membrane-bound ligand ephrin-B2 (Efnb2) and interferes with the binding of Efnb2 to its native receptors, including EphB4 and EphA3 (NCT02495896).

The TGF-beta/TGF-beta receptor type 1 (TGFBR1) signaling module is highly expressed in many PDACs and plays a major role in tumor formation and metastases. A phase Ib trial evaluates safety, tolerability, and exploratory efficacy of vactosertib (TEW-7197) in combination with FOLFOX in the second-line treatment of patients with mPDAC (NCT03666832). Vactosertib is an orally bioavailable inhibitor of TGFBR1 (also known as activin receptor-like kinase 5 (ALK5)) serine threonine kinase activity. Since activation of the TGFBR1 can also suppress the response of the host immune system to tumor cells, another trial examines safety and tolerability of the anti-TGF-beta antibody NIS793 either alone or in combination with an immune checkpoint inhibitor, PDR001 (NCT02947165).

The receptor tyrosine kinase Axl also plays a role in invasion and metastasis of PDAC. Bemcentinib is a small molecule tyrosine kinase inhibitor that inhibits Axl by binding to its intracellular catalytic kinase domain [4]. It is examined in combination with nab-paclitaxel/gemcitabine/cisplatin in patients with mPDAC. A goal of this study is to determine the complete response rate of bemcentinib plus chemotherapy in these patients (NCT03649321).

Another drug that targets the Axl pathway is BA3011. BA3011 is a conditionally active biologic AXL-targeted antibody drug conjugate (CAB-AXL-ADC) that has been designed to reversibly bind to recombinant AXL and AXL-expressing cells under conditions that are only present in the tumor microenvironment, but not in normal tissues. The study evaluates safety, tolerability, pharmacokinetics (PK), immunogenicity, and antitumor activity of BA3011 in patients with advanced solid tumors including PDAC (NCT03425279).

Fusions involving one of the three tropomyosin receptor kinases (TRK) rarely occur in pancreatic cancer but make the respective tumors highly susceptible to TRK inhibitors [5]. However, during treatment with a TRK inhibitor, acquired resistance can occur, particularly due to kinase domain mutations. LOXO-195 can overcome resistance in TRK fusion-positive cancers with an acquired kinase domain mutation [6]. A current phase 1/2, multicenter, open-label study evaluates safety and efficacy of LOXO-195 in patients with NTRK fusion cancers including PDAC treated with a prior TRK inhibitor (NCT03215511).

The glucocorticoid receptor is frequently overexpressed in PDAC [7]. Furthermore, dexamethasone that is regularly used as supportive treatment during chemotherapy has been implicated in tumor proliferation, chemotherapy resistance, and metastasis [8]. CORT125134 is a glucocorticoid receptor (GR) antagonist that is examined in combination with nab-paclitaxel in patients with solid tumors including PDAC to determine safety and efficacy of this combination (NCT02762981).

Apart from receptor tyrosine kinases, there are multiple intracellular pathways that contribute to tumor progression, invasion, metastasis, and the communication between PDAC cells and their microenvironment.

Protein Kinase Inhibitors

Focal adhesion kinase (FAK) is overexpressed and active in pancreatic cancer [9]. Recently, it could be demonstrated that FAK plays a key role in the regulation of the fibrotic and immunosuppressive microenvironment [10]. Inhibition of FAK is hypothesized to make tumors responsive to checkpoint inhibitors and could delay tumor progression in combination with chemotherapy and checkpoint inhibitors. A current phase I trial examines the combination of the FAK inhibitor defactinib in combination with the checkpoint inhibitor pembrolizumab and gemcitabine in patients with advanced solid tumors including pancreatic cancer (NCT02546531).

The Ras-MEK-ERK cascade is active in PDAC, partly due to the constitutively active KRAS^{G12D}, partly due to overexpression of receptor tyrosine kinases and their respective ligands and other factors, respectively. Therefore, interfering with this signaling cascade may have antiproliferative effects. Several phase I trials examine novel ERK inhibitors such as BVD-523 in combination with nab-paclitaxel and gemcitabine in patients with mPDAC (NCT02608229) or the ERK inhibitor ASN007 in patients with advanced solid tumors including PDAC (NCT03415126).

GSK-3β is a potentially important therapeutic target in human malignancies. The kinase is involved in energy metabolism, neuronal cell development, and body pattern formation [11]. Aberrantly active GSK3b can mediate tumor invasion and treatment resistance [12]. This has led to the design of GSK3b inhibitors for clinical use. A phase I/II study evaluates the safety and efficacy of 9-ING-41, a potent GSK-3β inhibitor, as a single agent and in combination with cytotoxic agents in patients with refractory cancers including PDAC (NCT03678883).

ABTL0812 is a small molecule that activates the nuclear receptors PPARα/γ and thereby induces the pseudokinase TRIB3 which in turn leads to inhibition of the Akt/mTORC1 axis and induces autophagy-mediated cancer cell death [13]. A current trial examines the efficacy and safety of ABTL0812 in combination with gemcitabine and nab-paclitaxel in patients with mPDAC (NCT03417921).

The mTOR pathway is also target of another phase I study that evaluates MLN0128 or sapanisertib, an experimental small molecule inhibitor of mTOR, in combination with ziv-aflibercept (NSC# 724770) in patients with advanced cancers including PDAC (NCT02159989).

Phosphoinositide-3 kinases (PI3Ks), upstream regulators of AKT and mTOR, play a key role in tumor-associated immune responses, tumor cell growth, survival, proliferation, angiogenesis, and dissemination as well as tumor-stroma cross talk [14]. INCB050465 inhibits the delta isoform of PI3K and is currently examined alone and in combination with the checkpoint inhibitor pembrolizumab in advanced solid tumors including pancreatic cancer (NCT02646748).

Wnt signaling also plays a role in certain pancreatic cancers [15]. A phase I trial investigates LGK974, a potent and specific inhibitor of porcupine, a central component of the Wnt pathway, in patients with various malignancies dependent on Wnt ligands (NCT01351103).

Inhibiting Mutated Kras

The small GTP binding protein KRAS is frequently mutated in pancreatic cancer but as yet regarded as not druggable. Recently, a novel approach has been described using modified small extracellular vesicles, so-called exosomes, that are produced by mesenchymal stromal cells and have been engineered to contain shRNA against KRAS with a G12D mutation (iExosomes). These exosomes have been shown to be delivered to the tumor and block growth of Kras[G12D]-mutated PDACs [16]. A current phase I trial examines side effects and the best dose of iExosomes in treating patients with metastatic Kras[G12D]-mutated PDAC (NCT03608631).

Inhibition of Mutated KRAS Signaling by Protein Phosphatase Inhibitors

Apart from protein kinases, their counterparts, protein phosphatases, emerge as interesting targets in PDAC. Recent data show that mutant KRAS-driven cancers depend on PTPN11/SHP2 phosphatase [17]. A current phase I study examines oral RMC-4630, a protein tyrosine phosphatase non-receptor type 11/SHP2 antagonist [18], as monotherapy in patients with advanced relapsed or refractory solid tumors harboring mutations/rearrangements that result in hyperactivation of the RAS-MAPK pathway (NCT03634982).

Targeting Heat Shock Proteins (HSPS)

Heat shock proteins act as molecular chaperones responsible for proper folding and activation of their substrate proteins. They are ubiquitously expressed and have been implicated in tumor cell proliferation, invasion, metastasis, and cell death [19]. Therefore, HSPs constitute promising targets.

Minnelide is a prodrug of triptolide and has been derived from the thunder God vine (*Tripterygium wilfordii*) [20]. One of its mechanisms of action is inhibition of HSP70. A phase I trial evaluates dose, safety, pharmacokinetics, and pharmacodynamics (PD) of this compound in patients with advanced solid tumors including PDAC (NCT03129139). A further phase I trial examines an HSP90 inhibitor, XL888, when given together with the checkpoint inhibitor pembrolizumab in treating patients with advanced metastatic gastrointestinal cancers including PDAC (NCT03095781).

Cell Cycle Inhibitors

The cell cycle is an attractive target in cancer. Various clinical trials investigate the use of cell cycle inhibitors in order to improve the treatment of patients with PDAC. A phase I/II clinical trial assesses the maximum tolerated dose, safety, and efficacy of BEY1107, an inhibitor of the CDK1 protein kinase, as monotherapy and in combination with gemcitabine in patients with locally advanced or metastatic PDAC (NCT03579836).

LY3143921 hydrate inhibits the serine/threonine kinase CDC7 that regulates chromosomal DNA replication. CDC7 is overexpressed in pancreatic cancer and inhibition of CDC7 results in apoptosis of pancreatic cancer cells [21]. The compound is examined in patients with advanced solid tumors including PDAC (NCT03096054).

Another phase I study evaluates safety, tolerability, and pharmacokinetics of SBP-101 in combination with nab-paclitaxel and gemcitabine in patients with mPDAC (NCT03412799). SBP-101 is a polyamine (PA) analogue that displaces endogenous PAs from PA-binding sites on the cell surface and thereby prevents internalization of PA which in turn blocks cell cycle progression. This may be even a tumor-specific mechanism of action since PA uptake is upregulated in various tumor types and increased levels of PA result in enhanced tumor cell growth.

Furthermore, combinations of selective inhibitors targeting different signaling pathways are evaluated. A current phase I study assesses safety and MTD of the ERK inhibitor ulixertinib (BVD-523) combined with the CDK4/6 inhibitor palbociclib (NCT03454035). Palbociclib is also combined with the PI3K/mTOR inhibitor gedatolisib (PF-05212384) for patients with advanced solid tumors including PDAC (NCT03065062).

DNA Damage Repair as Target

Targeting DNA damage repair has become an interesting approach in cancers with particular vulnerabilities such as mutations in the BRCA1 and BRCA2 genes. These tumors respond well to platinum-based chemotherapies and to poly(ADP-ribose) polymerase (PARP) inhibitors. PARP1 thereby is highly relevant in repairing DNA single-strand breaks. BRCA1 and BRCA2 mutations are comparatively rare in PDAC being detectable only in 1–4% of PDACs in a general population.

BTP-114 is a cisplatin prodrug with a maleimide moiety that strongly and selectively binds human serum albumin in the bloodstream prolonging the half-life and improving the biodistribution of the drug [22]. A phase I trial evaluates BTP-114 in patients with advanced solid tumors and BRCA or other DNA repair mutation (NCT02950064).

A single-arm phase I/II study examines the clinical activity of a novel PARP inhibitor, ABT-888, in combination with modified FOLFOX-6 (5-fluorouracil plus oxaliplatin) in patients with metastatic PDAC (NCT01489865). Another trial investigates the effectiveness, safety, and antitumor activity of the PARP inhibitor niraparib with either ipilimumab, a mAb against CTLA-4, or the PD-1 mAb nivolumab in patients with PDAC whose disease has not progressed on a platinum-based therapy (NCT03404960).

Also combinations of PARP inhibitors with chemotherapy are evaluated. A randomized phase II study assesses the combination of gemcitabine, cisplatin +/−, the PARP inhibitor veliparib in patients with PDAC, and a known BRCA/PALB2 mutation. In a second part of this trial, veliparib is examined as monotherapy (NCT01585805).

Histone Deacetylase (HDAC) Inhibitors

Targeting epigenetic regulation in solid tumors is an upcoming strategy that is studied in various tumor entities including PDAC. The majority of trials examines class I HDAC inhibitors either alone or in combination with chemotherapy or immunotherapy, respectively: The HDAC inhibitor CG200745 PPA is evaluated in combination with gemcitabine and erlotinib (NCT02737228), the HDAC1 and HDAC3 inhibitor entinostat in combination with FOLFOX (NCT03760614).

Super-Enhancers (SEs) as Targets

SEs are unique areas of the genome that are densely bound by numerous transcription factors. SEs often drive high-level transcription. Many genes that play an important role in cancer biology are likely to be SE-driven oncogenes [23, 24]. A phase I trial investigates the SE inhibitor GZ17-6.02 in patients with advanced solid tumors including PDAC (NCT03775525). GZ17-6.02 is a synthetic formulation of *Arum palaestinum* extracts that has shown antitumor activity against PDAC [24].

Targeting Tumor Metabolism

Due to the high genomic heterogeneity of PDAC, approaches have been sought in order to allow efficient treatment of these heterogeneous tumors. One of these approaches is addressing key metabolic pathways in PDAC.

RGX-202-01 is a small molecule inhibitor of the creatine transporter solute carrier family 6, member 8 (SLC6a8). RGX-202-01 reduces the intracellular levels of phosphocreatine available for ATP synthesis in tumor cells, thereby limiting tumor cell growth and metastasis [25]. The compound is examined with or without FOLFIRI (NCT03597581).

Tumor cell pyruvate dehydrogenase and alpha-ketoglutarate of the TCA cycle are inhibited using a lipoate analog, CPI-613, in a clinical trial. The compound mimics lipoate, a catalytic cofactor for both enzymes, and thereby inactivates the two enzymes. Tumor specificity is thought to result from the fact that many tumor cells overexpress a distinct set of lipoate-sensitive regulators. CPI-613 is examined in combination with gemcitabine and nab-paclitaxel in PDAC (NCT03435289).

The enzyme NAD(P)H dehydrogenase [quinone] 1 is encoded by the *NQO1* gene that encodes the enzyme 2-electron reductase. The NQO1 inhibitor ARQ 761, an intravenously administered analogue of naturally occurring β-lapachone, is examined in a phase I/Ib trial in combination with gemcitabine plus nab-paclitaxel in metastatic and locally advanced PDAC (NCT02514031).

Induction of Apoptosis

RX-3117 is an oral, small molecule nucleoside prodrug that is activated/phosphorylated by uridine-cytidine kinase 2 (UCK2). UCK2 is predominantly expressed in cancer cells. Once activated, it is incorporated into the DNA or RNA of cancer cells and induces apoptotic cell death. Because UCK2 is overexpressed in multiple human tumors, RX-3117 may be a comparatively selective nucleoside analogue. In a phase I trial, RX-3117 is examined in combination with gemcitabine plus nab-paclitaxel (NCT03189914).

A phase Ib/II trial studies the side effects and best dose of the Bcl-2 inhibitor navitoclax in combination with the MEK1/MEK2 inhibitor trametinib in patients with metastatic solid tumors including PDAC (NCT02079740).

GEN1029 (HexaBody®-DR5/DR5) is an agonistic hexamer formation-enhanced mixture of two antibodies (HexaBody) that target two separate epitopes on death receptor type 5 (DR5; TNFRSF10B; tumor necrosis factor-related apoptosis-inducing ligand receptor 2; TRAILR2) and has potential antineoplastic activity [26]. Upon administration, DR5 HexaBody agonist GEN1029 specifically binds to and activates DR5. A current first in human phase I trial examines this compound also in patients with advanced PDAC (NCT03576131).

Targeting the Cytoskeleton

Fascin is an actin filament bundling protein that is also a biomarker of invasive and advanced PDAC and regulates PDA cell migration and invasion in vitro. NP-G2-044 is a fascin inhibitor that is examined in a first-in-human phase I study to determine its safety when given orally (NCT03199586) [27].

Anetumab ravtansine or BAY 94-9343 is an antibody-drug conjugate consisting of a human anti-mesothelin antibody conjugated to the maytansinoid tubulin inhibitor DM4. The antibody binds selectively to mesothelin on cancer cells, and upon internalization the DM4 moiety disrupts microtubule assembly/disassembly dynamics, thereby inhibiting cell division. A phase Ib study examines this compound in patients with mesothelin expressing advanced or recurrent malignancies including PDAC (NCT03102320).

Targeting the Microenvironment

Stroma

The human cytokine leukemia inhibitory factor (LIF) is overexpressed in PDAC and drives PDAC-associated neural remodeling. In addition, LIF has immunosuppressive properties in cancer. MSC-1 is a first-in-class, humanized monoclonal antibody (IgG1) that binds LIF [28]. A current trial evaluates the safety and antitumor activity of MSC-1 in patients with solid tumors including PDAC (NCT03490669).

Hyaluronic acid is a major component of the tumor stroma in PDAC. Pegylated hyaluronidase (PEGP20) can improve permeability of the tumor stroma as well as tumor vascularization in PDAC, thereby improving the penetration of chemotherapeutic agents [29]. A current trial examines pharmacodynamics, safety, and efficacy of PEGPH20 in combination with the anti-PD-L1 mAb avelumab in adult patients with chemotherapy-resistant, advanced PDAC (NCT03481920).

The vitamin A derivative all-trans retinoic acid (ATRA) may also have the ability to break down stroma allowing chemotherapy to reach the cancer. A study examines the combination of ATRA, gemcitabine, and nab-paclitaxel in patients with locally advanced or metastatic PDAC (NCT03307148).

Immunotherapeutic Approaches

Chimeric Antigen Receptor (CAR) T Cells

Chimeric antigen receptor T cell (CAR-T) therapy is beginning to be explored in solid tumors. Numerous trials examine various antigens as a CAR-T cell approach in PDAC including CEA-targeted CAR-T cells (NCT02349724); anti-HER2

CAR-modified T cells (NCT02713984); EpCAM-specific CAR-T cells for EpCAM-positive cancers (NCT03013712); CAR-T cells that target mesothelin, given as single agent or in combination with a lymphocyte depleting dose of cyclophosphamide (NCT03323944); or anti-KRAS G12V mTCR cells (NCT03190941). There are also trials testing various antigens such as mesothelin, PSCA, CEA, HER2, MUC1, and EGFRvIII for CAR-T cell immunotherapy for PDAC (NCT03267173).

Further Immunotherapies

Oleclumab (MEDI9447) is a human mAb that binds to CD73/5′-nucleotidase and inhibits the production of adenosine and its immunosuppressive properties [30]. A phase I trial evaluates safety, antitumor activity, and immunogenicity of oleclumab with or without the checkpoint inhibitor durvalumab in combination with chemotherapy (gemcitabine plus nab-paclitaxel or mFOLFOX) in patients with mPDAC in the first and second line setting (NCT03611556).

CPI-006 is a type 2 humanized IgG1 antibody that inhibits the enzymatic activity of CD73 and adenosine production. A trial investigates safety, tolerability, and antitumor activity of CPI-006 as a single agent, in combination with CPI-444, a small molecule targeting the adenosine-A2A receptor on immune cells, and in combination with pembrolizumab, an anti-PD1 antibody against various solid tumors (NCT03454451).

Receptor-interacting serine/threonine-protein kinase 1, or RIPK1, regulates macrophages. Inhibition of RIPK1 results in a doubling of killer T cell activation and a fivefold decrease in the macrophage-influenced T cell type that suppresses the immune system [31]. A phase I/II study examines safety, clinical activity, pharmacokinetics, and pharmacodynamics of the RIPK1 inhibitor GSK3145095 alone and in combination with pembrolizumab in advanced solid tumors including PDAC (NCT03681951).

ADCT-301 or camidanlumab tesirine combines HuMax®-TAC™, a monoclonal antibody targeting CD25 (the alpha chain of the IL-2 receptor) with a highly potent pyrrolobenzodiazepine (PBD)-based warhead. In preclinical in vivo models, ADCT-301 exhibits strong dose-dependent antitumor activity against CD25-positive cell lines including cancer cells at low single doses [32]. A phase Ib trial evaluates safety, tolerability, pharmacokinetics, and antitumor activity of ADCT-301 in patients with advanced solid tumors including pancreatic cancer (NCT03621982).

FATE-NK100 is a first-in-class natural killer (NK) cell cancer immunotherapy comprised of adaptive memory NK cells, a highly specialized and functionally distinct subset of natural killer cells. A phase I study examines FATE-NK100 as monotherapy in patients with advanced solid tumors and also in combination with trastuzumab in case of HER2+ or in combination with cetuximab in patients with EGFR1+ advanced solid tumors (NCT03319459).

Immune checkpoint inhibitors, especially PD1/PD-L1 inhibitors, have only very limited efficacy as single agents in PDAC unless the tumors exhibit high microsatellite instability. Nevertheless, novel anti-programmed cell death ligand 1 (PD-L1) checkpoint antibodies such as LY3300054 are examined in patients with advanced refractory solid tumors including PDAC in phase I trials (NCT02791334).

Alternatively activated (M2-type) macrophages may protect tumor cells from cytotoxic T cells and thereby confer resistance to PD1/PD-L1 targeted agents in PDAC. Blocking CSF1R to deplete the tumor microenvironment of M2 macrophages may enable a more robust cytotoxic antitumor T cell response following PD-L1 blockade and sensitize PDAC to this approach. A phase I trial examines the combination of an anti-CSF1R (pexidartinib) with an anti-PD-L1 mAb (durvalumab) in patients with advanced/metastatic PDAC (NCT02777710).

Another sensitizing approach is the combination of immune checkpoint inhibitors with co-stimulatory molecules. T cell activation induces co-stimulatory molecules, including the ICos (inducible co-stimulator). ICos belongs to the CD28 family and is only expressed at low levels on naive T cells. ICos-mediated signals contribute mainly to the regulation of activated T cells and to effector T cell functions [33]. A phase I trial examines XmAb23104, a bispecific anti-PD1 and anti-ICOS antibody in subjects with selected advanced solid tumors including PDAC (NCT03752398).

It has been demonstrated that CD40 agonists can alter the stroma and inhibit growth of PDAC. RO7009789 is a novel CD40 agonist antibody with potential antineoplastic and immunostimulatory properties [34]. A clinical trial examines neoadjuvant RO7009789 alone or in combination with nab-paclitaxel and gemcitabine followed by adjuvant RO7009789 plus nab-paclitaxel and gemcitabine for patients with newly diagnosed, resectable PDAC (NCT02588443).

Another approach to reverse immunosuppression in pancreatic cancer is targeting macrophage infiltration mediated by the CCL2/CCR2 axis. The CCR5/CCL5 chemokine axis also promotes migratory and invasive properties of PDAC [35]. A phase I trial evaluates safety, PD, and preliminary efficacy of the CCR2/CCR5 antagonist BMS-813160 alone or in combination with chemotherapy or nivolumab in patients with metastatic colorectal and pancreatic cancers (NCT03184870).

Therapeutic Viruses

A phase I study examines intravenous administration of the VCN-01 oncolytic adenovirus with or without gemcitabine and nab-paclitaxel in patients with advanced solid tumors including PDAC. VCN-01 is a replication-competent adenovirus that expresses PH20 hyaluronidase that targets hyaluronic acid, a major component of the PDAC stroma (NCT02045602) [36].

Another phase I trial examines of the tolerability and safety of a replication-competent adenovirus-mediated double suicide gene therapy (Ad5-yCD/mutTKSR39rep-ADP) in combination with chemotherapy for locally advanced PDAC (LAPC) (NCT02894944).

TBI-1401(HF10) is a replication-competent HSV-1 oncolytic virus that is studied in combination with chemotherapy (gemcitabine + nab-paclitaxel or TS-1) in Japanese patients with stage III or IV unresectable PDAC (NCT03252808).

A phase I/IIa trial evaluates intratumoral injection of LOAd703, an armed oncolytic adenovirus, in combination with gemcitabine and nab-paclitaxel in patients with PDAC (NCT02705196).

Targeting Specific Antigens and Vaccination Strategies

TAK-164 is an antibody-drug conjugate comprising a full-length, fully human IgG1 monoclonal antibody (mAb) directed toward the extracellular domain of guanylyl cyclase C (GCC) [37]. TAK-164 binds to antigen-expressing cells resulting in a GCC-dependent uptake and cytotoxicity. A phase I study examines TAK-164 in patients with advanced GI malignancies including PDAC (NCT03449030).

NEO-201 is a humanized IgG1 mAb derived from an immunogenic preparation of tumor-associated antigens from pooled allogeneic colon tumor tissue extracts. It reacts against a wide variety of human tumor tissues, but is largely nonreactive against normal tissues [38]. NEO-201 binds to members of the CEACAM family and can activate innate immune mechanisms such as antibody-dependent cellular cytotoxicity and complement-dependent cytotoxicity. A first-in-human phase I trial determines safety and DLT of NEO-201 in patients with advanced solid tumors including PDAC (NCT03476681).

A phase Ib/II trial examines the NANT vaccine as treatment for patients with advanced PDAC. A combination of agents will be administered to subjects in this study: aldoxorubicin HCl, ALT-803, ETBX-011 (CEA), ETBX-021 (HER2), ETBX-051 (brachyury), ETBX-061 (MUC1), GI-4000, GI-6207, GI-6301, haNK for infusion, avelumab, bevacizumab, capecitabine, cyclophosphamide, fluorouracil, leucovorin, nab-paclitaxel, oxaliplatin, and stereotactic body radiation therapy (SBRT) (NCT03586869).

CV301 is a targeted MUC1 and CEA vaccination strategy that is examined in a phase I/II study in combination with durvalumab and maintenance chemotherapy in patients with metastatic PDAC whose disease is stable on or responding to first-line therapy for metastatic disease (NCT03376659).

The combination of cyclophosphamide, pembrolizumab, GVAX, and IMC-CS4, a CSF1R blocking antibody, is examined in patients with borderline resectable pancreatic cancer (NCT03153410).

MVT-5873 is a fully human IgG1 monoclonal antibody (mAb) that targets sialyl Lewis A (sLe^a), an epitope on CA19-9 which is expressed in PDAC and other GI cancers, plays a role in tumor adhesion and metastasis, and is a marker of an aggressive tumor phenotype [39]. A phase I trial evaluates MVT-5873 as monotherapy and in combination with a standard of care chemotherapy in patients with PDAC (NCT02672917).

A carboanhydrase IX (CAIX) inhibitor, SLC-0111, is examined in combination with gemcitabine in CAIX-positive mPDACs (NCT03450018).

Mesothelin is targeted in PDAC by various approaches. A phase Ib/II study examines the mesothelin-targeted immunotoxin LMB-100 alone or in combination with nab-paclitaxel in patients with advanced PDAC and mesothelin-expressing solid tumors (NCT02810418).

APN401 is an autologous cellular therapy consisting of ex vivo cbl-b-silenced PBMCs using siRNA. Silencing of the cbl-b ubiquitin ligase in PBMCs enhances T cell and NK cell antitumor activity in mouse tumor models and in vitro in human immune cells [40]. APN401 is evaluated in patients with solid tumors including PDAC (NCT03087591).

The data presented above demonstrate that all state-of-the-art concepts currently available for cancer treatment are nowadays examined in PDAC. Of course, the phase I/Ib design is merely focused on safety, PK, and PD, and therefore many trials do not focus in this setting on biomarker or particular PDAC subgroups. However, there is an increasing number of trials that already take specific properties of PDAC such as immunosuppression into account and try to target it, focus on specific antigens, or examine a concept only in a particular subgroup (e.g., BRCA mutated tumors). This shows that even at the level of phase I/Ib studies data from basic science and translational research are much more taken into account, and we are moving into "targeted strategies" examining safety, PD, and PK of compounds or their respective combinations in specific PDAC subgroups that have a higher chance of responding to a particular treatment. This will speed up drug research and safe costs and most importantly bring true innovations faster to our patients.

References

1. Harder J, et al. Multicentre phase II trial of trastuzumab and capecitabine in patients with HER2 overexpressing metastatic pancreatic cancer. Br J Cancer. 2012;106:1033–8.
2. Tan EH, et al. Phase 1b trial of ficlatuzumab, a humanized hepatocyte growth factor inhibitory monoclonal antibody, in combination with gefitinib in Asian patients with NSCLC. Clin Pharmacol Drug Dev. 2018;7:532–42.
3. Shi S, et al. Biophysical characterization and stabilization of the recombinant albumin fusion protein sEphB4-HSA. J Pharm Sci. 2012;101:1969–84.
4. Lorens J, et al. Phase II open-label, multi-centre study of bemcentinib (BGB324), a first-in-class selective AXL inhibitor, in combination with pembrolizumab in patients with advanced NSCLC. J Clin Oncol. 2018;36:3078.
5. Drilon A, et al. Efficacy of larotrectinib in TRK fusion-positive cancers in adults and children. N Engl J Med. 2018;378:731–9.
6. Drilon A, et al. A next-generation TRK kinase inhibitor overcomes acquired resistance to prior TRK kinase inhibition in patients with TRK fusion-positive solid tumors. Cancer Discov. 2017;7:963–72.
7. Bekasi S, Zalatnai A. Overexpression of glucocorticoid receptor in human pancreatic cancer and in xenografts. An immunohistochemical study. Pathol Oncol Res. 2009;15:561–6.
8. Liu Y, et al. Amlexanox, a selective inhibitor of IKBKE, generates anti-tumoral effects by disrupting the Hippo pathway in human glioblastoma cell lines. Cell Death Dis. 2017;8:e3022.
9. Kanteti R, et al. Focal adhesion kinase a potential therapeutic target for pancreatic cancer and malignant pleural mesothelioma. Cancer Biol Ther. 2018;19:316–27.

10. Jiang H, et al. Targeting focal adhesion kinase renders pancreatic cancers responsive to checkpoint immunotherapy. Nat Med. 2016;22:851–60.
11. Marchand B, Arsenault D, Raymond-Fleury A, Boisvert FM, Boucher MJ. Glycogen synthase kinase-3 (GSK3) inhibition induces prosurvival autophagic signals in human pancreatic cancer cells. J Biol Chem. 2015;290:5592–605.
12. Domoto T, et al. Glycogen synthase kinase-3beta is a pivotal mediator of cancer invasion and resistance to therapy. Cancer Sci. 2016;107:1363–72.
13. Erazo T, et al. The new antitumor drug ABTL0812 inhibits the Akt/mTORC1 Axis by upregulating tribbles-3 pseudokinase. Clin Cancer Res. 2016;22:2508–19.
14. Birtolo C, Go VL, Ptasznik A, Eibl G, Pandol SJ. Phosphatidylinositol 3-kinase: a link between inflammation and pancreatic cancer. Pancreas. 2016;45:21–31.
15. Zhan T, Rindtorff N, Boutros M. Wnt signaling in cancer. Oncogene. 2017;36:1461–73.
16. Kalluri R. The biology and function of exosomes in cancer. J Clin Invest. 2016;126:1208–15.
17. Ruess DA, et al. Mutant KRAS-driven cancers depend on PTPN11/SHP2 phosphatase. Nat Med. 2018;24:954–60.
18. Dempke WCM, Uciechowski P, Fenchel K, Chevassut T. Targeting SHP-1, 2 and SHIP pathways: a novel strategy for cancer treatment? Oncology. 2018;95:257–69.
19. Lianos GD, et al. The role of heat shock proteins in cancer. Cancer Lett. 2015;360:114–8.
20. Banerjee S, Saluja A. Minnelide, a novel drug for pancreatic and liver cancer. Pancreatology. 2015;15:S39–43.
21. Huggett MT, et al. Cdc7 is a potent anti-cancer target in pancreatic cancer due to abrogation of the DNA origin activation checkpoint. Oncotarget. 2016;7:18495–507.
22. Moreau B, et al. Abstract 4484: BTP-114: an albumin binding cisplatin prodrug with improved and sustained tumor growth inhibition. Cancer Res. 2015;75:4484.
23. Ghosh C, et al. Abstract 1398: super-enhancers: possible target in pancreatic cancer for therapeutic approaches. Cancer Res. 2018;78:1398.
24. Rodela E, et al. Abstract LB-B27: Novel antitumor agent GZ17-6.02 exerts discrete effects on transcriptional regulation in pancreatic cancer cells and cancer associated fibroblasts. Mol Cancer Therap. 2018;17:LB–B27.
25. Kurth I, et al. Abstract 5863: RGX-202, a first-in-class small-molecule inhibitor of the creatine transporter SLC6a8, is a robust suppressor of cancer growth and metastatic progression. Cancer Res. 2018;78:5863.
26. van der Horst HJ, et al. Potent ex vivo anti-tumor activity in relapsed refractory multiple myeloma using novel DR5-specific antibodies with enhanced capacity to form hexamers upon target binding. Blood. 2017;130:1835.
27. Li A, et al. Fascin is regulated by slug, promotes progression of pancreatic cancer in mice, and is associated with patient outcomes. Gastroenterology. 2014;146:1386–1396.e1–17.
28. Bressy C, et al. LIF drives neural remodeling in pancreatic cancer and offers a new candidate biomarker. Cancer Res. 2018;78:909–21.
29. Hingorani SR, et al. Phase Ib study of PEGylated recombinant human hyaluronidase and gemcitabine in patients with advanced pancreatic cancer. Clin Cancer Res. 2016;22:2848–54.
30. Overman MJ, et al. Safety, efficacy and pharmacodynamics (PD) of MEDI9447 (oleclumab) alone or in combination with durvalumab in advanced colorectal cancer (CRC) or pancreatic cancer (panc). J Clin Oncol. 2018;36:4123.
31. Wang W, et al. RIP1 kinase drives macrophage-mediated adaptive immune tolerance in pancreatic cancer. Cancer Cell. 2018;34:757–774.e7.
32. Nagayama A, Ellisen LW, Chabner B, Bardia A. Antibody-drug conjugates for the treatment of solid tumors: clinical experience and latest developments. Target Oncol. 2017;12:719–39.
33. Dong C, et al. ICOS co-stimulatory receptor is essential for T-cell activation and function. Nature. 2001;409:97–101.
34. Beatty GL, et al. CD40 agonists alter tumor stroma and show efficacy against pancreatic carcinoma in mice and humans. Science. 2011;331:1612–6.

35. Singh SK, et al. CCR5/CCL5 axis interaction promotes migratory and invasiveness of pancreatic cancer cells. Sci Rep. 2018;8:1323.
36. Rodriguez-Garcia A, et al. Safety and efficacy of VCN-01, an oncolytic adenovirus combining fiber HSG-binding domain replacement with RGD and hyaluronidase expression. Clin Cancer Res. 2015;21:1406–18.
37. Abu-Yousif AO, et al. Abstract B120: TAK-164, a GCC-targeted antibody-drug conjugate (ADC) for the treatment of colorectal cancers and other GI malignancies. Mol Cancer Ther. 2018;17:B120.
38. David JM, Fantini M, Annunziata CM, Arlen PM, Tsang KY. Abstract 3821: the neoantigen-targeting antibody NEO-201 enhances NK cell-dependent killing of tumor cells through blockade of the inhibitory CEACAM5/CEACAM1 immune checkpoint pathway. Cancer Res. 2018;78:3821.
39. O'Reilly EM, et al. Single agent HuMab-5B1 (MVT-5873), a monoclonal antibody targeting sLea, in patients with pancreatic cancer and other CA19-9 positive malignancies. J Clin Oncol. 2017;35:4110.
40. Loibner H, et al. Adoptive cellular immunotherapy with APN401, autologous cbl-b silenced peripheral blood mononuclear cells: data from a phase I study in patients with solid tumors. J Clin Oncol. 2018;36:3055.

Chapter 16
Translational Approaches in Surgical Treatment

Manish S. Bhandare, Vikram A. Chaudhari, and Shailesh V. Shrikhande

Pancreatic ductal adenocarcinoma (PDAC) carries one of the poorest overall prognosis of all human malignancies. The 5-year survival in patients with PDAC, for all stages, remains as low as 6–7%. The low survival rate is attributed to several factors, of which the two most important are aggressive tumor biology and late stage at which most patients are diagnosed. Only 10–20% of patients are eligible for resection at presentation, 30–40% are unresectable/locally advanced, and 50–60% are metastatic [1].

Pancreatic cancer without distant metastasis can be divided into three categories: resectable, borderline resectable, and locally advanced. In absence of metastatic disease, the most important factor for improving survival and possibly offer cure is to achieve a margin-negative resection. Even after potential curative resection, most patients develop recurrences eventually, and 5-year survival of completely resected patients is only up to 25% [1]. The aggressive tumor biology and its inherent resistance to chemotherapy and radiotherapy contributes to early recurrence and metastasis.

Surgical Advances/Techniques

Pancreatic cancer surgery has evolved over the past few decades and remains the cornerstone of treatment of resectable and borderline resectable tumors. Advances in modern imaging give precise information on disease extension and vascular involvement that aids in surgical planning in order to achieve a margin-negative resection.

M. S. Bhandare · V. A. Chaudhari · S. V. Shrikhande (✉)
Gastrointestinal and Hepato-Pancreato-Biliary Surgical Service,
Department of Surgical Oncology, Tata Memorial Hospital, Mumbai, India

© Springer Nature Switzerland AG 2020
C. W. Michalski et al. (eds.), *Translational Pancreatic Cancer Research*,
Molecular and Translational Medicine,
https://doi.org/10.1007/978-3-030-49476-6_16

Surgical techniques for pancreatic cancer include pancreaticoduodenectomy, distal pancreatectomy with splenectomy, and total pancreatectomy. Standard lymphadenectomy for pancreatoduodenectomy should include removal of lymph node stations 5, 6, 8a, 12b1, 12b2, 12c, 13a, 13b, 14a, 14b, 17a, and 17b.

Involvement of superior mesenteric vein (SMV)/portal vein(PV) was previously considered as a contraindication for resection. However, curative resection along with SMV/PV with vascular reconstruction has now become a standard practice in specialized high-volume centers. To improve margin-negative resections, specially in borderline resectable tumors with proximity to vascular structures, SMA first approach (six different approaches) was proposed as a new modification of standard pancreaticoduodenectomy [2]. In a systematic review, SMA first approach was shown to be associated with better perioperative outcomes, such as blood loss, transfusion requirements, pancreatic fistula, delayed gastric emptying, and reduced local and metastatic recurrence rates [3, 4].

In case of arterial involvement, there is no good evidence at present to justify arterial resections for right-sided pancreatic tumors [5]. However, the modified Appleby procedure, which includes en bloc removal of celiac axis with or without arterial reconstruction, when used in appropriately selected patients, offers margin-negative resection with survival benefit for locally advanced pancreatic body and tail tumors and should be performed in high-volume centers [6].

Most evidence does not support advantage of more extended resections such as removal of the para-aortic lymph nodes and nerve plexus and multivisceral resections routinely [7–9]. Such extended resections are associated with compromised quality of life because of associated higher perioperative morbidity and intractable diarrhea. However, in highly selected patients, with preserved performance status and stable or nonprogressive disease on neoadjuvant treatment, such extended resections can provide survival advantage over palliative treatments [10]. Radical surgery in the presence of oligometastatic disease has also been reported to prolong survival in highly selected patients [11].

Translational Approaches in Surgery

Currently, the AJCC (American Joint Committee on Cancer) TNM staging is the only prognostic factor used in clinical practice to assess the survival of a resected PDAC and guide treatment decisions. However, this clinicopathological staging fails to consistently predict the outcomes after pancreatic resection. Due to the large genomic heterogeneity within PDAC tumors, prognostic gene expression signatures may be useful to predict outcome.

Earlier studies had shown that the most frequently altered genes in PDACs are KRAS, SMAD4, TP53, and CDKN2A/B (one oncogene and three tumor suppressor genes) [12–14]. Many genes were later found altered by using comprehensive genomic approaches including array-comparative genomic hybridization [15, 16].

Molecular Classification of PDAC

More recently, molecular classification according to gene expression and genomic alterations has been proposed [17–19]. The first such profiling of PDAC was published in 2011 based on microdissection performed on surgically resected specimens [17]. According to the results, PDAC was classified into three different subtypes (Collison's subtypes: "classical," "quasi-mesenchymal," and "exocrine-like"). These subtypes had different clinical outcomes and therapeutic responses and were also validated externally. The classical tumor subtype had a better survival, whereas the quasi-mesenchymal subtype had worst survival. Subtype classification was the only independent prognostic factor for overall survival (OS) in multivariate analysis and the chemosensitivity also varied among the subtypes. In another study, Moffitt et al. [18] separated the stromal component from the malignant epithelial component and identified different subtypes, based on the observation that PDAC is comprised of a dense peritumoral stroma. Two specific stromal subtypes, "normal" and "activated" stroma, were identified, with the latter showing the worst prognosis (median survival of 15 months vs. 24 months). The malignant component was further classified as "classical" and "basal-like" tumor-specific subtypes. Classical tumor and normal stroma subtypes correlated with best prognosis, and prognosis was worst with basal-like tumor and activated stroma subtypes. More recent transcriptional classification for PDAC by Bailey et al. [19] distinguished four tumor subtypes associated with different molecular pathways as "squamous," "pancreatic progenitor," "immunogenic," and "aberrantly differentiated endocrine exocrine (ADEX)." This classification is based on the differential expression of transcription factors and downstream targets important for lineage specification and differentiation during pancreas development and regeneration. Correlating with outcomes, the squamous subtype was an independent poor-prognostic factor.

Indeed, identifying such genetic signatures and their expression profiling is presently the most promising approach for identifying new prognostic tools and tailoring individualized treatment in PDAC, possibly independent of the AJCC staging.

Early Detection

Late stage at diagnosis is one of the most important factors for overall dismal outcomes in PDAC. Early detection at stage I or II can provide a window of opportunity when the disease can be eradicated by high-quality surgery and together with adjuvant chemotherapy and can result in cure [20]. Development of promising molecular biomarkers for early detection of PDAC is hence the need of the hour. For this purpose, blood-based molecular biomarkers, which include proteins, nucleic acids, autoantibodies, aberrantly glycosylated antigens, exosomes, circulating tumor cells, and metabolites, have been studied. The ideal, noninvasive biomarkers should be universally present in precancerous lesions (PanIN, pancreatic intraepithelial neoplasia; IPMN, intraductal papillary mucinous neoplasm with dysplasia; carcinoma in situ) and should have a high sensitivity and specificity which is inexpensive, rapid, and practical to perform. Current clinical practice uses CA19-9, which is a carbohydrate antigen found on multiple carrier proteins [21]. However, it is not detectable in 5–10% of patients and lacks specificity as it is often elevated in biliary obstruction with or without malignancy. Hence, it is useful for monitoring response to therapy, but it is not a useful tool as an early detection biomarker. With molecular profiling of PDAC, a number of novel biomarkers have been discovered and are under evaluation. Also, with development of organoids recapitulating PDAC, new biomarker discovery is enhanced [22].

Circulating tumor cells (CTCs) could represent another source of blood-based molecular profiles. CTCs are tumor cells that are shed off from a primary tumor into the circulation and can be detected in the blood samples (liquid biopsy) [23]. Recently, CTCs have been studied as a potential biomarker for PDAC [24]. In this study, the authors evaluated CTC subtypes (triploid, tetraploid, or multiploid cells) and their total number and found that both were upregulated in the peripheral blood of PDAC patients when compared with healthy controls, serving thus as a diagnostic tool for the disease.

Although at present these biomarkers have not been able to make a great clinical impact, the progress made to date in finding biomarkers for early detection specially in high-risk individuals (e.g., family history of PDAC, recent-onset diabetes, chronic pancreatitis, etc.) provides optimism to the field.

Chronic Pancreatitis

Chronic pancreatitis (CP) represents a risk factor for pancreatic cancer and is a frequent differential diagnosis as well [25]. CP can involve the whole pancreatic gland or can result in development of an inflammatory head mass, which can become a considerable source of diagnostic confusion, as even high-quality CT/MRI scans fail to conclusively differentiate between the two. A positive endoscopic ultrasound (EUS) or image-guided biopsy confirms presence of a cancer; however, a negative report does not conclusively rule out malignancy. In order to enhance the diagnostic accuracy of PDAC in the background of CP, molecular markers on EUS-FNA samples have been evaluated in recent years. Utilities of DNA mutations such as kras [26], p53 [27], telomerase activity with a ribonucleoprotein enzyme [28], and a broad panel of microsatellite allele loss markers [29] have been shown to improve diagnostic accuracy in such situations.

Recently metabolic biomarkers have also been studied and introduced in this field. One such study evaluated nine metabolites [proline, sphingomyelin (d18:2,C17:0), phosphatidylcholine, isocitrate, sphinganine-1-phosphate, histidine, pyruvate, ceramide, sphingomyelin (d17:1,C18:0)] along with CA 19.9 in patients with CP having high risk for PDAC and were found to have a sensitivity of 89.9% and a specificity of 91.3% for detection of malignacy [30].

Utilization of these molecular and metabolic biomarkers may reduce the diagnostic delay and early diagnosis of PDAC in CP and can result in early initiation of treatment and surgery in resectable patients leading to improved overall outcomes.

Summary

Given the potential clinical correlation of PDAC molecular subtyping and long-term survival, the emphasis now should be on defining a universally accepted PDAC molecular subtyping which can guide personalized therapy including surgery, irrespective the AJCC stage of the disease. Also, the focus should be on formulating an ideal biomarker for early detection of PDAC, at least in high-risk population and those with chronic pancreatitis, in order to offer early curative treatment resulting in overall improved outcomes.

References

1. Gillen S, Schuster T, Zum Büschenfelde CM, Friess H, Kleeff J. Preoperative/neoadjuvant therapy in pancreatic cancer: a systematic review and meta-analysis of response and resection percentages. PLoS Med. 2010;7(4):e1000267.
2. Sanjay P, Takaori K, Govil S, Shrikhande SV, Windsor JA. "Artery-first" approaches to pancreatoduodenectomy. Br J Surg. 2012;99(8):1027–35.
3. Negoi I, Hostiuc S, Runcanu A, Negoi RI, Beuran M. Superior mesenteric artery first approach versus standard pancreaticoduodenectomy: a systematic review and meta-analysis. Hepatobiliary Pancreat Dis Int. 2017;16(2):127–38.
4. Ironside N, Barreto SG, Loveday B, Shrikhande SV, Windsor JA, Pandanaboyana S. Meta-analysis of an artery-first approach versus standard pancreatoduodenectomy on perioperative outcomes and survival. Br J Surg. 2018;105(6):628–36.
5. Bockhorn M, Uzunoglu FG, Adham M, Imrie C, Milicevic M, Sandberg AA, Asbun HJ, Bassi C, Büchler M, Charnley RM, Conlon K. Borderline resectable pancreatic cancer: a consensus statement by the International Study Group of Pancreatic Surgery (ISGPS). Surgery. 2014;155(6):977–88.
6. Latona JA, Lamb KM, Pucci MJ, Maley WR, Yeo CJ. Modified Appleby procedure with arterial reconstruction for locally advanced pancreatic adenocarcinoma: a literature review and report of three unusual cases. J Gastrointest Surg. 2016;20(2):300–6.
7. Evans DB, Farnell MB, Lillemoe KD, Vollmer C, Strasberg SM, Schulick RD. Surgical treatment of resectable and borderline resectable pancreas cancer: expert consensus statement. Ann Surg Oncol. 2009;16(7):1736–44.
8. Nimura Y, Nagino M, Takao S, Takada T, Miyazaki K, Kawarada Y, Miyagawa S, Yamaguchi A, Ishiyama S, Takeda Y, Sakoda K. Standard versus extended lymphadenectomy in radical pancreatoduodenectomy for ductal adenocarcinoma of the head of the pancreas: long-term results of a Japanese multicenter randomized controlled trial. J Hepatobiliary Pancreat Sci. 2012;19(3):230–41.
9. Jang JY, Kang MJ, Heo JS, Choi SH, Choi DW, Park SJ, Han SS, Yoon DS, Yu HC, Kang KJ, Kim SG. A prospective randomized controlled study comparing outcomes of standard resection and extended resection, including dissection of the nerve plexus and various lymph nodes, in patients with pancreatic head cancer. Ann Surg. 2014;259(4):656–64.

10. Mitra A, Pai E, Dusane R, Ranganathan P, DeSouza A, Goel M, Shrikhande SV. Extended pancreatectomy as defined by the ISGPS: useful in selected cases of pancreatic cancer but invaluable in other complex pancreatic tumors. Langenbecks Arch Surg. 2018;403(2):203–12.
11. Hackert T, Niesen W, Hinz U, Tjaden C, Strobel O, Ulrich A, Michalski CW, Büchler MW. Radical surgery of oligometastatic pancreatic cancer. Eur J Surg Oncol. 2017;43(2): 358–63.
12. Wood LD, Hruban RH. Pathology and molecular genetics of pancreatic neoplasms. Cancer J. 2012;18(6):492.
13. Jones S, Zhang X, Parsons DW, Lin JC, Leary RJ, Angenendt P, Mankoo P, Carter H, Kamiyama H, Jimeno A, Hong SM. Core signaling pathways in human pancreatic cancers revealed by global genomic analyses. Science. 2008;321(5897):1801–6.
14. Hidalgo M. New insights into pancreatic cancer biology. Ann Oncol. 2012;23(suppl_10): x135–8.
15. Birnbaum DJ, Adelaide J, Mamessier E, Finetti P, Lagarde A, Monges G, et al. Genome profiling of pancreatic adenocarcinoma. Genes Chromosomes Cancer. 2011;50(6):456–65.
16. Birnbaum DJ, Birnbaum D, Bertucci F. Endometriosis-associated ovarian carci-nomas. N Engl J Med. 2011;364(5):483–4, (author reply 4–5).
17. Collisson EA, Sadanandam A, Olson P, Gibb WJ, Truitt M, Gu S, Cooc J, Weinkle J, Kim GE, Jakkula L, Feiler HS. Subtypes of pancreatic ductal adenocarcinoma and their differing responses to therapy. Nat Med. 2011;17(4):500.
18. Moffitt RA, Marayati R, Flate EL, Volmar KE, Loeza SG, Hoadley KA, Rashid NU, Williams LA, Eaton SC, Chung AH, Smyla JK. Virtual microdissection identifies distinct tumor-and stroma-specific subtypes of pancreatic ductal adenocarcinoma. Nat Genet. 2015;47(10):1168.
19. Bailey P, Chang DK, Nones K, Johns AL, Patch AM, Gingras MC, Miller DK, Christ AN, Bruxner TJ, Quinn MC, Nourse C. Genomic analyses identify molecular subtypes of pancreatic cancer. Nature. 2016;531(7592):47.
20. Matsuno S, Egawa S, Fukuyama S, Motoi F, Sunamura M, Isaji S, Imaizumi T, Okada S, Kato H, Suda K, et al. Pancreatic Cancer Registry in Japan: 20 years of experience. Pancreas. 2004;28:219–30.
21. Lennon AM, Wolfgang CL, Canto MI, Klein AP, Herman JM, Goggins M, Fishman EK, Kamel I, Weiss MJ, Diaz LA, et al. The early detection of pancreatic cancer: what will it take to diagnose and treat curable pancreatic neoplasia? Cancer Res. 2014;74:3381–33819.
22. Kleeff J, Korc M, Apte M, LaVecchia C, Johnson CD, Biankin AV, Neale RE, Tempero M, Tuveson DA, Hruban RH, et al. Pancreatic cancer. Nat Rev Dis Primers. 2016;2:16022.
23. Pantel K, Speicher MR. The biology of circulating tumor cells. Oncogene. 2015;35:1–9.
24. Liu H, Sun B, Wang S, Liu C, Lu Y, Li D, Liu X. Circulating tumor cells as a biomarker in pancreatic ductal adenocarcinoma. Cell Physiol Biochem. 2017;42(1):373–82.
25. Shrikhande SV, Barreto G, Koliopanos A. Pancreatic carcinogenesis: the impact of chronic pancreatitis and its clinical relevance. Indian J Cancer. 2009;46(4):288.
26. Pellisé M, Castells A, Ginès A, et al. Clinical usefulness of KRAS mutational analysis in the diagnosis of pancreatic adenocarcinoma by means of endosonography-guided fine-needle aspiration biopsy. Aliment Pharmacol Ther. 2003;17:1299–307.
27. Itoi T, Takei K, Sofuni A, Itokawa F, Tsuchiya T, Kurihara T, Nakamura K, Moriyasu F, Tsuchida A, Kasuya K. Immunohistochemical analysis of p53 and MIB-1 in tissue specimens obtained from endoscopic ultrasonography-guided fine needle aspiration biopsy for the diagnosis of solid pancreatic masses. Oncol Rep. 2005;13(2):229–34.
28. Mishra G, Zhao Y, Sweeney J, Pineau BC, Case D, Ho C, Blackstock AW, Geisinger K, Howerton R, Levine E, Shen P. Determination of qualitative telomerase activity as an adjunct to the diagnosis of pancreatic adenocarcinoma by EUS-guided fine-needle aspiration. Gastrointest Endosc. 2006;63(4):648–54.

29. Salek C, Benesova L, Zavoral M, Nosek V, Kasperova L, Ryska M, Strnad R, Traboulsi E, Minarik M. Evaluation of clinical relevance of examining K-ras, p16 and p53 mutations along with allelic losses at 9p and 18q in EUS-guided fine needle aspiration samples of patients with chronic pancreatitis and pancreatic cancer. World J Gastroenterol: WJG. 2007;13(27):3714.
30. Mayerle J, Kalthoff H, Reszka R, Kamlage B, Peter E, Schniewind B, Maldonado SG, Pilarsky C, Heidecke CD, Schatz P, Distler M. Metabolic biomarker signature to differentiate pancreatic ductal adenocarcinoma from chronic pancreatitis. Gut. 2018;67(1):128–37.

Index

© Springer Nature Switzerland AG 2020
C. W. Michalski et al. (eds.), *Translational Pancreatic Cancer Research*,
Molecular and Translational Medicine,
https://doi.org/10.1007/978-3-030-49476-6

Printed in the United States
by Baker & Taylor Publisher Services